The Physician and Sexuality in Victorian America

THE PHYSICIAN
AND SEXUALITY
IN VICTORIAN
AMERICA

John S. Haller, Jr.,
and
Robin M. Haller

The Norton Library
W·W·NORTON & COMPANY·INC·
NEW YORK

Books That Live
The Norton imprint on a book means that in the publisher's
estimation it is a book not for a single season but for the years.
W. W. Norton & Company, Inc.

Library of Congress Cataloging in Publication Data

Haller, John S
  The physician and sexuality in Victorian
America.

  (The Norton library)
  Bibliography: p.
  Includes index.
    1. United States—Moral conditions. 2. Women—
United States—Social conditions. 3. Women—Health
and hygiene—United States. 4. Physicians—United
States. I. Haller, Robin M., joint author.
II. Title.
HN90.M6H34   1977   301.41′7973   76-49082
ISBN 0-393-00845-1

              1 2 3 4 5 6 7 8 9 0

for Peter

Contents

Introduction

THE VICTORIAN men and women who approached maturity in post–Civil War America have been variously described as fittest men, founts of purity, molders of men's souls, brainworkers, blessed homemakers, white men of the white man's burden, neurasthenics, mannish maidens, and aggressive suffragettes. If they could have been any of these caricatures, they could have been all, for the men and women in late nineteenth-century America faced a bewildering and conflicting array of roles forced upon them by a newly industrialized society seeking to formulate a middle-class ethic from the ashes of pre–Civil War traditions and the challenges of postwar technology. Nowhere were these roles more brazenly drawn than in the area of sexuality, a term describing the complexity of relations between the sexes, the roles each sex played, and the functions, purposes, capacities, and behavior of men and women. Most of the external influences which acted upon the Victorian woman, for example, cautioned her to remain at home and continue the vicarious life assigned to her by tradition. This "ideal" role, as it were, conflicted with the reality of postwar inventions which emancipated her from household drudgery. At the same time there was an obvious effort to make the cultured woman into a status symbol in a society of new mobility and growing urban affluence, the advances in industrialism, transportation, and communication offered her the opportunity for becoming a more complete social being, active in affairs no longer limited to the home. The dilemma facing the Victorian woman represents a microcosm of the effects of these old and new forces acting upon American society, and her relationship with the male-dominated culture offers an illuminating focus on the creation and perpetuation of those values.

Not only because of the formalities of etiquette which surrounded personal relationships, but also because of the uprooting of family life which had accompanied the industrialization and urbanization of society, growing numbers of Victorians found themselves unable to confide in husbands, wives, parents, or relatives on personal matters. Increasingly, they turned to advice columns in newspapers, etiquette books, philanthropic organizations, marriage manuals, and an assortment of "private" counselors who dealt with personal problems. Increasingly, too, Victorians turned to the physician who, through the professional distance his office imposed, assumed a neutrality in which they felt secure. Like the priest's confessional, the minister's study, or the lawyer's office, the doctor's consultation and examination rooms became a sacred setting in which confidential conversation might take place, and the Victorians could give vent to feelings, emotions, fears, and anxieties that afflicted them. The peculiar relationship which existed between the physician and his patient enabled the medical profession to exert a moral influence that could not be circumscribed in terms of its healing abilities alone. And as the medical profession became more and more aware of the link between mental state and physical well-being, and recognized the significance of psychosomatic illness, the doctor, through his diagnostic and healing skills, soon found himself with the additional responsibility of acting as the arbiter of fashion, the watchman of morals, and the judge of personal needs. This study, therefore, is not only concerned with nineteenth-century sexuality, but is also, by implication, a social history of the medical profession —those doctors, homeopaths, and eclectics who administered to the sexual fears and problems of Victorian society.

In an era when the generalist as opposed to the specialist dominated in many areas of the sciences, the physician gradually assumed the roles and duties heretofore reserved to the minister. He had more opportunity than any other person outside the family circle to enter it on terms of intimacy and become a party to family secrets in the natural course of his duties. Indeed, the physician often gained entrance where the minister was denied, and his responsibility to attend first to his patient's physical state in no way hindered his obligation to be "instrumental in saving a soul from death, and thus adding another jewel to the Redeemer's crown." The physician's moral influence extended further, however, than the soul of his patient; he used his standing as a medical man to exert influence on the community as well. For the community had a right to expect "a dignified and firm expression of his sentiments, and a decided influence for good upon every great moral question [from] one who has so great a share . . . in moulding the character of society."[1] While ostensibly exponents of reason and science, most medical men recoiled, like much of the middle class, from any great change in society's value structure, only to emerge as eloquent defenders of the status quo.

While this is not a study of the feminist movement, it does necessarily touch upon it in more than a tangential way. Because the medical profession held itself responsible for the moral and spiritual, as well as the physical, health of the nation, doctors felt it necessary to bring all their professional authority to bear against those elements which threatened the stability, if not the very existence, of society. And this certainly included the women's rights movement. Doctors attempting to deal with all areas of human health found themselves facing the problem of sexuality, and increasingly, woman's awareness of her position. Neurasthenia, the harbinger disease of urban America, very early became tied to the question of woman's new mobility. The problems of drug abuse, personal hygiene, marriage relations, contraception, the corset, and even the bicycle became embroiled in the larger question of sexuality. As Victorian men and women struggled with their faster moving world, and with the passing away of old traditions and roles and the coming of new ones, they faced the dilemma of themselves as men and women in a new social structure.

Response by more conservative elements of society, including the medical profession, to the attempts by women to fulfill themselves as human beings, both in the nineteenth century and today, have been markedly similar. The reaction to the "new woman" in the late nineteenth century was to suggest creative home economics, which would ensure that the time and energy of this newly activated middle-class woman would be safely expended within the home circle. Echoes of this are

1. Worthington Hooker, *Physician and Patient; Or, a Practical View of the Mutual Duties, Relations and Interests of the Medical Profession and the Community* (New York, 1849), 391, 429.

heard in our own day for women to concern themselves with those areas most closely connected to their roles as wife and mother. Magazine advertisements and media commercials exhort the American woman to have the cleanest wash, the cleanest kitchen, the cleanest children. Glorification of the American housewife is used to sell almost any product.

Yet there is a danger in contrasting today's movement for sexual freedom with the stereotypes of Victorian America. Because of the myths which pervade our popular culture concerning the so-called prudery of the nineteenth century, we tend to look upon the women who manifested that prudishness as somehow more akin to a backward age, introverted, and sexually repressed. Although it is obvious that many Victorians suffered from sexual repression, it appears on closer observation that those women who contributed to the concept of prudishness were far closer to today's feminists than most are willing to admit. The options open to the Victorians were few. Respectable ladies, even in the privacy of their own homes, had to remain ladies. They could not become promiscuous without attracting the wrath of society; they went the other way, and abstained from sex except for procreation. In other words, the Victorian woman sought to achieve a sort of sexual freedom by denying her sexuality, by resorting to marital continence or abstinence in an effort to keep from being considered or treated as a sex object. Her prudery was a mask that conveniently hid her more "radical" effort to achieve freedom of person. No doubt sexual abstinence turned many husbands to prostitution and mistresses, in order to gratify their own sex needs while still perpetuating the sanctity of the home, but abstinence may well have answered the problems existing for many women in the Victorian marriage. Although out of character in our own twentieth-century culture, sexual asceticism has nonetheless served the needs of earlier societies. Today when sexual restraints are less binding, the woman can express her sexuality as she pleases, without risking social ostracism, or loss of job, husband, or standing in the community. The woman today flaunts her sexuality to achieve the same end that many Victorian women could only achieve by denying theirs. The seeming paradox between these two almost contradictory behaviors can be explained by the fact that each was acting within the bounds of her society and each was taking a radical departure from existing mores. It is erroneous to accept the popular dictum that the Victorian period was an aberration in the ascent of women to greater sexual freedom. Despite appearances, both the Victorian woman and the modern feminist reflect responses to the disparity of roles between the sexes, and both reflect a demand for greater freedom of person.

Historians who discuss the revolution of middle-class morals in America commonly turn to the period after World War I for its most pronounced manifestations. Others have suggested that the sexual freedom of the postwar period had begun to emerge during the years from 1912 to 1917, when changes in divorce rates, the crusades of the muckrakers, and the efforts of Margaret Sanger were already challenging the manners and mores of the day. Both these ideas are founded on the premise that sexual freedom was at its nadir during the late nineteenth century, a period of sexual repression with all the symptoms of sexual neuroses. However, it is important to realize that the Victorian period never was a monolithic culture in terms of its sexual standards, and that throughout the period some rather novel ideas blossomed amid the virtues of hard work, discipline, and self-denial—ideas which ran the gamut from Zugassent's Discovery and animal magnetism to ethical marriage and strict continence. The social norms which prevented the Victorian woman from public display of her sexuality did not prevent her from attempting to challenge her traditional role in the home circle. To judge the Victorian era merely on the basis of its attitudes toward romantic novels, boy-girl parties, contraception, and prostitution is to mistake Victorian sexuality as an atavism rather than as a transitional period in the evolution of middle-class morality. To pronounce as retrogressive the notion of marital continence or separate bedrooms is to misunderstand what was actually an effort by many Victorian women to challenge their role as sex objects in marriage without at the same time destroying the image of Victorian stability and the goals of racial and national progress. Until contraception could be taken from the streets and used in the home, and until woman won the right to greater mobility outside the home circle, her effort to define—and restrict—her sexual role in the marriage was the only sexual freedom available to her and her behavior should be considered an important step in the transition to modern womanhood. The Victorian era, not simply a bland sexual regression, was rather a time of molding new sex mores, which even when compared to the permissive society sparked by World War I marked significant departures from the ultra-masculine world.

We wish to express our sincerest thanks to Dick and Samilda Reich, Pat Havalice, Betty Shaw, Susan Jo Thompson, Larry Fortado, Agota Kuperman, Elaine Hansen, Jim Self, Becky Kennedy, and Karen Freeman, research librarians and assistants at Indiana University. We are equally grateful to Dorothy T. Hanks, Lucinda Keister, K. Janelle Wilson, and Otis A. Parman of the National Library of Medicine. Without the help from the library staff of these two great institutions, the many difficulties which we faced in writing this book would surely have proved insurmountable. Our debts also go to Frank O. Williams, Richard L. Wentworth, and Bruce A. McDaniel (Ms.) of the University of Illinois Press; to our colleagues Paul Kern, James Newman, and James Lane for their many helpful suggestions; to Rosalie Zak for her typing of the several drafts; to Roger Daday, Judith Smith, Barbara Skubish, Judith Grandfield, Gail Dailey, Diane Holom, Linda Dougherty, Darlene Licinda, Priscilla Smith, Vicky Skorish, Ana Maria De La Rosa, and Karen Farabaugh, students whose questions and observations helped to clarify numerous conceptional problems; and to the encouragement extended by Judy Hughes, Dick Austin, Bill Kane, Margaret Winske, and Sheldon Cohan.

We also appreciate the courtesies extended by the librarians and staff of the Institute for Sex Research at Indiana University, the Midwest Regional Medical Library, John Crerar Library, Library of Congress, Vanderbilt University Medical Center Library, Billings Medical Library at the University of Chicago, Oberlin College Library, New York Academy of Medicine Library, University of California at Los Angeles—Bio-

Medical Library, University of Wisconsin Library, Indiana University School of Medicine Library, Rutgers University Library, New York Medical College Library, University of Iowa Medical Library, University of Tennessee Library, University of Kentucky Medical Center Library, University of Louisville—Kornhause Memorial Medical Library, University of Michigan Medical Center Library, University of Minnesota —Bio-Medical Library, Northwestern University—Archibald Church Medical Library, Ohio State University Medical Center Library, Yale University Medical Library, University of British Columbia—Woodward Bio-Medical Library, Tulane University —Rudolph Matas Medical Library, College of Physicians of Philadelphia Library, Enoch Pratt Free Library of Baltimore, Purdue University Library, St. Louis Public Library, Boston Public Library, and the Louisville Free Public Library. Most important, we thank Indiana University, the Indiana Foundation, and the Office of Research and Advanced Studies for the many services which facilitated the progress of this book.

The Physician and Sexuality in Victorian America

[S]ome communication with the external world is indispensable to animal existence, but this communication can take place only through the Nervous pulp. But in the very lowest orders of creation, that pulp is so equably diffused throughout the membranaceous creature, that a polypus may be turned inside out, without being thereby incommoded. Gradually, however, the nervous matter is collected into distinct chords, and then into a central mass, with the elongation generally termed the spinal marrow. The higher the grade, the greater the inequality between the concentrated cerebral substance, and the filaments of which it forms the focus, until the disproportion attains its acme in woman, who, in this respect, surpasses those sometimes called the Lords of Creation. And furthermore, as you ascend the scale of organization, in addition to this general improvement, one distinct organ of sense after another is conferred—the window of the mind, the eye, being the last. Lastly, parts intended in some measure, at least, for adornment, are superadded, until finally, the work is completed. And thus, with the original type of nervous communication preserved throughout, there emerges, as the crowning act, the most elaborate and most perfect form and model of beauty, human eyes have yet beheld—THE CAUCASIAN FEMALE BUST.

John A. Smith, M.D.
The Mutations of the Earth, 1846

Chapter I

THE NERVOUS CENTURY

No good and wise man can possibly dispute, or be indifferent to, or unconcerned at, the increase of invalid females. What is the cause? It is the march of civilization and over-refinement. It is the cultivation of the mental powers: of the sentiments and passions, the refinements, the indulgences, the luxuries, ay, even the character, of social intercourse. It is the want of light, pure air, proper food, and healthful exercise . . . instead of being confined within doors, studying absurd accomplishments and romantic nonsense. It is the uninterrupted rounds of excitement consequent upon balls, parties, the opera, etc., with the liability to cold imposed by these amusements; protracted vigils sacrificed at the shrine of folly, luxury, and fashion; pampering with stimulating food, injuring by modes of dress which unduly compress most important viscera. . . . the perusal of prurient books, passion-stirring pictures, statues, etc., obtruding their seductions on the youthful imagination, provoking flights of vivid fancy, and arousing impulses of desire and yearnings after unknown gratifications.

W. W. Bliss, *Woman's Life: A Pen-Picture of Woman's Functions, Frailties, and Follies,* 1879

In 1869 in a speech before the New York Medical Journal Association, subsequently printed in the *Boston Medical and Surgical Journal*, physician George M. Beard used the word "neurasthenia" to explain a condition or state of nervous exhaustion which he believed was inundating the urban middle class of industrial America. A forerunner of Freud, a pioneer in psychological medicine, and a specialist in electrotherapy, Beard had taken the word from Fordyce Barker, M.D., who used the term "nervous asthenia" to express the condition of nervous disease common to the northeast section of the United States. Neurasthenia or "nervelessness," the deficiency of nerve force in the human body, subsequently became in the eyes of many late nineteenth-century physicians the predominant malady of modern culture. In no past society, wrote Beard, not even in the years of Rome's greatest glory, had such a disease existed. Neurasthenia had only accompanied the increased activity of industrialized man: the use of steampower, the press, the telegraph, the achievements of science, and the entrance of the alienated woman into the "outside world." The growth of the disease, argued Beard, not only marked a new watershed in the history of mankind but also unfolded a very complex and suggestive theory for the proper understanding of man and his national character, and even hinted at some of the future problems of sociology.[1]

Portions of this chapter were previously published as "Neurasthenia: Medical Profession and Urban 'Blahs'" and "Neurasthenic Women: The Medical Profession and the 'New Woman' of the Nineteenth Century," in the *New York State Journal of Medicine*, LXX (1970), 2489–97, and LXXI (1971), 473–82.

1. George M. Beard, "Neurasthenia, or Nervous Exhaustion," *Boston Medical and Surgical Journal*, III (1869), 217; George M. Beard, *American Nervousness, Its Causes and Consequences* (New York, 1881), vii–viii; Joseph M. Aiken, "Neurasthenia," *Medical News*, LXXI (1902), 970–74; Edward Wakefield, "Nervousness: The National Disease of America," *McClure's Magazine*, II (1893–94), 302–7; T. C. Allbutt, "Nervous Diseases and Modern Life," *Contemporary Review*, LXVII (1895), 210–31; Charles E. Rosenberg, "The Place of George M. Beard in Nineteenth Century Psychiatry," *Bulletin of the History of Medicine*, XXVI (1962), 245–59; Henry Alden Bunker, Jr., "From Beard to Freud. A Brief History of the Concept of Neurasthenia," *Medical Review of Reviews*, XXXVI (1930), 109–14; Philip P. Weiner, "G. M. Beard and Freud

As a Spencerian social-Darwinist, Beard applauded neurasthenia as one of the cardinal traits of evolutionary progress
marking the increased supremacy of brain force over the more
retarded social classes and barbarous peoples. In his analysis,
American society contained the finest brain-worker in history.
Characterized by "fine, soft hair, delicate skin, nicely chiselled
features, small bones, tapering extremities, and frequently by
a muscular system comparatively small and feeble," the urban
brain-worker had evolved beyond the phlegmatic constitution
of the working class and the "slow easy-going nations of the
old world." The New York specialist, however, distinguished between the urban business class and those who composed the
lower orders of the cities as well as the peasant class of rural
America. These latter groups rarely exhibited the nervous disorders evident in the brain-worker. "As would logically be expected," he wrote, neurasthenia "is oftener met with in cities
than in the country, is more marked and more frequent at the
desk, the pulpit and in the counting-room than in the shop or
on the farm."[2]

While America experienced the first "epidemic" of nervous
exhaustion, Beard saw evidence that it was also occurring in
certain favored countries of Europe. The nations of England
and Germany showed signs of similar nervous debility which,
as in America, marked the highroad of advanced industrialism.
In the Catholic countries of Europe, however, there were no
traces of this marvelous burden. Unlike those nations with a
Reformation heritage, Catholic Europe lacked the individual-
ism, intellectual confrontation, and enhanced social intercourse
necessary for race excellence.[3] In the savage races, nervous
exhaustion was almost nonexistent. Beard viewed the barbar-
ian, the Negro, and the Indians of North and South America
as so many children "who have never matured in the higher

on 'American Nervousness,' " *Journal of the History of Ideas,* XVII (1956),
269–74.
    2. Beard, *American Nervousness, Its Causes and Consequences,* 26; William
Snow, "The Electro-Static Treatment of Neurasthenia," *Transactions,* American
Electro-Therapeutic Association (1899–1900), 338.
    3. Beard, *American Nervousness, Its Causes and Consequences,* 126.

ranges of intellect," and as a result, were "living not for science or ideas, but for the senses and emotions."[4] Those nervous diseases that existed in these "backward races," he wrote, were not examples of neurasthenia, but occurred as a result of their contact with higher civilizations and their inability to cope with the consequent race struggle.[5] Nervous diseases of this type were simply occupational or race-contact neuroses and not marks of race achievement and consequent brain development. Like many Spencerians in his day, Beard conceived a unilinear scale of evolution in which social achievement correlated directly with biological development. The human brain was the combined register of past evolution and present experience which, strengthened or weakened from use or disuse, became an index for measuring race character. Beard's rationalization was a reflection of the nineteenth-century racial belief in national growth and Anglo-Saxon brain power. It was also a reflection of American nationalism and of the material prosperity that had accompanied achievements in industrialization and modernization.[6]

As a result of man's psychological evolvement, neurasthenia became an inevitable prospect facing all advanced civilized societies. As the quiet, sedentary life changed into the perilous social, political, and economic struggle for survival, nervous exhaustion became a natural by-product. Physicians like Carlin Phillips and Joseph Collins of New York believed that there was little likelihood that the evolutionary process would, by itself, correct the phenomenon, but that man must adopt measures that would "contribute to the fortification of his neural resistance and equilibrium." As civilization advanced, society

4. *Ibid.*, 131.
5. *Ibid.*, 186; Daniel G. Brinton, "Nervous Disease in Low Races and Stages of Culture," *Science*, XX (1892), 339–40; A. D. Rockwell, "Nervous Diseases and Civilization," *Science*, XX (1892), 373; Irving C. Rosse, "Brief Mention of a Few Ethnic Features of Nervous Disease," *American Journal of Social Science*, XXXVII (1900), 239–40.
6. Grace Peckham, "The Nervousness of Americans," *American Journal of Social Science*, XXII (1887), 41; Edward C. Towne, "American Climate and Character," *Popular Science Monthly*, XX (1881), 109; (Anony.), "Americans and Their Civilization, a Product of Climate," *Sanitarian*, VIII (1880), 200; N. S. Shaler, "Nature and Man in America," *Scribner's Magazine*, VIII (1890), 361–64.

collectively had to set up preventive treatment of neurasthenia.[7]

There was an obvious distinction to being identified as a neurasthenic. In a certain sense, it classified the individual as one of the brain-workers of civilization and, if not that, possibly the product of the new breed of civilization's nervous people. If one had a sufficient number of nervous symptoms, wrote William Marrs, M.D., in his *Confessions of a Neurasthenic,* he could "move in neurasthenic circles."[8] Furthermore, although the neurasthenic suffered grievously from his malady, he could enjoy, at least vicariously, the feeling of satisfaction that came in knowing he was in the best of company, including George Eliot, Charles Darwin, Herbert Spencer, Schiller, Kant, Bacon, Montaigne, Rousseau, and others. The list of eminent neurasthenic persons was inspiring, to say the very least, and not only gave evidence that the neurasthenic could live a long life, but also that he was kin to the most original thinkers society had to offer.[9] "We neurasthenics," wrote Marrs, "have slumbering within our bosoms ambitions and possibilities that, if set in motion, would move mountains and revert the course of rivers. But we can't work up enough energy to consummate our aims and carry things to a finish. Perhaps we may be able to do so some day. Oh, Some Day, you are a mirage on the desert of life and ever lure us on to things that can only be attained in the land where dreams come true!"[10]

The symptoms of neurasthenia were almost unlimited. By the end of the nineteenth century, the disorder had become the pathological dumping ground for moralists within and outside the medical world. Tenderness of the scalp, the spine, the teeth and gums, itching, abnormal secretions, "flying neuralgias," flushing, "fidgetiness," palpitation of the pulse, "sudden

7. Carlin Phillips and Joseph Collins, "The Etiology and Treatment of Neurasthenia. An Analysis of Three Hundred and Thirty-Three Cases," *Medical Record,* LV (1899), 415.

8. William Taylor Marrs, *Confessions of a Neurasthenic* (Philadelphia, 1908), 2.

9. George M. Beard, *Sexual Neurasthenia, Its Hygiene, Causes, Symptoms, and Treatment with a Chapter on Diet for the Nervous* (New York, 1884), 59; W. W. Johnston, "On the Evils Arising from the Failure to Recognize the True Nature of Neurasthenia, and Some Cases of This Failure," *Transactions,* Association of American Physicians, XVI (1901), 198–207.

10. Marrs, *Confessions of a Neurasthenic,* 114.

giving away of general or special functions," sensitiveness to weather changes, ticklishness, need for stimulants, insomnia, dyspepsia, forgetfulness, spermatorrhea, and distaste for certain foods were the most noted symptoms. But there were also indications which included impotency, "changes in the expression of the eyes," depression, timidity, morbid fears, astraphobia, headaches, chills, heat flashes, and muscle spasms, as well as "deficient thirst," dryness of skin, sweaty hands, "atonic voice," yawning, dilated pupils, hopelessness, writer's cramp, and even the "appearance of youth." Many other clinicians believed that few neurasthenics had normal sexual experiences, and that at the basis of most worry, overstrain, and anemia lay a sexual problem.[11]

Theory of Nervous Energy

Explanations for the physiological and psychological changes occurring in nervous exhaustion were never adequately stated. The difficulty appeared to stem from the fact that neurasthenia was a "state" of disease rather than a "special, limited, and geometrically defined disease."[12] For this reason, explanations were metaphorical, allowing the patient to relax in a simplistic comprehension of his problems, and permitting the clinician to conceal his own ignorance behind an all-encompassing prognosis. "The neurasthenic is a dam with a small reservoir behind it, that often runs dry or nearly so through the torrent at the sluiceway, but speedily fills again from many mountain streams; a small furnace, holding little fuel, and that inflammable and combustible, with strong draught, causing quick exhaustion of materials and imparting unequal, inconstant warmth; a battery with small cells and little potential force, and which with little internal resistance quickly becomes actual

11. George M. Beard, *Other Symptoms of Nervous Exhaustion* (Chicago, 1879), 1–2; G. M. Hammond, "Nerves and the American Woman," *Harper's Bazaar*, XL (1906), 592–93; R. M. Ladova, "The Nature of Neurasthenia: A Study of the Recent Literature," *Medicine*, VI (1900), 183–84; (Anony.), "The Confessions of a Nervous Woman," *Post-Graduate; a Monthly Journal of Medicine and Surgery*, XI (1896), 364–68; George M. Beard, "The Symptoms of Sexual Exhaustion (Sexual Neurasthenia)," *Independent Practitioner*, I (1880), 221, 271.

12. Beard, *Sexual Neurasthenia, Its Hygiene, Causes, Symptoms, and Treatment with a Chapter on Diet for the Nervous*, 75.

force, and so is an inconstant battery, evolving a force sometimes weak, sometimes strong, and requiring frequent repair-
ing and refilling."[13]

These metaphorical explanations did little to define the exact
changes that brought on the manifestations of nervous exhaustion. Beard, using the researches of Dubois-Reymond on molecular change, suggested that the nervous system, in becoming
"dephosphorized" during the process of use, underwent "morbid changes in its chemical structure" that frequently impaired
the nervous system of the brain-worker.[14] The chemical content of the nervous system varied, according to Beard, with the
race and class of a particular individual. The proportion of
water, phosphorus, fat, and other constituents in the nervous
system, the elements which had a direct relationship to the
intellectual capacity of an individual, were guided by the law
of evolution. "If we know what a nation eats," he wrote, "we
know what a nation is or may become."[15] The most vigorous
brain-workers in society had food demands far different from
the "inactive, phlegmatic, and stationary" peoples of the
earth.[16] The races of man stood in a hierarchical scale, the sensitive Caucasian at the top and the blunted insensitivity of the
savage at the other end. Much nearer "to the forms of life from
which they feed," the savages could subsist on foods that were
repulsive or even poisonous to the higher races. Both physically and intellectually inferior to the Caucasian, the savages
could live comfortably on vegetables or fruits. As races grew
in intellectuality, however, they consumed more and more
meat.[17] The difference between the savage and the civilized
man, evident in the richness of brain convolutions and brain
matter, required a correspondingly different diet. It was
Beard's belief that as man became civilized or susceptible to

13. *Ibid.,* 61.
14. Beard, "Neurasthenia, or Nervous Exhaustion," 218; Hugh Campbell, *A Treatise on Nervous Exhaustion and the Diseases Induced by It* (London, 1874), 26–27.
15. Beard, *Sexual Neurasthenia, Its Hygiene, Causes, Symptoms, and Treatment with a Chapter on Diet for the Nervous,* 260.
16. George M. Beard, *Eating and Drinking; a Popular Manual of Food and Diet in Health and Disease* (New York, 1871), 59.
17. Beard, *Sexual Neurasthenia, Its Hygiene, Causes, Symptoms, and Treatment with a Chapter on Diet for the Nervous,* 256.

nervous exhaustion, he should "diminish the quantity of cereals and fruits, which are far below him on the scale of evolution, and increase the quantity of animal food, which is nearly related to him in the scale of evolution, and therefore more easily assimilated."[18] While the savage and lower classes of a society might live exclusively on coarser foods, the brain-workers required lean meat as their main meal, except during times when the brain was at rest, when fish was allowed to take the place of meat.[19] This relationship of food to intellectual capacity became an essential part of the neurasthenic patient's treatment, for, in many instances, he was required to consume extracts of animal brain to replenish the molecular constitution of his own exhausted brain.

The pathological condition which brought on the various types of neurasthenia was expressed as an excessive expenditure of nervous energy by the nervous system, in which "the force-generating element of the nerve centres is reduced to a condition approaching complete exhaustion." This condition, due to a molecular defect in the constitution of the protoplasm of the cells of the gray neurine, caused a molecular disintegration of this substance in excess of integration by the reparative process.[20] Sanger Brown of Chicago coined the word "neur-energen" to define the form which organic matter took in the neurons, through which organic matter converted to nervous energy and waste products. According to Brown, a healthy individual had a continuous flow of neurenergen current into the neurons which he used as occasion demanded. For the neurasthenic, however, there was a deficiency in the recuperative power of the neurons to maintain a healthy quantity of neurenergen. Perhaps there was even a weakness in the neurons themselves which made them unable to continue proper metamorphosis.[21] It was not without reason then, with all the talk about neurenergen and nervous expenditure, that physi-

18. *Ibid.*, 250.
19. Beard, *Eating and Drinking; a Popular Manual of Food and Diet in Health and Disease*, 134.
20. James Brown, "Neurasthenia, or Nervous Exhaustion," *Transactions, Wisconsin State Medical Society*, XII (1878), 106–7; (Anony.), "The Pathology of the Partial Neurasthenias," *Journal, American Medical Association*, XXV (1895), 547.
21. Sanger Brown, "Neurasthenia," *Medicine*, VII (1901), 458.

cians discussed the nervous activity of the human body in terms of "current," "electricity," "nerve molecules," "conductibility of the neuron," "transmission of impulses," and "fluid theory." In describing the brain and nervous system, physicians frequently compared them to a galvanic battery "whose duty it is to provide a certain and continuous supply of its special fluid for consumption within a given time."[22]

Nineteenth-century physicians pointed out that, like electricity, the nervous energy in the human body was a compound fluid, one negative and the other positive. The natural balance in quantity of these fluids in a particular substance was known as "natural electricity," while the liberation of fluids produced a phenomenon of "active electricity." These same currents of electricity which flowed through the earth and were influenced by seasonal changes, the tides, and other natural phenomena, affected both quantitatively and qualitatively those individuals whose nervous systems were impressionable.[23] Hugh Campbell, in his *Treatise on Nervous Exhaustion* (1874), suggested that the earth's currents were affected strongly by daily tides of positive electricity, one occurring between nine and twelve in the morning and the other between six and nine in the evening, and that it was during these periods of greatest electrical flow that nervous individuals were most susceptible. The condition of nervous debility was subject to this natural earth phenomenon, and changes in the latter produced corresponding changes in the "microscopic molecules of which the nerve substance is composed, whereby their healthy balance is lost and the proper generation of nerve and muscle currents interfered with." This "molecular perturbation," Campbell wrote, gave rise to the nervous condition of neurasthenia as well as hysteria, dyspepsia, chlorosis, and other states of severe prostration.

The presence of this positive electricity has a sustaining and exhilarating effect on the nervous, who it is well known can as a rule employ their mental faculties with more clearness and precision, and with less effort, during the periods of high positive electric tides—the morning and early

22. Campbell, *A Treatise on Nervous Exhaustion and the Diseases Induced by It,* 6.
23. *Ibid.,* 51.

evening—while at the other periods there is a sensible declension of mental and bodily power. Negative electric currents, on the other hand, have a depressing and exhausting effect on the nervous; and this is evidenced in the unpleasant sensations felt by them before a thunderstorm, when negative electricity abounds. As there are daily tides of positive electricity, so are there also seasons. Autumn and winter are the periods when it is in the largest volume in the atmosphere, and these are the times when it is usual for the neurasthenic to enjoy the best health and spirits; while in the late spring and summer, when the opposite condition of atmosphere prevails, they are usually at the lowest point of health and spirit.[24]

Because of the relationship of electrical energy to the theory of nervous prostration, the use of electrical gadgetry became widely accepted in the late nineteenth century for alleviating the ills of neurasthenia. The tonic effect of electricity was both physical (causing muscular contractions of the tissues) and chemical (increasing the absorption of oxygen, modifying endosmosis and exomosis, and changing the form and color of the red corpuscles). The use of electricity on the neuron, it was believed, restored "conductibility" which, due to prostration, had become resistant to the nerve current. By exciting the nerve tissue, a condition of "electrotonos," or a change in nerve excitability, occurred, in which the neuron found newer paths of transmission for its nervous impulses. The "greater the number of ties or connections developing out of the protoplasmic body," wrote electrotherapist Beard, "the richer and more substantial becomes the mentality of the individual."[25]

Physicians experimented with two distinct types of electrization for the neurasthenic individual. One method, called central galvanization, was used chiefly on the central nervous system. It consisted of placing the feet of a patient on a sheet of copper which was attached to a negative pole. A positive pole attached to a sponge or the operator's hand was then applied to the patient, moving across the head, the back of the neck, the spine, arms, stomach, liver, bowels, and lower extremities.

24. *Ibid.*, 9.
25. George M. Beard, *A Practical Treatise on Nervous Exhaustion* (5th ed.; New York, 1905), 283–84, and his *Electricity in the Treatment of Diseases of the Skin* (New York, 1872); Alphonso D. Rockwell and George M. Beard, *A Practical Treatise on the Medical and Surgical Uses of Electricity Including Localized and General Electrization* (New York, 1871), 297.

Special emphasis, however, was given to the head and spine. According to Beard, the use of this procedure improved the "vital force" of the nerve in accordance with Herbert Spencer's theory of the correlation and conservation of forces, and the muscular contractions which accompanied its use increased the processes of waste and repair in those nerves which had become sluggish in their prostrated state.[26] Under a milder treatment, called general faradization, the electrical current was applied locally to a wider range of symptoms. Faradization was thought to impart a qualitative difference to the patient due to the use of bromide of potassium in faradic current rather than hydrate of chloral in the galvanic current. Quite often physicians suggested alternating general faradic with central galvanization in the belief that a combination of the two currents would aid those neurasthenic patients whose malady acted "with strange caprice."[27]

Physicians divided neurasthenia into several categories or varieties, including cerebral, spinal, digestive, traumatic, hysterical, and sexual. The human body, according to Beard, was a "reservoir of force constantly escaping, constantly being renewed from the centre of force—the sun." There was little nerve force in reserve in the neurasthenic and during those instances of excessive exhaustive mental, emotional, or physical labor, he found himself without the reserve or imput of nervous energy necessary to keep a healthy balance.[28] Irritations which arose in one part of the body frequently moved to other more

26. Beard, "Neurasthenia, or Nervous Exhaustion," 219; B. B. Massey, "Electro-Therapeutic Technique in the Treatment of Neurasthenia and Nervous Prostration," *Journal*, American Medical Association, XXV (1895), 974; S. Leduc, "Electrical Treatment of Neurasthenia," *Practitioner*, LXXXVI (1901), 151–65; F. H. Humphris, "Neurasthenia and Its Treatment by Electricity," *Journal of Advanced Therapy*, XXX (1912), 58–67.

27. George M. Beard, *Recent Researches in Electro-Therapeutics* (New York, 1872), 11; Alphonso D. Rockwell and George M. Beard, *The Medical Use of Electricity with Special Reference to General Electrization as a Tonic in Neuralgia, Rheumatism, Dyspepsia, Chorea, Paralysis, and Other Affections Associated with General Debility* (New York, 1867); J. H. Branth, "The Treatment of Neurasthenia," *New York Medical Journal*, LXXXIX (1909), 114.

28. Beard, *Sexual Neurasthenia, Its Hygiene, Causes, Symptoms, and Treatment with a Chapter on Diet for the Nervous*, 58; (Anony.), "Treatment of Neurasthenia," *Journal*, American Medical Association, XLII (1904), 1395; George M. Beard, "Traumatic Neurasthenia," *New England Medical Monthly*, I (1881–82), 246–49; B. C. Loveland, "Some General Considerations on the Treatment of Hysteria and Neurasthenia," *Medicine*, VI (1900), 6.

vulnerable parts. Nervous prostration due to brain work could quite easily affect the digestive as well as the reproductive system. Just as the sensitive nerve supply could cause "waves of hyperemia" that brought congestion and headache to the brain, so it often passed "from one organ to another under the influence of a myriad of exciting causes." The paths of current through the body created a situation in which symptoms would come and go and even substitute one form of disorder for another.[29]

The sexual organs were frequently the seat of nervous exhaustion, and there was almost no end to the variety of medicines and applications to aid the sexually neurasthenic person. Practitioners applied both galvanic and faradic electrization. One electrode was inserted in the rectum and the other in the urethra, or an electrode was inserted in the rectum and the other placed at the perineum or between the penis and scrotum, or on the inner sides of the thighs. External applications of electricity were given along the spine, inner sides of the thighs, and the nerves connected to the genital organs. Physicians also employed a form of general electrization called franklinization, in which static electricity was applied along the spine and genital region. The patient sat on an insulated chair and the physician, applying a variety of electrodes, made "frequent use of electric wind" in treating the bankrupt nervous system.[30]

Confessions of neurasthenics added little to the symptoms already mentioned, except, perhaps, the nearly frantic efforts to which they went seeking a cure. Obsessed with the fear of losing his masculinity as a result of a nocturnal emission (an obsession acquired after reading a "sex-in-life" manual), one desperate subject threw himself into the hands of physicians

29. Beard, *Sexual Neurasthenia, Its Hygiene, Causes, Symptoms, and Treatment with a Chapter on Diet for the Nervous,* 367.

30. *Ibid.,* 277; F. X. Dercum, "The Diagnosis of Neurasthenia," *Medicine,* XII (1906), 27; Louis J. Kahn, *Nervous Exhaustion: Its Cause and Cure* (New York, 1876); Daniel G. Brinton, *The Basis of Social Relations* (New York, 1902), 118; Richard J. Ebbard, *How to Restore Life-Giving Energy to Sufferers from Sexual Neurasthenia and Kindred Brain and Nerve Disorders* (London, 1923); R. W. Miller, "Static Electrical Treatment of Neurasthenia," *Old Dominion Journal of Medicine,* IV (1905–1906), 154–56; Clara E. Gray, "Static Electricity in Neurasthenia," *Journal of Electrotherapeutics,* XVI (1898), 293.

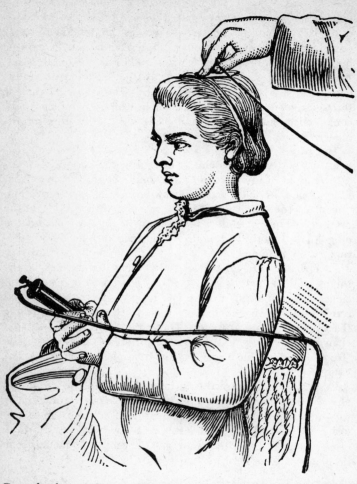

Central galvanization, as illustrated in G. M. Beard and A. D. Rock-well, *A Practical Treatise on the Medical and Surgical Uses of Electricity,* 1881. One pole was placed on the epigastrium, the other on the center of the cranium, the hair at that point being moistened. National Library of Medicine, Bethesda.

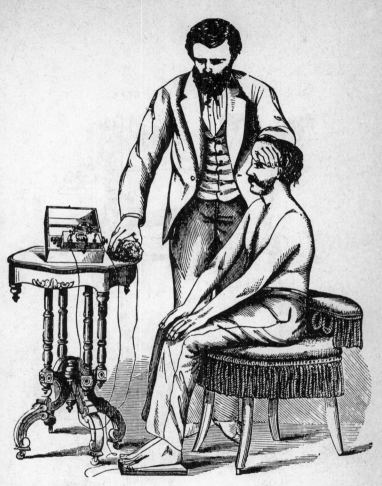

General faradization, as illustrated in G. M. Beard and A. D. Rockwell, *A Practical Treatise on the Medical and Surgical Uses of Electricity*, 1881. The patient is shown "without any covering" but generally patients were "protected by a shawl or wrapper, and frequently the underclothing" was not removed. National Library of Medicine, Bethesda.

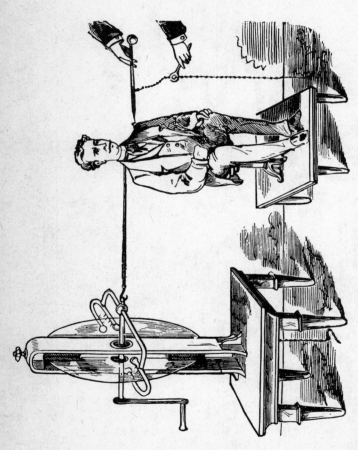

A method of franklinization, as illustrated in G. M. Beard and A. D. Rockwell, *A Practical Treatise on the Medical and Surgical Uses of Electricity*, 1881. National Library of Medicine, Bethesda.

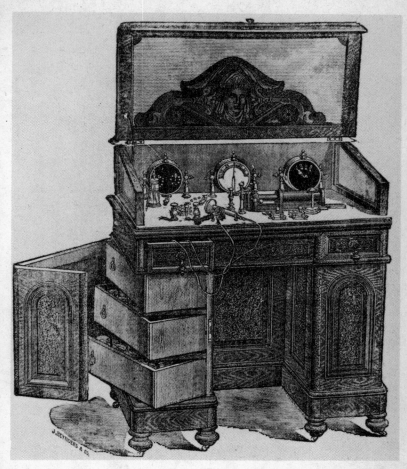

A galvano-faradic machine, with rheostatic coil, as shown in G. M. Beard and A. D. Rockwell, *A Practical Treatise on the Medical and Surgical Uses of Electricity,* 1881. National Library of Medicine, Bethesda.

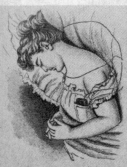
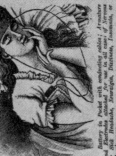
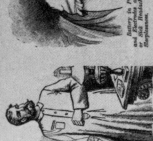

An advertisement from *Harper's Weekly*, June 15, 1889. National Library of Medicine, Bethesda.

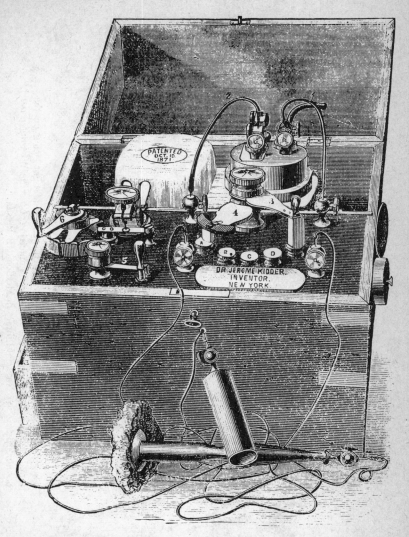

A faradic machine, with a tip arrangement, as illustrated in G. M. Beard and A. D. Rockwell, *A Practical Treatise on the Medical and Surgical Uses of Electricity*, 1881. National Library of Medicine, Bethesda.

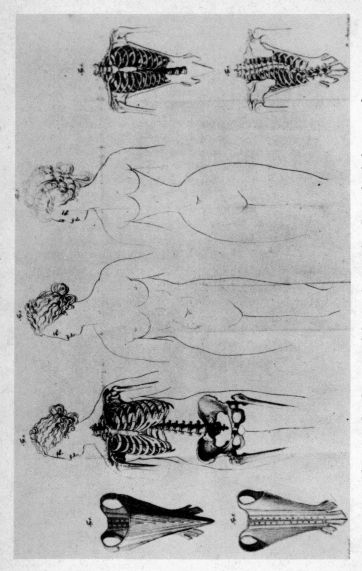

The corseted and uncorseted figure, showing the effects of tight-lacing on the female anatomy, as illustrated in S. T. von Sömmering, *Über die Wirkungen der Schnürbrüste*, 1793. National Library of Medicine, Bethesda.

and quacks who introduced him to electric belts, "crayons inserted in the urethra," rectum medication, magnetism, galvanism, sanitariums, drugs, and baths. He spent months taking animal extracts, and finally, because of his enormous medical bills, bought books on electrization, purchased batteries, and made the electrical applications himself.[31] One case of sexual nerve weakness received notoriety because of the apparatus used to correct "a most obstinate case of impotence" in a patient who had been in the hands of several prominent New York neurologists. The apparatus consisted of a zinc cylinder filled with Rhine wine or weak alcohol and built to enclose the penis. A positive pole was attached to a large electrode and placed over the spine, while the negative pole was connected to the cylinder. The patient used the device three times a day for five or six minutes and was assured of obtaining the sedative effects of the galvanic current.[32]

There were any number of "cures" for neurasthenia, ranging from patent medicines such as Arsenauro and Celernia to prescriptions suggested by concerned physicians and published in the *Journal* of the American Medical Association. The Goat Lymph Sanitarium Association advertised its product, Lymphoids, as a brain and nerve tonic made from animal extracts. The association reported that their tonic stimulated nerve-cell activity and restored the diseased structures to a healthy condition.[33] Another common treatment, called "nervous transfusion," consisted of sheep brain which was macerated, mixed in a glycerin solution, and then injected into the abdomen of the neurasthenic.[34] In addition there were any number of galvanic belts, self-administered electrical stimulators, and a host of "rest cures" or retreats such as the J. H. Kellogg Sanitarium in Battle Creek, Michigan, and Oakwood Springs Sanitarium on Lake Geneva, Wisconsin, where urban society's brain-workers could relax from their hectic pace.

31. (Anony.), "The Autobiography of a Neurasthenic," *Post-Graduate; a Monthly Journal of Medicine and Surgery,* IX (1896), 269.
32. C. L. Dana, "On the Pathology and Treatment of Certain Forms of Nerve-Weakness," *Medical Record,* XXIV (1883), 61.
33. [Advertisement], *Medicine,* X (1904), 2.
34. (Anony.), "A New Cure for Neurasthenia," *Medical Record,* XLII (1892), 343; R. E. Evans, "Case of Neurasthenia Treated by Hypodermic Injections of Nerve Extract," *British Medical Journal,* II (1893), 1321.

The Nervous Woman

Accompanying the medical discovery of neurasthenia was a parallel effort on the part of the urban woman to break from her traditional role as guardian of the home circle and become an active participant in political, business, and reform-minded concerns. Feminists heretofore restricted by political and legal disabilities had, through their efforts in the abolitionist movement before and during the Civil War, begun to look for more egalitarian positions in society than those designated simply by sex. And it was in the abolitionist movement, moreover, that women learned the skills which they would apply to their own cause in the postwar decades. Years of experience in gathering petitions, addressing lecture halls, and holding meetings prepared them in their struggle for recognition in the professions, in the trades, and in areas of society previously closed to them. The decades of the 1850s and 1860s saw the steady rise of women's rights groups which at first could do little but discuss their problems, but which later, through organizing skills learned from abolitionism, actively engaged in fighting for rights before legislative bodies, church boards, university regents, and state bar associations. These women were concerned with their legal position in marriage (eased by the passage in most states by 1850 of married women's property acts), guardianship of children, lack of educational and employment opportunities, divorce laws, and the whole concept of the inferiority of women. Their more militant sisters, led by Elizabeth Cady Stanton and Susan B. Anthony, pressed for women's suffrage, while others (women who formed one-fourth of the total labor force in manufacturing by 1850) organized to secure better working conditions and equal pay. The postwar decades saw women enter colleges and universities more easily and begin to be accepted into the professions—albeit reluctantly and in token numbers only. Elizabeth Blackwell, who in the early 1850s was barred from practicing in New York City hospitals, opened a medical school for women in 1868. Maria Mitchell, the first woman to be elected to the American Academy of Arts and Sciences, came to newly opened Vassar to teach in 1865.

With these ever increasing roles in a society outside the home, however, many women fell victim to the plethora of nervous disorders affecting the urban businessman. The tension between the conservative traditional life-style heretofore expected of women, and the new vistas opening before them, led to anxiety, hysteria, depression, and expressions of insecurity which doctors and laymen in the late nineteenth century noted with rising alarm. No cultured lady of the century, wrote the editor of the *Spectator*, indulged in the hysterics of fainting any more. An unpopular device no longer accepted as a proper drawing-room phenomenon, it was relegated to the kitchen-maid.[35] But while the female of the country swooned less, she compensated for her lack of fainting spells by any number of other complaints which drew even greater attention to her. She burdened those around her with the worry and anxiety that accompanied her nervousness—symptoms which indicated that her adolescence had come to an end, and that she, like the male, was encountering the demands of modern life imposed upon the "better sort."[36]

As cultivated urban women began to see themselves as important participants in the future development and quality of American society, they also began to look upon the evidence of nervous exhaustion as a consequence of their greater intellectuality, and themselves as sufferers for humanity's sake. Conscious of their real as well as imagined contributions to society, they turned to a rather subtle self-flattery by suggesting that society become indulgent to their intoxication with themselves and their own estimation of their talents. Women talked about their nervous conditions in a way they certainly would have avoided a generation before. This was not because there was an element of shamefacedness in the telling, but because their previous illnesses did not have the social acceptability that neurasthenia merited in the late nineteenth century. Furthermore, like the male who had found it more satisfying to seek the emulation of the society around him for the efforts of his brain work, so the "new woman," peering from behind the curtains of domesticity for the first time, found the nervous traffic

35. Editorial, "Nerves and Neurasthenia," *Spectator*, LXXII (1894), 12.
36. Wakefield, "Nervousness: The National Disease of America," 305.

more pleasing outside the home. The "new woman" was mannish enough to demand equal time for discussing her nervous problems, a situation which resulted, according to one critic, in both sexes attempting "to chant nerves together, to compare symptoms, to speculate together on physiological problems and to worry out their cures hand in hand."[37]

What followed was a deluge of neurasthenic men and women who transported their irritable spines across Europe and America to any number of socially accepted health resorts and rural "recovery" homes, filling doctors' offices and hospitals, demanding specialists, tasting nearly every drug from bromide to opium, wearing plates on their feet and magnetic belts around their waists and foreheads, converting to Christian Science, going on "nerve food" diets, and trying innumerable quack devices to alleviate the suffering they endured for the sake of progress.[38] These world-weary jeremiads had an inward satisfaction in presenting the tortured mien of worry, of misfortune, and of morbid heredity, as the stock-in-trade of the brainworker of American society. Yet their maladies, however severe, marked the line between genius and the common sort, between culture and depravity, between mental superiority and mere mechanical activity. The only element that displeased the physician and the class-conscious neurasthenic was the appalling evidence that the malady had spread (by unconscious emulation?) to the working classes. "The much larger class who prate of their nerves without due cause," wrote one disgusted society doctor, "advance them as a reason for holding back from the rough fight of everyday life." Nine-tenths of the neurasthenics in society who eagerly discussed their weak nerves, he went on, "ought never to have been conscious that they had any." As for the American woman, neurasthenia became a cloak behind which she not only made her claim to equality, but also, in many instances, justified her lack

37. Allbutt, "Nervous Diseases and Modern Life," 217; Marrs, *Confessions of a Neurasthenic*, 2.

38. Allbutt, "Nervous Diseases and Modern Life," 217; P. C. Knapp, "Nervous Diseases—Are They Necessary?," *Century Magazine*, LII (1896), 147; (Anony.), "The Autobiography of a Neurasthenic," *American Magazine*, LII (1910), 230; (Anony.), "The Age of Nerves," *Living Age*, CCLXVII (1910), 505; Humphris, "Neurasthenia and Its Treatment by Electricity," 58–60.

of achievement. And the medical profession, while grudgingly recognizing the existence of neurasthenia in the woman, nonetheless took the opportunity to translate her prevailing concern over nerves into a medium seeking to rectify the "woman question."[39]

In one sense, the medical profession interpreted woman's symptoms of nervous exhaustion as a product of the role she played in society. Encumbered with "old worries and irritations," she had allowed her life to become too much of a habit. Woman, unlike man who could go outside the home to release his nervous energy, had "no such taste or opportunity." Trapped in an occupational role she neither accepted nor could find relief in, and fearful of the outside world of which she was still unsure, she languished in a condition of constant nervousness.[40] Because of centuries of dependence upon the male, women tended to lack not only incentive but the will power to develop their own natural feelings. Women were victims of "habit-fatigue" because of the lack of diversification in their work. A psychophysical change thus occurred, a change which affected "the centers of sensation of the brain and [gave] rise to feelings of lassitude and tension."[41] Forced into a life requiring flattery, women had deprived their faculties of legitimate and rewarding emotions.[42] By withholding their feelings because of the strictures of a particular culture, women became victims of nervous debility, and when they ventured outside the home they saw their nerve centers lose control and go astray, traveling along "forbidden channels."[43] This condition was frequently rationalized by the woman as a cross to be borne for civilization's sake, but it was also used, particularly by the practitioner,

39. Editorial, "Nerves and Neurasthenia," 12; (Anony.), "Science and Women," *Medical Record*, XLII (1892), 46.

40. H. J. Hall, "The Systematic Use of Work as a Remedy in Neurasthenia and Allied Conditions," *Boston Medical and Surgical Journal*, CLII (1905), 30; F. B. Bishop, "The Cause of Some Cases of Neurasthenia, and Their Treatment by Electricity," *Transactions,* American Electro-Therapeutic Association (1889–1900), 327.

41. Samuel McComb, "Nervousness—A National Menace," *Everybody's Magazine*, XX (1910), 259.

42. Cyril Bennett, *The Modern Malady; or, Sufferers from "Nerves"* (London, 1890), 166.

43. Peckham, "The Nervousness of Americans," 46; Ferdinand Lundberg and Marynia F. Farnham, *Modern Woman: The Lost Sex* (New York, 1947), chap. 6.

to explain her natural inferiority (like the "inferior races") and her susceptibility to nervous disease when she took on too many duties, moved out of the home, or just presumed too much in a man's world. A perceptive remark by a young victim of neurasthenia, Jane Addams, seems to support this argument. In a state of nervous depression that lasted for years after her graduation from college, and heightened by the awareness of her inability to bear children, a loss, as it were, of femininity, she remarked that perhaps the newly emancipated young women had suffered too much by forsaking the "emotional" life led by their grandmothers and great-grandmothers.[44]

Many doctors argued that fashionable women sufferers saw in neurasthenia a certain status and social accomplishment—a feeling of intellectuality and high culture. This group of women, wrote Margaret Cleaves, M.D., of Des Moines, often delighted in their illnesses. They floundered amid "an endless round of social dissipations and a thousand and one indiscretions." Conscious of their plight, yet with little or no distraction to turn their heads to other things, they lived "upon the sweet counsel of their physicians and the daily ministration of loving friends." It was to them that the "house physician like a house fly is in chronic attention."[45] Unlike man, the fashionable sufferer found it difficult to divert attention away from herself. The monotony of her life turned "her mind back upon itself," and she tended to dwell upon her mental and physical troubles if for no other reason than "because she [had] little else to think of." While man's pursuits, wrote Harry Campbell, M.D., led him away from the agonizing role of self-pity and contemplation, woman, being less developed than man, sought comfort in the intensity of her condition and her suffering.[46]

44. Jane Addams, *Twenty Years at Hull House* (New York, 1910), 71; Merle Curti, "Jane Addams on Human Nature," *Journal of the History of Ideas,* XXII (1961), 240–44.

45. Margaret Cleaves, "Neurasthenia and Its Relation to Diseases of Women," *Transactions,* Iowa State Medical Society, VII (1886), 166–67; Anne Bryan McCall, "The Girl Who Is Nervous," *Woman's Home Companion,* XXXIX (1912), 27.

46. Harry Campbell, *Differences in the Nervous Organization of Man and Woman: Psychological and Pathological* (London, 1891), 190; D. R. Brower, "Cerebral Neurasthenia, or Failure of Brain-Power, with Special Reference to Its Electro-Therapeutics," *Transactions,* American Electro-Therapeutic Association (1899–1900), 335.

But there were reasons beyond self-pity that explained the fashionable sufferers. Neurasthenia, added Cleaves, frequently beset those women who carried their sex to a greater plateau of learning—"those women occupying the higher social plane, women of intelligence, education and culture." Their ambitions for intellectual, social, and financial success, their constant strain to exceed the accomplishments of those who came before them, their desire for improving the lot of other women, were "predisposing or exciting causes of neurasthenia."[47] Throughout her book, *The Autobiography of a Neurasthene* (1910), Cleaves depicted herself as a "mannish Maiden." Her father's closest companion in her youth, she said of herself often: "I was my father's boy." As a result of a masculinity complex in her childhood, the driving force of male-dominated cultural values, and her father's wish that she enter the professional world, Cleaves went into medicine. But saddened by the sense of deficiency and inferiority that her sex and society had prepared for her, and feeling chronically exhausted by the mental tensions and disappointments that her chosen career in medicine had given her, she exhibited feelings of castration, depression, and all manners of hypochondriacal ideas.[48] She had been brought up to assume a man's role in society, when, in fact, the society was still unprepared to accept such an identity. The result, as she diagnosed it, was a "sprained brain."[49] Prepared for a greater, more intellectual role than her sex had been permitted to assume, she felt "alone, shut out from the active whirl of the world."[50] "Victory will come to the few," she wrote, "but shattered nerves to the most. Women, more than men, are handicapped at the outset, not necessarily because they are women, but because, suddenly and without the previous preparations that men for generations have had, they attempt to fulfill certain conditions and are expected to qualify themselves for certain work and distinctions. . . . It may be

47. Cleaves, "Neurasthenia and Its Relation to Diseases of Women," 165.

48. Margaret Cleaves, *The Autobiography of a Neurasthene* (Boston, 1910), 119–20; C. Thompson, "Penis Envy in Women," *Psychiatry*, VI (1943), 123–25; K. Horney, "The Flight from Womanhood: The Masculinity Complex in Women," *International Journal of Psychoanalysis*, VII (1925), 324–39.

49. Cleaves, *The Autobiography of a Neurasthene*, 109.

50. *Ibid.*, 225, 239.

true, as emphasized by [Samuel Weir] Mitchell and others, that girls and women are unfit to bear the continued labor of mind because of the disqualifications existing in their physiological life."[51]

For women like Margaret Cleaves and Jane Addams, neurasthenia was a manifestation of the insecurity felt by the Victorian woman in her efforts to challenge the mores of a male-dominated society. Yet despite the obstacles they encountered, one receives the impression that these women had the satisfaction of believing that society thought them better women for their neurasthenia. But for most practitioners, the insecurity which women felt was more real than imagined since a fundamental difference existed between the mental aptitudes of the sexes. As civilization advanced, as it developed greater minds and strained to newer heights of technology, so the woman in society, "the companion or ornamental appendage to man," was forced to come to terms with the complexities of the age. Because the woman used her brain "but little and in trivial matters," argued George Beard, and because the capacity of her brain was but nine-tenths that of man, the efforts to change her life-style amounted to a thorough challenge to her physical and mental constitution.[52]

According to many clinicians who treated neurasthenia, women who inherited weakened nervous systems were less able to resist the state of tension that accompanied urban life. The weakened nerve force did not by itself cause neurasthenia, but it did prevent women from developing normal strength needed to ward off constitutional ailments. The weakened nervous system of the young girl or harassed housewife annoyed with household and family cares was a sufficient catalyst for the development of any number of organic problems.[53] Implying that women were innately inferior to men in their nervous development, Graeme M. Hammond, M.D., professor of mental

51. Cleaves, "Neurasthenia and Its Relation to Diseases of Women," 166.

52. Beard, *Eating and Drinking; a Popular Manual of Food and Diet in Health and Disease*, 103; E. P. Hayward, "Types of Female Castration Reaction," *Psychoanalytical Quarterly*, XII (1943), 45–66.

53. H. B. Deale and S. S. Adams, "Neurasthenia in Young Women," *Transactions*, Obstetrical and Gynecological Society of Washington, IV (1892), 109–110.

and nervous diseases at the New York Post-Graduate School, suggested that while "ample in all probability to meet the requirements of an even, placid, and uneventful existence," women were absolutely unable "to stand against a strong current of misfortune, care or overwork."[54] "We live in the midst of eternal and never ending vibrations," added neurasthenic Margaret Cleaves, "and our myriads of chemical cells are ceaselessly vibrating to the end that nerve energy may be stored, transmitted and recorded." But for the urban woman, the "neurotic wires are down and the higher vibrations fail to reach us."[55] No matter how much the urban woman achieved in a day's work, she would always experience a feeling of having "ignominiously failed" in life's duties.[56] She bore through life "a fundamental nutritive lack of the nerve centres," and was unable to confront the harsh realities of the city without giving evidence of major constitutional disorders.[57]

Physicians pointed to a number of constitutional problems affecting women that grew out of the environmental influences of urban development in America. Between the urban woman and the rural housewife there were obvious differences in the capacity of the chest, the quality of lung tissue, the amount of oxygen and carbonic acid in the blood, and the accumulation of waste products in the body. Furthermore, the urban woman's greater confinement in the home, her lack of exercise and fresh air, the disuse of arm and chest muscles, the substitution of an "artificial shape" for a simple dress, and the burden of carrying large amounts of heavy clothing and ornament suspended from the waist rather than from the shoulders added to her constitutional deficiencies. The cultured woman of the city dressed in the height of fashion wore an average of thirty-seven pounds of street costume in the winter months, of which nineteen pounds suspended from her waist.[58] To complicate her situation even more, she suffered from the irritating noises of the city's life, and the constant "jarring of the brain and

54. Hammond, "Nerves and the American Woman," 590–91.
55. Cleaves, *The Autobiography of a Neurasthene*, 208.
56. *Ibid.*, 236.
57. *Ibid.*, 18.
58. A. L. Smith, "What Civilization Is Doing for the Human Female," *Transactions,* Southern Surgical and Gynecological Association, II (1890), 355.

spinal cord by continual treading upon the stone and brick"
pavements tended to exaggerate her physical and mental deterioration.[59]

Despite the repeated contrasts made between the urban and
rural woman, few physicians gave rural life anything more
than a remote mythical importance—a vague reminder of the
nation's pastoral origins in the age of machines. The rural environment could scarcely meet the technological needs of the
new age, and physicians seemed to prefer the urban reality
with all its assorted problems to the charm of rural life. At best,
Victorian doctors created a middle ground where they sought
to join an enthusiasm for urban life with a romantic appeal to
race origins. But included in that middle ground was an obvious contempt for the rural type. The physician's middle ground
was a pastoral land tilled by a vague, prelapsarian rustic whom
they admired and compared to the industrial brain-worker.
Essentially then, the urban brain-worker, despite physical deficiencies in lung size, strength, chest dimensions, and endur-
ance, was the direct descendant of the prelapsarian rustic. The
rural "hayseeds," on the other hand, while retaining many of
the physical attributes of the rustic types, were nonetheless
mental atavisms further remote than the urban brain-worker
from their rural cousins. With this sort of balance, physicians
indulged in rural analogy. The industrial age was not so much
a counterforce to the pastoral myth as a progressive evolution
out of it.

The social complexities of neurasthenia, and in particular
the proper role of the American woman, aggravated the political spleen of medical prognosticators. Given the fact that the
urban woman was delicate and nervous, and that she reacted
in a more severe way to the environment of city life, doctors
were nonetheless conspicuously glib about the prospects of a
solution to the problem. For some, it meant that the woman
must return to the home (though surely not the "home" of the
rural American), and find values in a new threshold of domesticity. This group argued that while modern conveniences such
as baker's bread, canned foods, and ready-made clothes had

removed much of the traditional role of women in the home, there remained many avenues of self-satisfaction through the new science of home economics. Only in admitting her true nature in the home circle and then seeking respectability within that circle could woman avoid the misfortunes of neurasthenia.

Those physicians who thought that the neurasthenic disorders of the urban woman were the product of her wanderings outside domesticity were also quick to point out that her subsequent mental and physical problems threatened not only to destroy her sexual instincts but democratic institutions as well. The nervous exhaustion of those cultured women who left the home circle gave a birth advantage to alien stocks in America, a fact which some suspected had caused a socialistic undermining of the American way of life. While an increased number of ignorant and poor inundated the birth rolls of the census bureau, the educated and cultured American woman seemed to prefer no family at all.[60] Indeed, one doctor believed that the nervous exhaustion evidenced in the middle-class woman was a sign of her growing distaste for her sexual role. The young woman who entered the professions accepted a life of spinsterhood to marriage, or at best, became a poor wife and mother to a numerically smaller family.[61] It seemed apparent to some doctors that the civilized woman cared little for sexual relations, "that the higher one rises in the grade of civilization, the less the sexual instinct remains."[62] Moses T. Runnels, M.D., warned men not to marry such a woman because the mode of her dress, which was destructive of natural physical development, and the career-mindedness of her intentions, made her less than a companion in marriage. Dwarfed, nervous, and constantly demanding in her delicate ailments, she became a continual disappointment to happy wedlock.[63]

Doctors splashed medical journals with lurid accounts of bluestockings who entered into the business world in competition with men. Woman's efforts, acted out rashly and foolishly, wrote one physician, made her ultimately unfit for marriage

60. M. T. Runnels, "Physical Degeneracy of American Women," *Medical Era*, III (1886), 302.
61. Brinton, *The Basis of Social Relations*, 118–19.
62. Smith, "What Civilization Is Doing for the Human Female," 359.
63. Runnels, "Physical Degeneracy of American Women," 297.

due to the perilous injury brought on by the "deleterious irritation" of the outside world upon her system. Desiring to demonstrate her ability in the business world, the bluestocking did too much too quickly. It should be remembered, admonished Cyril Bennett, M.D., that those women who entered the professions held by men and who succeeded in showing that they were equal to the occasion were usually mistaken in their capacity. Women who proved mentally capable for particular professions did not really show that, like men, they were "highly organized." Rather than enlarging the scope of their relationships, such women "seem to have shot out a long angle on one side of their natures at the expense of drawing to a corresponding extent on the other side." In the long run, the advent of women into the professions would only increase their emotional disorder, since their "sensitive organizations . . . are more easily injured by [the professions] than are the tougher organizations of men." High-strung women merely prolonged and intensified an inevitable nerve deterioration in a business-world environment.[64]

Arabella Kenealy, M.D., suggested additional evidence to the theory of listlessness as a cause for the urban woman's neurasthenia. It seemed to her that the female of the nineteenth century had been left with few chores because of the variety of conveniences available to her. She no longer spent hours over the stove or made her own clothes. Paid hirelings now nursed, clothed, and taught her children, and professional performers entertained her guests. Left to a life of boredom because of a lack of those duties which formerly defined her womanly role, she became neurasthenic. Yet Kenealy did not advocate a business orientation for the woman. Outside the home, where "the sole business wherewith the mightiest forces of the universe and evolution are concerned," was no place for woman to find her "nobler sphere." Preserving her essential femininity and womanhood was the best of all vocations. Woman had to re-

64. Bennett, The Modern Malady, or, Sufferers from "Nerves," 169–70; Louise Fiske-Bryson, "Woman and Nature," New York Medical Journal, XLVI (1887), 628; Otto Juettner, "The Place of Woman in the Modern Business World as Affecting the Future of the Race," Bulletin, American Academy of Medicine, IX (1908), 349; Norman Bridge, "The Place of Woman in the Modern Business World as Affecting Health and Morals," ibid., 343–48.

orient herself in the home. This did not mean that she had to give up the idea of education and self-support; only that her noblest sphere could be found in the home in roles yet undefined.[65] Similarly, Minerva Palmer, M.D., of Rochester, in an article in the *Medical News* in 1890, remarked disparagingly that whenever women left the home, or bettered their opportunities through education and the professions, they were inevitably met "by disagreement from one of the best informed and most philanthropic class of citizens—the doctors." Their usual remarks, she pointed out, were that such a step was impossible, that women could not equal the brain work of men, and that further, in those cases where women were not yet married, they would "probably be deprived of happy marriage" through a weakened mental and physical constitution. But while Palmer disagreed with the degree of this old-fashioned moralism, she betrayed no impulsive sentiment for the completely liberated female. Her remarks, like those of Kenealy, tended to suggest that women's future still lay in the home, perhaps obtaining a new respectability through the home economics movement which offered a "safe" and noncompetitive education and career for women, still centered in the home circle.[66]

As the female constitution was frail, those physicians (both male and female) who argued for a role of domesticity believed that the woman required increased protection from the "march of civilization and over-refinement." Though she should remain in the protective atmosphere of the home, doctors cautioned her to avoid those elements that threatened her delicate position even in the home environment—over-excitement, stimulating reading, and improper food and dress. She was advised to bathe frequently in order to stimulate her skin, get proper amounts of open-air exercise, abstain from all undue mental

65. Quoted in (Anony.), "A Lady Doctor on the Girl of To-Day," *Medical Record*, LV (1899), 719; James Weir, Jr., "The Effects of Female Suffrage on Posterity," *American Naturalist*, XXIX (1895), 824–25; Andrew S. Lobingier, "The Place of Women in the Modern Business World as Affecting Homelife and Marriage," *Bulletin*, American Academy of Medicine, IX (1908), 335–42; J. S. Weatherly, "Woman; Her Rights and Her Wrongs," *Transactions,* Medical Association of Alabama (1872), 67–68.

66. Minerva Palmer, "Co-Education and the Higher Education of Women," *Medical News,* LVI (1890), 77.

excitement, avoid horseback riding, bicycle riding, and alcohol, and take generous amounts of rest. She was told to travel abroad, and spend a portion of her vacation in a camp-life environment "where [she] may be free from sympathizing friends and indulgent parents." And most important, she was to control her sexual desires.[67]

Even more destructive of health, thought G. M. Hammond, M.D., was the fashionable practice of eating out in restaurants for luncheon. Women caused physical and mental harm to their delicate constitutions by making a habit of eating rich foods, drinking numerous cups of tea, and sometimes taking what was termed "light refreshment." Hammond also advised women against the game of cards. Too many society women were "making a dissipation out of what should be harmless amusement." Excessive bridge playing was taking its toll upon the nervous centers of women. "Nature will have her pound of flesh," he warned, "and generally demands usurious interest as well."[68] The whole nature of woman's constitution, wrote another doctor, was not only "more delicate," but was more easily disturbed by exposure to the outside world. For that reason, nature had prescribed for her a "life of ease and comparative inactivity." Both men and women had well-defined roles. A romantic melodramatist, he described them as two distinct rivers seeking an outlet in the same sea.

They flow through different channels, but the aim of both is the same. Her course like the stream which flows through meadows of grass and flowers; his the wild mountain torrent, dashing through gorges and leaping precipices, causing the mild roar of the cataract, but bearing everything before it by main force. For the work peculiarly appropriate to woman, she of course is far superior to man. Her work, however, does not tend toward massive strength either of body or mind, but rather to a gentle modelling of both. Purely mental culture in her, yielding to the affections, which, being more stimulated, predominate. Where these go hand in hand, both the affections and mind receiving the best culture,

67. W. W. Bliss, *Woman's Life: A Pen-Picture of Woman's Functions, Frailties, and Follies* (Boston, 1879), 7; Deale and Adams, "Neurasthenia in Young Women," 112–13; H. B. Combs, "Sexual Neurasthenia Resulting from Posterior Urethritis," *Transactions,* State Medical Association of Texas (1904), 362; H. M. Jones, "The Sexual Element in the Neurasthenia of Women," *Practitioner,* LXXXVI (1911), 61–75; J. A. Holloway, "Sexual Neurasthenia," *Texas Medical News,* XII (1902–1903), 51–54.

68. Hammond, "Nerves and the American Woman," 591–92.

we find the highest type of womanhood—I might say the highest type of humanity.[69]

A large number of physicians regarded education as a factor in the rising number of neurasthenic girls. Young women "whose mental powers are overtaxed before their brains are sufficiently developed" were easily susceptible to nervous exhaustion. The young girl needed to conserve the powers of the brain during her formative years. While mental labor was necessary to strengthen the mind, too much labor forced the brain beyond its natural capacity. William A. Hammond, M.D., who directed a private hospital for nervous disorders in Washington, pointed out that cerebral hyperemia was more frequent among girls who indulged in mental pursuits beyond their capacity.[70] Some clinicians argued that education beyond high school was both physically and mentally destructive for women. The smaller brain weight was proof enough of a striking natural limitation to intellectual attainment. The "struggle for existence on deficient nerve capital," wrote another skeptic, brought early bankruptcy to the woman's system. Having loosened the moorings of her past life-style and drifting "faithlessly in the sea of doubt, with no respect for authority," the educated woman fell an easy victim to nervous disease.[71] One doctor in his study of 187 high school girls found that 137 of them constantly complained of headaches—evidence, he concluded, of their inability to cope with the complexities of intellectual life beyond a minimum level.[72] A Boston physician's study of school girls in 1902 indicated that girls were worse off physically when leaving school than when they arrived.[73] Another medical practitioner in 1903 suggested that

69. Weatherly, "Woman; Her Rights and Her Wrongs," 67.

70. William A. Hammond, *Cerebral Hyperaemia, the Result of Mental Strain or Emotional Disturbance; the So-Called Nervous Prostration or Neurasthenia* (Washington, 1895), 71.

71. Brower, "Cerebral Neurasthenia, or Failure of Brain-Power, with Special Reference to Its Electro-Therapeutics," 335.

72. (Anony.), "Sexual Brain Differences and High-School Education," *Medical Record*, XLII (1892), 46.

73. R. W. Lovett, "The Health of School Girls," *Boston Medical and Surgical Journal*, CXLVI (1902), 376–78; A. L. Smith, "Are Modern School Methods in Keeping with Physiologic Knowledge," *Bulletin*, American Academy of Medicine, VI (1905), 871–79; John Duffy, "Mental Strain and 'Overpressure' in the Schools: A 19th Century Viewpoint," *Journal of the History of Medicine*, XXIII (1968), 63–79.

trained medical people should thoroughly examine those women who chose to enter college, study both personal and family health history, and classify their school curriculum "in accordance with their physical condition."[74]

Those doctors who advised a life of domesticity for the American woman were also the ones whose arguments for woman's inferiority in the late nineteenth century were almost identical with the century's rationalization for the inferiority of the blacks. Arguing for the inferior position of women, these physicians used statistics that suggested a direct comparison with the Negro. Harry Campbell, M.D., for example, in his *Difference in the Nervous Organization of Man and Woman: Physiological and Pathological* (1891), pointed out that just as black children showed an early precocity and atrophy ("their mental evolution seeming to come to a stand-still") so the white woman's mental evolution appeared to blossom early, frequently achieving bright success during her early years, then declining after a short span of time. The mental development of the white male, on the other hand, while slower, continued to mature beyond puberty. More conventional and more a creature of routine, the female (like the Negro) had innate limitations on her capacities. At best she was imitative and generally lacked the spark of originality.[75]

In general, doctors admonished the nineteenth-century woman against forcing her intellect beyond the bounds of her natural capacity. Furthermore, by delaying or prolonging her education she threatened to undermine her marriageable status. Out of 705 women who went to college, wrote Runnels of Kansas City, only 196 married, and of those 66 had no children, and of those who did have children, there was a high percentage of still-born births. It seemed clear that the cause was

74. D. L. Wilkinson, "Some Remarks Concerning Education and the Results of the Examination of over 2,000 Young College Women," *Transactions,* Medical Association of Alabama (1903), 114; Stephen H. Weeks, "Is Equal Treatment of the Sexes Best, or Do Girls Require the Same Treatment as Boys," *Bulletin,* American Academy of Medicine, VI (1905), 887–96; James H. McBride, "The Life and Health of Our Girls in Relation to Their Future," *Bulletin,* American Academy of Medicine, VI (1903), 321–42.

75. Campbell, *Differences in the Nervous Organization of Man and Woman: Psychological and Pathological,* 172, 232.

higher education.[76] "Women beware," wrote R. R. Coleman, M.D., of Birmingham, "You are on the brink of destruction: You have hitherto been engaged in crushing your waists; now you are attempting to cultivate your mind: You have been merely dancing all night in the foul air of the ball-room; now you are beginning to spend your mornings in study. You have been incessantly stimulating your emotions with concerts and operas, with French plays, and French novels; now you are exerting your understanding to learn Greek, and solve propositions in Euclid. Beware!! science pronounces that the woman who studies is lost."[77]

There were, of course, physicians less disposed to seeing women continue to live within the narrow confines of domesticity. Yet the woman's role remained largely undefined in their writings. The proper role and how the woman should pursue it caused endless argument among them. At best, they agreed that the new role would be outside the home; but they also believed that the woman must recognize her "natural" inclinations and aptitudes before attempting to more completely enter into the man's world. The suggestion had the effect of encouraging women to leave the home if they must, but maintain the femininity of the domesticated housewife. Women were advised to carry with them all the paraphernalia of the home virtues. Indeed, these nineteenth-century doctors advised women to perpetuate the fantasy of their home circle in the outside world, a request which if complied with would have made them noncompetitive, ministering angels to the less fortunate of the city. Physicians, like the society around them, could not accept the "mannish maiden." Women personified an ideal and the "new woman" was sacrified to that ideal: she was made to perpetuate the myth outside the home. Her position in the community could only mirror that of her domestic life-style. The "new woman" portrayed by this group of practi-

76. Runnels, "Physical Degeneracy of American Women," 297; C. Pope, "Vi ginity of Twenty Years Standing in a Married Woman Suffering from Neurasthenia," *American Journal of Urology*, XI (1915), 250–60.

77. R. Coleman, "Woman's Relations to the Higher Education and Professions, as Viewed from Physiological and Other Standpoints," *Transactions*, Medical Association of Alabama (1889), 238.

tioners was surely not as timid or as quiet as those who remained at home, but she was nonetheless required to yield quickly to the domination of man, her natural protector. Her modesty, piety, physical weakness, and lack of intellectual training made hers a destiny of implicit compliance with the value system in which she would always be subordinate, venerated, admired, and ignored.

Charles L. Dana, M.D., wrote in the *Boston Medical and Surgical Journal* that in no instance had he ever found a woman who suffered from neurasthenia to be a victim of overwork or mental exhaustion. Both he and Herbert J. Hall, M.D., of Massachusetts thought the cause of women's neurasthenia lay more in their idleness than anything else. "When neurasthenia in almost any degree is established," wrote Hall, "a feeling of fatigue is often brought on by the mere thought of exertion or by the anticipation of any task." Neurasthenic women were those who led "faulty lives" and correction required a radical change in life-style. Old worries, irritations, and a life guided by habit had been the cause of their difficulties. The great need for neurasthenic women, suggested Hall, was not in "prolonged rest," but rather in "bringing about a gradual progress in the conditions of a normal life, a life of pleasant and progressive occupation, as different as possible from the previous life and resulting in self-forgetfulness." He reminded the profession that most neurasthenics were more creative than average people; generally they were clever, artistic, and had a potentiality for more difficult problems. The condition of neurasthenia was not a result of attempting to change, but in remaining passive to the creative power and continuing to subsist on the meager and unchallenging life.[78]

But the degree to which these physicians hesitated in encouraging fully emancipated women is more than evidenced in their suggestions that women seek altruistic vocations in the urban streets, rather than in the urban business houses. In Boston, New York, San Francisco, Chicago, and other urban cen-

78. Quoted in H. J. Hall, "The Systematic Use of Work as a Remedy in Neurasthenia and Allied Conditions," 29–30; August Forel, *The Sexual Question; a Scientific, Psychological, Hygienic and Sociological Study for the Cultured Classes* (New York, 1906), 468.

ters, doctors and clergy cooperated to deal with the "mannish maiden." This self-centeredness of urban woman, wrote Samuel McComb of the Emmanuel Movement of Boston, left them "without any conscious purpose in life." Constructive work, and above all, altruistic work, had a healing character. If only urban women would transform the misery of their existence, their brooding, their worry, and vacillation into organizational work devoted to the redemption of others, the wretchedness of neurasthenia would become a passing phase. The solution to women's dilemma was a social gospel with roots in both medicine and religion. McComb's Emmanuel Movement, like other mind-cure urban agencies, sought to create ministering angels out of the neurasthenic sufferers who chose to leave their homes. Unhappiness came from "a disease of the soul," wrote McComb, a disease which did not need drugs, but a new view of life. Women's altruism would overcome "nerve-wasting emotions" and create individuals whose minds were sustained by "moments of physical and mental relaxation." Drugs, those crutches used by women to carry them through the depression of self-centeredness, would be supplanted by a social gospel of good works. Urban life for liberated women depended upon a harmony of brain, nerve, and religious aptitude.[79]

The so-called neurasthenic woman was never defined in any measurable way in the late nineteenth century. Too often the term stood for conflicting terms and ideologies. Woman was an enigma to the medical profession, an enigma that grew first from an imperfect apprehension of her disorder, and was confused even further by the dialectical skills of the physician-philosophers of the age and their efforts to deal with the implications of feminism in a male-oriented society. The origin of woman's neurasthenia was spurious—connected at one point to a romantic idea of herself and her impending suffering for the fruits of progress, and at another, to a banal, mechanical

79. Samuel McComb, "My Experience with Nervous Sufferers," *Harper's Bazaar*, XLIV (1910), 29; Ellwood Worcester, Samuel McComb, and Dr. Isidor H. Coriat, *Religion and Medicine; the Moral Control of Nervous Disorders* (New York, 1908); L. Gilbert Little, *Nervous Christians* (Nebraska, 1956). Similar organizations to that of the Emmanuel Movement were begun in Chicago by Samuel Fallowes and in San Francisco by Bishop Nichols. See Donald Meyer, *The Positive Thinkers* (New York, 1965), 250–52; Gilbert Seldes, *The Stammering Century* (New York, 1928), chaps. 22 through 25.

rejection of her accepted life-style. Neurasthenia, a reservoir of class prejudices, status desires, urban arrogance, repressed sexuality, and indulgent self-centeredness, was also an index, among other gauges, by which the nineteenth-century woman measured her right to recognition and her claim to equality. The will, the imagination, and a thousand concealed disorders of the body conspired to formulate an ethic for the urban woman. Perhaps the ambiguity concerning her malady explains the voluminous material on the neurasthenic woman. While few physicians questioned the greater intellectual brain force of the urban businessman as a cause for his neurasthenia, almost all were willing to dispute the similar implications that accompanied the signs of neurasthenia in women. Physicians conspicuously divided on the social implications of women's nervousness, a division that went to the very heart of the woman's role in the society of the nineteenth century.

In their etiology of neurasthenia, late nineteenth-century physicians took the opportunity to transpose the nervous disorders of middle-class society into a rationalization for the superiority of urban life, a belief in the greater brain force of the urban business class, a foundation for the nation's rapid development as a world power, and a justification for the superiority of urban culture over traditional rural values. Neurasthenia became, in a very real sense, a rationalization of America's new social order. Greedy for material wealth, yet sobered by the less wholesome aspects of the city's lure, urban society conveniently discovered in neurasthenia an ideology to counter the traditional values attributed to the countryside and the stereotyped evils of urban living. The seemingly objective observations made by practitioners on nervous exhaustion became an analysis of and a justification for the mores of the Gilded Age. Neurasthenia in this sense was part of a much larger self-evaluation of America's concept of civilization and an object of value attributed to certain members of that society. It reflected an essential ethic in the society, a certain social value in middle-class behavior. In diagnosing the malady, pre-Freudian clinicians brought meaning to the assumptions of that ethic, and drew a thread between the changes and demands of their culture and the image of the middle class as the embodiment of that society's values.

The word neurasthenia received respectful consideration by the medical profession in the Victorian period and only slowly was it challenged. In the early 1900s, however, physicians began to question whether both the physician and the patient might be better off without the term. J. L. Tracy, M.D., for example, wrote to the American Medical Association in 1904 that he refused to make a diagnosis of neurasthenia. "I would rather anytime say outright that I do not know," he wrote, than to use the term which, by its very vagueness, applied to almost any and all diseases. "To diagnose neurasthenia," he argued, "is to beg the question, and what is worse and still more unscientific, is to say that neurasthenia is the cause of some local trouble."[80] Yet the word continued in usage through World War I and applied to conditions arising from concussion, battle fatigue, and shell shock. In 1916 the French military, concerned that the word was spoken "rather too glibly [by] the lay tongue," abandoned the term altogether and created special examination boards for those individuals claiming to be the victims of the disease.[81] Although neurasthenia died a pauper's death in the 1920s, it nevertheless was an important documentary of America's (as well as Europe's) uneasy accommodation with the industrialized age. The tensions and problems of the urban man and woman were both feared and respected; indeed, the disease was an anomaly that puzzled those who did not suffer from it and frustrated those whose satisfaction it was to be its victim.

80. J. L. Tracy, "That 'Neurasthenia' Foolishness," *Journal,* American Medical Association, XLII (1904), 1034; Knapp, "Nervous Diseases—Are They Necessary?," 146; W. Browning, "Is There Such a Disease as Neurasthenia?," *New York State Journal of Medicine,* XI (1911), 7; C. H. Miles, "Neurasthenia: A 20th Century Neurosis, a Preventable and Curable Disease," *Medical Times,* LIII (1925), 46.

81. J. Collie, "The Management of Neurasthenia and Allied Disorders Contracted in the Army," *Journal of State Medicine,* XXVI (1918), 7; (Anony.), "Treatment of Neurasthenia at Golders Green," *Lancet,* I (1918), 723; A. J. Brock, "The War Neurasthenic; a Note on Methods of Reintegrating Him with His Environment," *Lancet,* I (1918), 436.

Chapter II

THE LESSER MAN

[Woman] does nothing as we do. She thinks, speaks, and acts differently. Her tastes are different from our tastes. Her blood even does not flow in her veins as ours does, at times it rushes through them like a foaming mountain torrent. She does not respire as we do. Making provision for pregnancy and the future ascension of the lower organs, nature has so constructed her that she breathes, for the most part by the four upper ribs. From this necessity, results woman's greatest beauty, and gently undulating bosom, which expresses all her sentiments by a mute eloquence. She does not eat like us—neither as much nor of the same dishes. Why? Chiefly, because she does not digest as we do. Her digestion is every moment troubled by one thing: She yearns with her very bowels. The deep cup of love (which is called the pelvis) is a sea of varying emotions, hindering the regularity of the nutritive functions.

Jules Michelet, *Woman's Love and Life*, 1881

A profoundly skeptical scientific commentary lay concealed beneath the penmanship and decorated canvasses glorifying the woman of the nineteenth century. Hidden under the lofty sentiment which depicted her as the "soul gardener" in the life of the nation lurked theories which hinted at other, more restrictive, occupations. The controversy in medical circles over the causes of neurasthenia was only one aspect of a larger ideology concerning the role of woman in society—a role which defined her as a "lesser man" and limited her to a position of dependence and subordination. In reinforcing these traditions, the medical community used a mixture of anthropometric studies, biblical references, medical evidence, and evolutionary law to explain woman's proper role and place in nature. Persuaded that she was sovereign only within the protected genteel environment of velvet swathings, lace doilies, tassels, and massive drapes, science dismissed any possibility of roles other than those which assured the stability of the home circle. While this advice sounded at times like pathetic exhortation rather than logical reasoning, it nonetheless contained a convenient combination of science, moralism, and statistical imagination. For many in the medical community, the task before them was crucial to the very future of the nation. The "new woman" had become so powerful, wrote one concerned physician in 1896, that society seemed "afraid of offending her, and, as a result, the true differences between men and women have never been pointed out, except in medical publications." While this assertion seemed somewhat facetious since both physicians and social scientists joined in denouncing the demands of the feminists, nonetheless the medical profession exercised a significantly disproportionate influence in discussing women's role by providing a wealth of scientific prognostication. By the end of the century, medical

The chapter title comes from Tennyson's "Locksley Hall." "Woman is the lesser man, and all thy passions matched with mine/Are as moonlight unto sunlight, and as water unto wine."

science had depicted women as creatures inferior to men yet somehow kin to the angels.[1]

Anthropometry of Race and Sex

A considerable portion of scientific opinion relating to the sexes originated in somatometric examinations carried out during the nineteenth century, which focused upon differences among the various races of man. Analyses of skull capacity, facial angle, and body dimensions provided weighty documentation to support the Caucasian's claim of racial superiority. These early examinations included statistics on women, and evidence amassed from the very beginning tended to relegate the female, with the Negro, to a subordinate position in race and sex development. The attitude of medical science was one of paternalistic guidance, demonstrating through the instruments of anthropometry and statistics the proper role and place of human life. Corresponding to the eighteenth-century's "Chain of Being," or for that matter, Aristotle's hierarchy of superior and subordinate forms, nineteenth-century medical science attempted to "fix" the races and sexes in a natural order of ascendancy. By the end of the century scientists and social scientists who had pored through the accumulations of these early studies, sifting the evidence and comparing and contrasting similar investigations, were able to construct pseudo-medical and social-scientific theories directly affecting the status of woman in society. The same quiet confidence with which science rendered judgment on the Negro and the non-Aryan races of the world was merely refined by rearranging the elements in a slightly different order. With arguments weighted by the value-laden statistics of medical science, society skirted the coarseness of contemporary racial language by constructing a shallow paternalism that not only placed woman under constant medical guardianship but also recast contemporary racial terminology to demonstrate her innate inferiority to the male.

Most investigations in the nineteenth century centered prin-

1. Lawrence Irwell, "The Competition of the Sexes and Its Results," *American Medico-Bulletin*, X (1896), 316; Thomas W. Higginson, *Common Sense about Women* (Boston, 1881), 342.

cipally on the study of the head—phrenology, facial angle, prognathism, cranial capacity, and brain weight. The researches of Hermann Welcker on German and Negro skulls, the observations of Rudolph Wagner on the brains of German men and women, and the study by Emil Huschke, *Skull, Brain and Mind in Men and Animals* (1854), pointed to differences in skull capacity of more than 220cc. between the sexes. Because early craniometrists assumed a direct correlation between skull capacity, facial angle, and intellectuality, the implications of somatometric differences between the sexes showed a striking resemblance to scientific indictments of the so-called inferior races.[2] Paul Topinard's claim that the Caucasian woman was more prognathous than the male, Albin Weisbach's measurements of the cubic content of the male and female skulls of Austrians, Christian Bischoff's research in Bonn, and similar studies by Joseph Barnard Davis on the weight of the brain merely reinforced the male-Caucasian–dominated structure of nineteenth-century society.[3] Topinard gave a listing in 1878 of the skull capacity of the sexes as accumulated by the century's leading scientists:[4]

MEN	GRAMMES
105 English and Scotch (Peacock)	1427
28 French (Parchappe)	1334
40 Germans (Huschke)	1382
18 Germans (Wagner)	1392
50 Austrians (Wiesbach)	1342
1 Annamite (Broca)	1233
7 African Negroes (various authors)	1239
8 African Negroes (Broca)	1289
1 Negro of Pondicherry (Broca)	1330

2. Ludwig Büchner, "The Brain of Women," *New Review,* IX (1893), 166; W. L. Distant, "On the Mental Differences between the Sexes," *Journal,* Royal Anthropological Institute of Great Britain and Ireland, IV (1874–75), 78–80; Alexander M. Hamilton, *The Anatomy of the Brain* (Edinburgh, 1831).

3. Büchner, "The Brain of Women," 167; (Anony.), "Science and Woman," *Medical Age,* XLII (1892), 46; Gaëtan Delaunay, "Equality and Inequality in Sex," *Popular Science Monthly,* XX (1881), 185; Albin Weisbach, "The Weight-Proportions of the Brains of Austrian Peoples, with Reference to Stature, Age, Sex, and Diseases," *Anthropological Review,* VII (1869), 92–95; Joseph B. Davis, "Contributions towards Determining the Weight of the Brain in Different Races of Man," *Philosophical Transactions,* Royal Society of London, CLVIII (1868), 505–27; Joseph B. Davis, "On the Weight of the Brain in the Negro," *Anthropological Review,* VII (1869), 190–2.

4. Paul Topinard, *Anthropology* (London, 1878), 311.

1 Hottentot (Wyman)	1417
1 Cape Negro (Broca)	974

WOMEN

34 English and Scotch (Peacock)	1260
18 French (Parchappe)	1210
22 Germans (Huschke)	1244
13 Germans (Wagner)	1209
19 Austrians (Wiesbach)	1160
2 African Negresses (Peacock)	1232
2 African Negresses (Broca)	1067
2 Bushwomen (Marshall, Flower, and Murrie)	974
1 Australian (Owen)	907

Nineteenth-century medical science indicated that women's inferiority was clearly evident in almost every analysis of the brain and its functions. For the sake of argument, however, medical men discounted as inaccurate the straight calculation of brain weights, such as those made by Robert Boyd and Vierordt between 1839 and 1847, which gave a 10 to 12 percent advantage to the male. The researches of Thomas B. Peacock, Joseph and Charles Wenzel, and Frederick Tiedemann had since demonstrated that the female brain, while lighter than that of the male, was proportionately heavier relative to body weight. Bischoff's examination of 426 men and 332 women, for example, gave the woman a brain-weight advantage of 6 percent.[5] In an effort to resolve the apparent statistical embarrassment in the light of the century's theory of male dominance, concerned scientists sought a new denominator from among alternative criteria. The frustration of craniometrists who found their conclusions challenged by advancements in anthropometric procedures, and the tempting political implication which the brain-body weight relation spelled for the feminist,

5. Alexander Sutherland, "Woman's Brain," *Nineteenth Century*, XLVII (1900), 804; Büchner, "The Brain of Women," 166; Robert Boyd, "Tables of the Weights of the Human Body and Internal Organs in the Sane and Insane of Both Sexes, Arranged from 2614 Post-Mortem Examinations," *Philosophical Transactions*, Royal Society of London, CLI (1861), 241–62; Frederick Tiedemann, *A Systematic Treatise of Comparative Physiology* (London, 1834); Joseph and Charles Wenzel, *De Penitiori Structura Cerebri Hominis et Brutorum* (Tubingae, 1812); Thomas B. Peacock, "On the Weight of the Brain and Capacity of the Cranial Cavity of the Negro," *Memoirs*, Anthropological Society of London, I (1863–64), 520–24; Thomas B. Peacock, *Tables of the Weights of the Brain and of Some Other Organs of the Human Body* (London, 1861).

were twin evils which forced medical science to take another look at its instruments. The validity of newer brain analyses suffered from the prejudices of domestic politics, and in the empirical search for more exacting techniques, medical science all but reinforced the century's a priori belief in male superiority. Craniometry became a medium through which medical science, in its desire for certainty, evaluated and attacked the demands of the "new woman." In pursuit of an alternative craniometric tool, Manouvrier turned to an ingenious yet questionable index which related brain weight to weight of the thigh bone. A more serious index constructed by Alexander Sutherland related brain weight to body height, and using Boyd's figures, he found that the male had .73 ounce of brain for every inch of height, while the woman fell behind with only .70 ounce. Similar measurements by French surgeon and anthropologist Paul Broca gave the male a 6.5 percent brain-weight advantage over the woman.[6] Comparing brain weight of men and women of the same height, Boyd, Broca, and Bischoff assigned the male a brain-weight (intellectuality) advantage of 12 percent, 9 percent, and 11 percent respectively. Here, they felt, lay sound confirmation of male superiority, and until science discovered qualitative differences in the neurons and brain elements, the evidence of male advantage seemed clearly proven.[7]

Actually craniometrists were fighting a straw issue with respect to brain-weight analysis, since those feminists who were aware of these medical conclusions preferred to argue for qualitative differences in tissue composition and development. Most feminists attempted to separate themselves from craniometric studies implying racial inferiority for the Negro, since those same studies suggested similar inferiority for the Caucasian woman. The remark by Carl Vogt, professor of natural history at the University of Geneva, for example, that "the grown up Negro partakes, as regards his intellectual faculties, of the nature of the child, the female, and the senile White," became a common maxim of medical and political prognosticators, and remained an irksome thorn in the side of the feminist.[8]

6. Sutherland, "Woman's Brain," 805.
7. *Ibid.*, 807–8.
8. Carl Vogt, *Lectures on Man, His Place in Creation, and in the History*

Suggestions by craniometrists that the Negro had a brain weight and intellectuality comparable to the Caucasian woman caused them to react defensively, arguing that it was unreasonable to assume a similarity between the two. Claiming that the white female was clearly more intelligent than the black man despite similar brain weights, feminists contended that a qualitative difference in brain structure existed between the female and Negro. Obviously, however, categorizing both the Negro and the Caucasian female in the same somatometric framework made it easier for scientists to carry conclusions of race inferiority into the area of sex differentiation. Arguments for justification of segregation and disfranchisement on the one hand, and refusal to extend suffrage on the other, derived from a common fund of somatometric data.

In most of their public utterances, feminists sided with the Negro in his quest for equality. Indeed, women had found in the slavery and Negro suffrage issues the grounds for their own plea for equal rights.[9] By the 1880s and 1890s, however, society had come full circle on the question of Negro voting rights, and vocally demanded that the race be disfranchised on the basis of alleged mental and physiological inferiority. The medical journals in the nineteenth century were filled with racial overtones that spelled disaster for the Negro and even intimated his "natural" extinction on the basis of race struggle.[10] The pervasive belief in the Negro's racial inferiority brought many feminists in the United States to the point of seeking not only to separate themselves from the Negro's civil

of the Earth (London, 1864), 192; J. McGrigor Allan, "On the Differences in the Minds of Men and Women," *Journal,* Anthropological Society of London, VII (1869), cciv.

9. See Benjamin Quarles, "Frederick Douglass and the Woman's Rights Movement," *Journal of Negro History,* XXV (1940), 35–44; James M. McPherson, "Abolitionists, Woman Suffrage and the Negro, 1865–1869," *Mid America,* XLVII (1965), 40–47; Gerda Lerner, *The Grimké Sisters from South Carolina: Rebels against Slavery* (Boston, 1967).

10. John S. Haller, Jr., "The Physician Versus the Negro: Medical and Anthropological Concepts of Race in the Late Nineteenth Century," *Bulletin of the History of Medicine,* XLIV (1970), 154–67; John S. Haller, Jr., "The Negro and the Southern Physician: A Study of Medical and Racial Attitudes, 1800–1860," *Medical History,* XVI (1972), 238–53. See also John S. Haller, Jr., *Outcasts from Evolution: Scientific Attitudes of Racial Inferiority, 1859–1900* (Urbana, 1971), chap. 6.

rights efforts, but to revise their own arguments for equal rights by suggesting that the women's vote could insure political supremacy of Anglo-Saxonism in America.[11] With "what feelings must a highly educated American woman view a dirty, idiotic negro shoe-black or street sweeper going to the ballot-box," remarked one writer, "while she herself remains excluded from it."[12]

By accepting the implications of science regarding racial inferiority, the women's rights movement followed a precarious line of argument, conceding the Negro's innate inferiority, but timidly admitting only an environmental handicap for their own sex. While society might judiciously restrict the rights of the blacks, it should permit women the opportunity of undoing the environmental inferiority which had occurred as a result of the divsion of labor in modern society. Although women might "improve" their intellectual powers stifled by an environmental inferiority, they did not extend the same opportunity to the Negro. The woman was "becoming the possessor of her brains and of an equipment that will facilitate her use of them"; but few in Victorian America, including Caucasian women, were willing to admit the same possibility for the Negro.[13]

We are told [wrote one feminist] by those who argue woman's intellectual inferiority that although next to nothing is known of qualitative differences of brain, there is sufficient reason for believing that man's brain is of superior quality. Yet, then, if the male Negro has the same brain-weight as the female European,—and being a man, a superior quality of brain—he ought to be expected on the argument of brain-weight, not only to produce the same intellectual achievements, but on the argument of quality, to produce superior ones. The fact is, he produces not even equal achievements. The intimation is that, if intellectual achievements depend at all upon a superior quality of brain, that must be accredited to the female.[14]

But even in the qualitative analysis of brain and its convolutions, feminists fared little better than before. Investigations

---

11. Anne Firor Scott, "The 'New Woman' in the New South," *South Atlantic Quarterly*, LXI (1962), 473–83.

12. Büchner, "The Brain of Women," 176.

13. Lucinda B. Chandler, "The Woman Movement," *Arena*, IV (1891), 708.

14. (Anony.), "The Intellectuality of Woman," *International Review*, XIII (1882), 126–27.

indicated that woman's skull was smaller, the base more contracted, and the crown (seat of the sentiments) larger than the male. Experiments carried out by Rudinger, Waldeyer, and Passet on newborn babies found major differences between the sexes in the formation and development of the brain. The frontal lobes in the male fetal brain were larger, wider, and higher, while the convolutions of the parietal lobe were significantly more developed than in the female fetal brain. Similarly, O. Schultze, Alexander Ecker, J. Crichton Browne, the Frenchman Jacquard, and Swedish anatomist Adolph Retzius pointed out the simplicity of structure in the woman's brain, and Pfitzner concluded from length, breadth, height, and circumference measurements that the woman's head was more infantile in quality than that of the male.[15] As Huschke wrote, "woman is a constantly growing child, and in the brain, as in so many other parts of her body, she conforms to her childish type."[16]

Despite the intentions of feminists to disassociate themselves from the implications of the century's ideas on race, their efforts proved generally ineffective. Thomas Peacock's research during the 1840s on the cerebrum and cerebellum, Lauret's measurements of more than 2,000 heads in 1861, and John Cleland's study of the frontal and temporosphenoidal lobes of the brain in 1870 established damaging evidence that the European female brain, like the Negro, was more childlike in development than the European male.[17] Hermann Schaffhausen in his article "On the Primitive Form of the Human Skull," pub-

15. George T. W. Patrick, "The Psychology of Women," *Popular Science Monthly*, XLVII (1895), 212; George J. Romanes, "Mental Differences between Men and Women," *Twentieth Century*, XXI (1887), 655; Iwan Bloch, *The Sexual Life of Our Time in Its Relations to Modern Civilization* (London, 1909), 63–64; Alexander Ecker, "On a Characteristic Peculiarity in the Female Skull and Its Significance for Comparative Anthropology," *Anthropological Review*, VI (1868), 350–56; August Forel, *The Sexual Question; a Scientific, Psychological, Hygienic and Sociological Study for the Cultured Classes* (New York, 1906), 67.

16. Quoted in Vogt, *Lectures on Man*, 183; Büchner, "The Brain of Women," 167; Felix L. Oswald, "Sexual Characteristics," *Open Court*, III (1899), 1814; Delaunay, "Equality and Inequality in Sex," 186; Topinard, *Anthropology*, 120–21.

17. John Cleland, "An Inquiry into the Variations of the Human Skull," *Philosophical Transactions*, Royal Society of London, CLX (1870), 117–74; John Cleland, *The Relation of Brain to Mind* (Glasgow, 1882).

lished in the *Anthropological Review* in 1868, remarked that "we so frequently find in ancient female skulls so decided a prognathism that they almost resemble the Ethiopian skulls, and have been mistaken for them."[18] Early suture closure in both the European female and the "lower races" coincided not only with the inferior mental organization of both, but also marked the female skull as retaining in its growth the last remaining vestiges of the race's earlier and imperfect development.[19] Welcker reinforced Schaffhausen's conclusions by observing that the skulls of men and women of the same race exhibited such notable differences that one could almost mistake them for two different species.[20]

Arguing that convolution differences as well as pronounced variations in the parietal and sphenoidal lobes stamped the woman with a mental apparatus radically divergent to the male's, medical scientists considered foolish the suggestion that women could ever be on the same intellectual footing, even if given the same educational opportunities. Referring to the multitude of past and contemporary brain studies, they regarded the more extensively developed cranial regions in the male as significantly more important than the emotional and sensory development in the woman's brain. Judged intellectually on the basis of the specific gravity of gray matter, or by texture or convolution development, man was more highly endowed "with judgment and creative power" than woman. Female intellectuals appeared occasionally in the history of the race, but the vast majority of intellectuals would continue to be males. Furthermore, while some women would acquire mental abilities equal to the male, their performance of intellectual responsibilities would continue only as long as they avoided their maternal duties. Thus, intellectual women would leave few heirs, and their occasional influence in the affairs of the world would remain negligible.[21] As one medical critic wrote in 1895, "neither the 'emancipated' woman at one end of

18. Hermann Schaffhausen, "On the Primitive Form of the Human Skull," *Anthropological Review*, VI (1868), 425.

19. *Ibid.*, 423; Topinard, *Anthropology*, 133–35; Herbert Spencer, *Education: Intellectual, Moral, and Physical* (New York, 1900), 288.

20. Vogt, *Lectures on Man*, 81; Topinard, *Anthropology*, 131.

21. Irwell, "The Competition of the Sexes and Its Results," 317–18.

the scale nor the prostitute at the other propagates her kind, and society has reason to be thankful in both cases."[22]

Even more embarrassing to the feminist cause were the findings of Carl Vogt and of English pathologist and anatomist Henry C. Bastian, which indicated that the differences in the cranial capacity of the sexes increased with the level of civilization; specifically, the differences in brain capacity between the European male and female was nearly twice that of the male and female inhabitants of ancient Egypt. Vogt wrote in 1864:

It has long been observed that among peoples progressing in civilization, the men are in advance of the women whilst among those which are retrograding, the contrary is the case. Just as, in respect of morals, woman is the conservator of old customs and usages, of traditions, legends, and religion; so in the material world she preserves primitive forms, which but slowly yield to the influence of civilization. We are justified in saying, that it is easier to overthrow a government by revolution, than alter the arrangements in the kitchen, though their absurdity be abundantly proved. In the same manner woman preserves, in the formation of the head, the earliest stage from which the race or tribe has been developed, or into which it has relapsed. Hence, then, is partly explained the fact, that the inequality of the sexes increases with the progress of civilization.[23]

Bastian's research in 1880, like the earlier studies of Vogt, Welcker, and Huschke, typified the close analogy between race and sex differentiation so commonly assumed by nineteenth-century anthropometrists. While there was little discrepancy between the male and female brains of the Negro or Australian (in some cases, the feminine sex, like females in certain species of cephalopods, cyprinoids, and reptiles, were more vigorous and intelligent than the male), the differences became more perceptible in the higher races and cultures. According to the tables published by French physician and sociologist Gustave Le Bon in 1879 and confirmed by Zametti of Sardinia, the scale of brain differences began with the Australians and moved slowly up through the Polynesians, ancient Egyptians,

22. Woods Hutchinson, "The Economics of Prostitution," *American Medico-Surgical Bulletin*, V (1895), 978.
23. Vogt, *Lectures on Man*, 82; Distant, "On the Mental Differences between the Sexes," 80–85.

Chinese, Italians, eventually culminating in the French and Germans. From evidence indicating the superiority of women among ancient and "inferior races" (principally due to the matriarchy system), nineteenth-century scientists concluded that evolution constantly advanced from "the supremacy of the female to that of the male." The tables furnished by Joseph B. Davis of the brain weights of 762 males and 377 females reinforced the findings of Vogt and Bastian[24] (see tables on pp. 58–59).

In a strikingly similar manner to the century's description of the Negro, medical scientists viewed the nervous system of woman, her needs, and her place in nature as part of a naturally restrictive physiology. In all civilized races, the woman was shorter and lighter than the male, her form was rounded and graceful, with more fat and less muscle, and with two-thirds the strength of man; in addition, woman (like the Negro) was flat-footed, with a prominent inclination of the pelvis making her appear less erect than man, and her gait was more unsteady. Her evolution resulted in a higher and shriller voice, a smaller larynx, a larger thyroid gland, a longer trunk compared with the arms and legs, less torsion in the humerus, fewer red corpuscles, and a faster pulse beat than man. Woman was more immune to disease although, like the "lower races," she was more susceptible to infantile illnesses such as anemia, diphtheria, phthisis, scarlet fever, and whooping cough. She endured surgery better than the male (because of her lack of complex nervous development) and recovered more easily and rapidly from wounds. Woman suffered less from senility, the loss of sight and hearing, and she generally had fewer physical abnormalities. Medical men warned, however, that feminism had destroyed much of woman's inherited immunity through efforts to imitate the male. General paralyses from overwork or prolonged worry, neurasthenia, insanity, crime, and alcoholism were making fear-

24. M. A. Hardaker, "Science and the Woman Question," *Popular Science Monthly*, XX (1882), 577–78; Delaunay, "Equality and Inequality in Sex," 184; Büchner, "The Brain of Women," 167–68; (Anony.), "The Intellectuality of Woman," 124; Franz Pruner-Bey, *De la chevelure comme caractéristiques des races humaines d'après des recherches microscopiques* (Paris, 1863); Davis, "Contributions towards Determining the Weight of the Brain in Different Races of Man," 510–13.

Tables of the Computed Weights of the Brains Contained in Skulls of
People of Different Races
(Expressed in Avoirdupois Ounces, and in Grammes)

BRAIN WEIGHTS OF THE SKULLS OF MEN

Races	Number	Heaviest		Lightest		Average	
I. European Races	299	52.68	1493	43.61	1236	48.25	1367
II. Asiatic Races	124	50.27	1425	41.57	1178	46.00	1304
III. African Races	53	47.37	1342	41.93	1188	45.63	1293
IV. American Races	52	48.16	1365	43.50	1233	46.17	1308
V. Australian Races	24	50.86	1441	36.96	1047	42.83	1214
VI. Oceanic Races	210	49.25	1396	42.90	1216	46.54	1319
Numbers and Averages	762	49.76	1410	41.74	1183	45.90	1301

ful inroads into the gentle sex.[25] Concern for the mental state
of the Caucasian woman closely paralleled medical interest in
the growing number of mental problems found among the
freedmen of the South. Doctors claimed that insanity had over-
taken the Negro race which, prior to emancipation, had enjoyed excellent mental health. As far as the medical profession
was concerned, feminism as well as the Negro civil rights movement had undermined the physical and mental stamina of
both the Caucasian woman and the Negro.[26]

Many physicians held the "periodical ordeal" responsible
for female inferiority by pointing to examples of hysteria, listlessness, and even stupidity that accompanied the menstrual

25. Patrick, "The Psychology of Women," 210–11; Delaunay, "Equality
and Inequality in Sex," 185; (Anony.), "Are Women Inferior to Men?,"
Knowledge, I (1881), 6–8; Irwell, "The Competition of the Sexes and Its Results," 319–20; Jean Finot, *Problems of the Sexes* (New York, 1913), chap. 4;
Bloch, *The Sexual Life of Our Time*, 60; R. E. Wrafter, "Peculiarities of the
Human Female," *Indian Medical Record*, XVIII (1900), 363–65; Vogt, *Lec-
tures on Man*, 120; Moritz Alsberg, *Anthropologie mit Berücksichtigung der
Urgeschichte des Menchen* (Stuttgart, 1888).
26. Patrick, "The Psychology of Women," 213–14; J. T. Walton, "The Comparative Mortality of the White and Colored Races in the South," *Charlotte
Medical Journal*, X (1897), 292; L. S. Joynes, "Remarks on the Comparative
Mortality of the White and Colored Population of Richmond," *Virginia Medical Monthly*, II (1875), 155; J. G. Rogers, "The Effects of Freedom upon the
Physical and Psychological Development of the Negro," *Proceedings*, American Medico-Psychological Association, VII (1900), 88–99.

	BRAIN WEIGHTS OF THE SKULLS OF WOMEN						MEAN OF SEXES		MEAN OF SERIES		
Number	Heaviest		Lightest		Average						Mean Internal Capacity
94	46.02	1304	39.56	1121	42.49	1204	45.73	1296	47.12	1335	92.3
86	45.95	1302	37.48	1062	42.13	1194	43.94	1245	44.44	1259	87.1
60	43.91	1244	39.59	1122	42.74	1211	43.66	1237	43.89	1244	86
31	45.44	1288	39.13	1109	41.89	1187	44.92	1273	44.64	1265	87.5
11	42.98	1218	34.77	985	39.22	1111	41.02	1162	41.81	1185	81.9
95	44.61	1264	41.01	1162	43.00	1219	44.52	1272	45.63	1293	89.4
377	44.81	1270	38.59	1094	41.91	1188	43.96	1246	44.58	1263	87.3

cycle. The onset of puberty ushered in the woman's distinctly separate destiny and implied a fundamental reappraisal of her educational, social, and political development. Because there was a diversion of blood as well as vital energy during the menstrual period, any excessive brain activity by the woman brought inevitable suffering and degeneration to the reproductive organs. While the male could withstand the rigors of healthy competition at all times, the female's education had to allow for periodical lapses to permit the construction of her reproductive organs. Overexertion in mental activity would cause females to suffer from "ovarian neuralgia," resulting in the inability of the body to supply both the brain and generative organs with sufficient blood.[27] "One shudders to think of the conclusions arrived at by female bacteriologists or histologists," wrote one doctor, "at the period when their entire system, both physical and mental, is, so to speak, 'unstrung,' to say nothing of the terrible mistakes which a lady surgeon might make under similar conditions."[28]

27. A. L. Smith, "Are Modern School Methods in Keeping with Physiological Knowledge?," *Bulletin,* American Academy of Medicine; VI (1905), 874; Henry N. Guernsey, *Plain Talks on Avoided Subjects* (Philadelphia, 1882), 72–73.

28. Irwell, "The Competition of the Sexes and Its Results," 319; Allan, "On

For the good of the race, medical men proposed that girls complete their education by the age of sixteen or seventeen and then marry, rather than wait until they were in their twenties. Not only did higher education and delayed marriage render "wifehood and motherhood distasteful owing to defective development of the sexual organs," but because education increased "the ability of the nerves to perceive pain more keenly," women easily fell victim to neurasthenic and hysterical disorders. The periodical ordeal, wrote A. Lapthorn Smith, M.D., was nature's warning to the mannish maiden that any effort to avoid her biological responsibilities was a crime against womanhood and the community.[29]

Girls, young ladies, to use the polite phrase, who are about leaving or have left school for society, dissipation, or self-culture, rarely permit any of Nature's periodical demands to interfere with their morning calls, or evening promenades, or midnight dancing, or sober study. Even the home draws the sacred mantle of modesty so closely over the reproductive function as not only to cover but to smother it. Sisters imitate brothers in persistent work at all times. Female clerks in stores strive to emulate the males by unremitting labor, seeking to develop feminine force by masculine methods. Female operatives of all sorts, in factories and elsewhere, labor in the same way; and, when the day is done, are as likely to dance half the night, regardless of any pressure upon them of a peculiar function as their fashionable sisters in the polite world. All unite in pushing the hateful thing out of sight and out of mind; and all are punished by similar weakness, degeneration and disease.[30]

Manly pursuits by women, such as higher education, lessened those sexual and maternal instincts so important to the perpetuation of the species. The duties of motherhood were "di-

the Differences in the Minds of Men and Women," cxcviii–cxcix; James E. Reeves, *Bad Health; Its Physical and Moral Causes in American Women* (Wheeling, W.Va., 1875), 25–29.

29. Smith, "Are Modern School Methods in Keeping with Physiological Knowledge?," 875–76; John H. Kellogg, *Ladies Guide in Health and Disease. Girlhood, Maidenhood, Motherhood* (Des Moines, Iowa, 1883), 156–57; John Thorburn, *Female Education from a Physiological Point of View* (Manchester, Eng., 1884), 4–5; Robert R. Rentoul, *The Dignity of Woman's Health and the Nemesis of Its Neglect* (London, 1890), 58–59; Gustavus Cohen, *Helps and Hints to Mothers and Young Wives* (London, 1880), 5.

30. Edward H. Clarke, *Sex in Education; or, a Fair Chance for Girls* (Boston, 1873), 130–31; William Goodell, *The Dangers and the Duty of the Hour* (Baltimore, 1881); M. S. Pembrey, "Woman's Place in Nature," *Science Progress*, VIII (1913–14), 138.

rect rivals of brain work, for they both require for their performance an exclusive and plentiful supply of phosphates." The demands made upon the pregnant woman by the unborn child were such that a secondary effort on her part for further brain development threatened physical degeneracy and insanity. Those who might recover their sanity would do so only "after the prolonged administration of phosphates, to make up for the loss entailed by the growth of the child." Smith believed that educated women physically disabled themselves in brain work, and their unusually late marriages not only limited potential offspring, but also prevented them from performing normal physiological functions. Urban middle- and upper-class women seldom enjoyed natural childbirth because of their lessened muscular power and tissue strength. Higher education, Smith argued, had been indirectly responsible for reducing the size of the pelvis.[31] He unwittingly revealed the tenacious foundation upon which the male-dominated society of Victorian America rested when he conjectured that while woman could attain the same mental aptitude as man, her pursuit of learning (or even the awareness of her own mental ability) encouraged "an aggressive, self-assertive, independent character" which made love impossible and forced the male to feel inferior. Modern businessmen, by refusing to marry educated females, subsequently became "ship-wrecked for life and for eternity by remaining single," or assuaged their egos by marrying women clearly their social inferiors.[32]

The Spencerians

Few men had greater impact on middle-class thinking in Victorian America than English philosopher Herbert Spencer.

31. A. L. Smith, "Higher Education of Women and Race Suicide," *Popular Science Monthly*, LXVI (1905), 467–68; Silas Weir Mitchell, *Doctor and Patient* (Philadelphia, 1888), 13, 138–39; Allan, "On the Differences in the Minds of Men and Women," cc–cci; T. S. Clouston, "Women from a Medical Point of View," *Popular Science Monthly*, XXIV (1883–84), 214–21; Harry T. Peck, "For Maids and Mothers; the Overtaught Woman," *Cosmopolitan Magazine*, XXVI (1898–99), 329–36.

32. Smith, "Higher Education of Women and Race Suicide," 471; Alfred R. Wallace, "Women and Natural Selection in Marriage," *Journal of Hygiene and Herald of Health*, XLIV (1894), 236–40; Silas L. Loomis, "Vitality in American Women," *National Medical Journal*, I (1870–71), 9–15.

Expressing optimism in the future, his philosophical observations imparted a quiet confidence to delicate minds whose mastery of life's problems had been rudely interrupted by the unsettling nature of Darwin's *Origin of Species* (1859). The uniqueness of his influence lay in his ability to support the foundations of the status quo while at the same time introducing to the middle class the revolutionary mechanism of evolutionary law and the discoveries of science. By promising stability amid change, laissez-faire along with determinism, and optimism despite struggle, Spencer cushioned Victorian society from the rigors of Darwin's dysteleology. He was a consummate systematist, and his passion for discovering nature's laws rested on a liberal use of the "comparative method" to bridge the social and scientific world, and an ingenious ability for endless extrapolation of previous writers. That he failed the test of time came as no surprise to his critics, who saw in his writings the casuist's zeal for obscuring truth. Yet for every person who questioned his theories, literally thousands read and studied his works with reverence and excused his lapses in logic with the indulgent air of devoted servants.

Reinforcing the century's conservative estimate of woman's role, the English philosopher argued that woman's physical evolution had terminated at an earlier stage than the male's in order to preserve those vital powers necessary for reproduction. At the same time, women had developed psychological peculiarities whose genesis lay in the struggle for existence and which had given the fittest women power to survive the aggressive and egoistic tendencies of the stronger male. For one thing, since women were the weaker sex, those who succeeded in pleasing the male survived and left children. This feminine peculiarity, the "special solicitude to be approved," became a common trait of successive generations. In addition, modern woman abstracted from her ancestors, through inheritance and selection, the power to disguise her feelings from the male. "Women who betrayed the state of antagonism produced in them by ill-treatment," Spencer wrote, were "less likely to survive and leave offspring than those who concealed their antagonism." More important, woman inherited intuition, which in barbarous times compensated for her weaker position by detecting the passions of her male consort. "A woman who could from a movement, tone of voice, or expression of face, instantly detect in her savage husband the passion that was rising," he wrote, "would be likely to escape dangers run into by a woman less skillful in interpreting the natural language of feeling." Although the woman's adaptation to the violent natures of primitive man had modified as a result of the social changes in civilized man, she nevertheless retained her mental and emotional characteristics—traits which could best serve society when directed toward her maternal capacity.[33]

According to Spencer, those advanced sentiments which developed in woman as a result of her maternal instincts—a sense of pity, and love of the helpless—were the very instincts which restricted her to the affairs of the home. Carrying such traits into social activity beyond the home circle threatened to undermine the state. Preferring generosity to justice, yielding to emotional appeals which had no basis in real needs, and anxious to provide immediate public good without any thought of more distinct public consequences, women would delay evolutionary progress by encouraging disastrous social upheaval. "Reverencing power more than men do," remarked Spencer, "women respected freedom less."[34] Retarded mentally as the small-brained races were, they tended to place their faith in whatever authority presented itself with the greatest strength, without a counterbalancing ability to doubt, criticize, or question. The thoughts of women and the "inferior races" were full of "special, and mainly personal, experiences, but with few general truths, and no truths of high generality." Neither were able to abstract ideas from concrete cases, and such things as framing a hypothesis, or reasoning from an hypothesis, were as incomprehensive as for either of them to suspend judgment or balance evidence.[35]

33. Herbert Spencer, *The Study of Sociology* (New York, 1896), 342–43.

34. *Ibid.*, 346–47; Romanes, "Mental Differences between Men and Women," 658–59.

35. Herbert Spencer, *Principles of Psychology* (2 vols.; New York, 1910), I, 581, 583, II, 537–38; Luke Owen Pike, "On the Claims of Women to Political Power," *Journal*, Anthropological Society of London, VII (1869), xlvii–lxi; Allan, "On the Differences in the Minds of Men and Women," ccxi.

While Spencer admitted that many of woman's political and domestic disabilities would diminish in the course of evolution, he objected to total emancipation. "If from that state of primitive degradation in which they were habitually stolen, bought and sold, made beasts of burden, inherited as property, and killed at will, we pass to the stage America shows us," he sarcastically observed, "in which a lady wanting a seat stares at a gentleman occupying one until he surrenders it, and then takes it without thanking him; we may infer that the rhythm traceable throughout all changes has carried this to an extreme from which there will be a recoil." While the position of women would undoubtedly improve, certain legal necessities would continue to demand the supremacy of the male, since he was by nature more judicious. Spencer likewise regarded any extensive change in the education of women to fit them for professions outside the home circle as only undermining the evolutionary laws of nature. "If women comprehended all that is contained in the domestic sphere," he wrote, "they would ask no other. If they could see everything which is implied in the right education of children, to the full conception of which no man has yet risen, much less any woman, they would seek no further function."[36]

Spencerians in the behavioral sciences utilized the "comparative method" to bridge gaps or suggest correlations among the various disciplines. Recognizing as had Spencer the artificial boundaries marking the division of the sciences, they maintained that generalizations derived from contemporary societal behavior could offer firm corroboration of what had appeared inconclusive or obscured in strictly biological studies. Theories which one could only suggest from biological grounds were readily documented by evidence from either psychology or sociology. The sciences affected one another in a "consentaneous" manner, each supporting and supplying facts to aid in the completion of the others. In response to feminist denial of the male's biological and psychological superiority, Spencerians responded by pointing to women's life history as

36. Herbert Spencer, *Principles of Sociology* (3 vols.; New York, 1910), I, 767–69.

"overwhelming external evidence of the existence of such differences."[37]

One argument used to support female inferiority analyzed food consumption and the ability of the sexes to transform food into energy. If both sexes were given a pound of bread to convert into "vital energy," the male, because of his larger organs and muscular development, would have an advantage in mastication and deglutition. Since scientists had the right to "insist on the legitimacy of judging brain-power by brain products," and because there was a direct ratio between food assimilation and energy, Spencerians argued that the male would not only do more thinking in an hour's time than the woman, but also that the lesser contributions of women to civilization historically merely proved the assumption.[38] If the facts were reliable, and reasoning correct, wrote Miss M. A. Hardaker in *Popular Science Monthly*, it should be obvious to all that the factor of size had given man an absolute superiority over woman, which he would always retain.

The absolute gain in time which his greater size has given him can not be set aside, unless he should cease to be the medium of transformation of energy, and should wait a few centuries for women to overtake him, as he might have waited for her to swallow her pound of bread. But even supposing such an impossibility, and granting that she should once overtake him (in the factor of time), so that the two sexes could start fairly in the race of progress, the man would immediately dart ahead again by virtue of his larger size and consequently greater capacity for transforming energy. But any such supposition as an even chance for the two sexes must remain an absurdity. Unless woman can devise some means for reducing the size of man, she must be content to revolve about him in the future as in the past. She may resist her fate, and create some aberrations in her course, but she will be held to her orbit nevertheless.[39]

Nineteenth-century advocates of woman's inferiority focused much of their attention upon the woman's role as perpetuator of the species. Maternal functions diverted nearly 20 percent

37. Hardaker, "Science and the Woman Question," 578.
38. *Ibid.*, 579–80; Alexander Bain, *Mind and Body. The Theories of Their Relation* (New York, 1873), 20; (Anony.), "The Intellectuality of Woman," 127–28.
39. Hardaker, "Science and the Woman Question," 581.

of women's vital energies from potential brain activity. Even if men and women began with an equal mental endowment, the energy required for maternity and its attendant duties would continually detract from that original supply. While males were most active intellectually between the ages of twenty and forty, women of the same age span were restricted in their roles as mothers. Consequently, the male's period of greatest intellectual development was in inverse ratio to the woman's duties as mother. The male had evolved further in the struggle for existence, and it appeared likely that the male's vital energy as well as his mental qualities would continue to gain over the female. Furthermore, since woman missed "the powerful intellectual stimulus which . . . competition creates among men," her chances for ever rivaling the male in the struggle for existence were remote.[40] Spencerians asserted that the laws of heredity, although imperfectly understood, had increased the mental endowment of the male at an almost geometric proportion over that of the female. Drawing from Darwin's law of transmission and from Spencer's inverse ratio between individuation and multiplication, they argued that not only would the intellectual mother have fewer daughters than the average mother, but also that "the chances of transmission of intellectual qualities in the female line will be lessened as culture increases among mothers."[41]

The principle of differentiation of labor, which extended by the use of the comparative method from ethnology to biology and psychology, proved to be an embarrassing problem for the feminist. In order to argue against it, she was forced to deny the mechanism of natural selection. Borrowing from craniometric evidence which indicated that the mass of the brain (meaning, of course, intellectuality) varied more between the sexes in the higher races as the sexes became more specialized in their labors, Spencerians concluded that as evolution advanced from pre-eminence of the female to that of the male, "equality of the sexes would thus be a stage in the natural

40. *Ibid.*, 581–82; Grant Allen, "Woman's Place in Nature," *Forum*, VI (1899), 258.
41. Hardaker, "Science and the Woman Question," 583.

transition between the two opposite phases of evolution."[42] And because the "advancement towards perfection is reached by differentiation," the feminists' efforts to avoid further differentiation were not only alien to the laws of natural selection but also threatened to encourage harmful atavistic tendencies.[43] Should the "women's rights viragoes" ever succeed in their social ideas, wrote one concerned Spencerian antifeminist, civilization will have come full circle and the once great attributes of Western culture would retrogress to barbarism.[44] In its worst form the feminist movement attempted to create through a process of "unnatural selection" a race of monstrosities hostile to men, women, society, and the future of the race.[45]

Feminist Olive Schreiner, a close friend of English sexologist Havelock Ellis, in an article published in *Cosmopolitan Magazine*, lamented the parasitism which civilization had encouraged in the American woman. "Year by year, day by day," she wrote, "there is a silently working but determined tendency for the sphere of woman's domestic labors to contract itself: and this contraction is marked exactly in proportion as that condition which we term modern civilization is advanced."

It is when this point has been reached, and never before, that the symptoms of female parasitism have in the past almost invariably tended to manifest themselves and have become a social danger. . . . Then, in place of the active laboring woman, upholding society by her toil, has come the effete wife, concubine or prostitute, clad in fine raiment, the work of other's fingers; fed on luxurious viands, the result of others' toil; waited on and tended by the labor of others. The need for her physical labor having gone, and mental industry not having taken its place, she bedecked and scented her person or had it bedecked and scented for her;

42. (Anony.), "The Woman's Rights Question Considered from a Biological Point of View," *American Journal of Science*, XV (1878), 473; D. P. Livermore, "Woman's Mental Status," *Forum*, V (1888), 93; Delaunay, "Equality and Inequality in Sex," 192.

43. (Anony.), "The Woman's Rights Question Considered from a Biological Point of View," 484; Bloch, *The Sexual Life of Our Time*, 76–77.

44. Henry T. Finck, *Romantic Love and Personal Beauty; Their Development, Causal Relations, Historic and National Peculiarities* (New York, 1887), 175–76; Pembrey, "Woman's Place in Nature," 133–36.

45. (Anony.), "The Woman's Rights Question Considered from a Biological Point of View," 484; Thomas W. Higginson, *Women and Men* (New York, 1888), 46.

she lay upon her sofa or drove or was carried out in her vehicle; and loaded with jewels, she sought by dissipations and amusements to fill up the inordinate blank left by the lack of productive activity. And as the hand whitened the frame softened, till, at last, the very duties of mother- hood, which were all the constitution of her life left her, became dis- tasteful and from the instant when her infant came damp upon her womb it passed into the hands of others, to be tended and reared; and from youth to age her offspring often owed nothing to her personal toil. . . . Finely clad, tenderly housed, life became for her merely the grati- fication of her own physical and sexual appetites, and the appetites of the male, through the stimulation which alone she could maintain her- self. And whether as kept wife, kept mistress or kept prostitute, she con- tributed nothing to the active and sustaining labors of her society.[46]

In their studies of the Victorian woman, Spencerians paid obsequious attendance to those psychological and anthropo- metric peculiarities which seemed to relate her to the "inferior races." They saw in woman's physical and mental character- istics a remarkable resemblance to the Negro in the nineteenth- century evolutionary framework, and their conclusions, like those regarding the politics of southern reconstruction, tended to project a similar foreboding to any change in the woman's station in life. Grounded in what the medical profession claimed were biological laws beyond the power of man (or woman) to question, let alone change, Spencerian antifeminists ruled out all those ameliorative tools of the women's rights movement which were directed outside the home circle. They viewed any effort which ignored woman's "natural" station as a reckless attempt to flout the laws of nature—an attempt which carried women beyond the pale of femininity and drove them relentlessly back to a more diseased and atavistic stage of sex development.

The Separatist Doctrine of the Sexes

In 1879, William K. Brooks, professor of zoology at Johns Hopkins University, published an article in *Popular Science Monthly* entitled "The Condition of Women from a Zoological Point of View." Like Hardaker, he not only believed in a pro- nounced division of labor and aptitude between the sexes in

46. Olive Schreiner, "The Woman Question," *Cosmopolitan Magazine*, XXVIII (1899), 184–85. Schreiner used the pseudonym "Ralph Iron."

the more advanced races, but also maintained that a clear recognition of this division "must form the foundation and superstructure of all plans for the improvement of women."[47] Science was responsible for determining the role of the sexes in both the lower and higher forms of life and applying the results to the issue of education for the present stage of women. Since every organism was the product of the laws of heredity and variation, the series of inherited structures and functions which determined the life of the organism were "constantly being extended by the addition of new features, which at first were individual variations, and [were] gradually built into the hereditary life history."[48] Reinforcing the complementary studies of Sabatier and Rolph on the function of the male zygote in sexual reproduction, Brooks concluded that the male was the progressive or variable factor in evolution. The sperm functioned to vitalize the ovum, and was actually the vehicle through which newer variations were implanted in the conservative ovum.[49] According to Brooks, nature had designed the female organism to transmit those features of the species which were established by heredity.[50] The female mind became "a storehouse filled with the instincts, habits, intuitions, and laws of conduct which have been gained by past experience." The male mind, on the other hand, because the male organism was the variable, originating element in the process of evolution, had the "power of extending experience over new fields, and by comparison and generalization, of discovering new laws of nature, which are in their turn to become rules of action, and to be added on to the series of past experiences."[51] In his support of this theory, evolutionary popularizer Grant Allen (1848–99), professor of mental and moral philosophy in a college for Negroes in Jamaica, remarked that women had no more to do with newer acquisitions than a Negress or mulattress had to do with the intellectual qualities

---

47. William K. Brooks, "The Condition of Women from a Zoological Point of View," *Popular Science Monthly*, XV (1879), 145.
48. *Ibid.*, 147.
49. *Ibid.*, 150–51.
50. *Ibid.*, 152.
51. *Ibid.*, 154.

in the offspring of miscegenation. "Any other belief," Allen argued, "seems to be pre-Darwinian and anti-biological."[52]

Differences in the hereditary structure and function of the sexes implied corresponding psychological and sociological disparities which profoundly affected their roles in society. In the world of change where instincts and intuitions were of little use in present conduct, the man had a distinct advantage over the woman. The innovative quality of his brain enabled him to "pursue original trains of abstract thought" and arrive at newer generalizations. Obviously, scientists argued, man had a special advantage over woman in those competitive professions where success depended upon inventiveness and ingenuity. On the other hand, in situations where experience determined proper conduct and circumstances did not entail judgment, comparison, or adjustment, the physiological factors which defined the female tended to predominate. Women were best suited for those skills "where ready tack and versatility are of more importance than the narrow technical skill which comes from apprenticeship or training, and where success does not invoke competition with rivals."[53] While Brooks's analysis of the sexes incorporated the most advanced techniques of physiology and zoology, his conclusions only preserved the century's conservative view of woman's role in society.

The positions which women already occupy in society and the duties which they perform are, in the main, what they should be if our view is correct; and any attempt to improve the condition of women by ignoring or obliterating the intellectual differences between them and men must result in disaster to the race, and the obstruction of that progress and improvement which the history of the past shows to be in store for both men and women in the future. So far as human life in the world is concerned there can be no improvement which is not accomplished in accordance with the laws of nature; and, if it is a natural law that the

52. Allen, "Woman's Place in Nature," 263; Irwell, "The Competition of the Sexes and Its Results," 316; Finot, *Problems of the Sexes,* 130–31; Allan, "On the Differences in the Minds of Men and Women," ccxiii.

53. Brooks, "The Condition of Women from a Zoological Point of View," 154–55; J. T. Searcy, "The Mental Characteristics of the Sexes," *Alienist and Neurologist,* IX (1888), 555–64; Patrick, "The Psychology of Women," 217–18; Thomas Davidson, "Ideal Training of the American Girl," *Forum,* XXV (1898), 472; Annie L. Mearkle, "The Woman Who Wants to Be a Man," *Midland Monthly,* IX (1898), 173–76; G. G. Buckler, "The Lesser Man," *North American Review,* CLXV (1897), 295–309.

parts which the sexes perform in the natural evolution of a race are complemented to each other, we can not hope to accomplish anything by working in opposition to the natural method. We may, however, do much to hasten advancement by recognizing and working in accordance with this method.[54]

Although feminists in the nineteenth century cited John Stuart Mill's essay on "Subjection of Women" (1867) in their demands for equality, antifeminists maintained that a more careful reading of Mill in light of zoology and psychology only corroborated the hereditary limitations of woman's place in nature. Even Mill, who had regarded woman's inferiority as originating in "accidental" rather than "natural" traits, had defined the highest type of woman as one distinguished by her power of intuition; the talents of women were oriented toward practicality and seemed to eschew speculative thinking for intuitive perception. For Brooks, this admission merely reflected what zoologists had so recently confirmed in their studies of sexual heredity.[55] Using Mill's own observations, the zoologist concluded that the dissimilar nature of the male and female mind precluded identical education; and that further, the peculiarities of the two minds indicated a division of labor based firmly on principles in nature rather than upon the whims of either male chauvinism or the factors of environment.[56] Because of woman's aptitude for "acquiring and applying the results of past progress, by empirical methods and without needs for proofs and reasons," women were far more suited to an education emphasizing culture over training. "The hard fate which compels the boy to sacrifice some of the delights of culture in order to fit himself for competition with men," Brooks wrote, "presses less heavily upon girls."[57]

Borrowing many of his ideas from Spencer's writings, Brooks indicated that development of the Anglo-Saxon constitutional

54. Brooks, "The Condition of Women from a Zoological Point of View," 349–50.

55. *Ibid.*, 350, 353; John Stuart Mill, *The Subjection of Women* (New York, 1874), 311–28; Romanes, "Mental Differences between Men and Women," 656–57; Allan, "On the Differences in the Minds of Men and Women," cxcvii.

56. Brooks, "The Condition of Women from a Zoological Point of View," 356.

57. William K. Brooks, "Women from the Standpoint of a Naturalist," *Forum*, XXI (1896), 287–88, 293–94.

government owed its success to the judicial frame of mind, the ability to deliberate on crucial issues, and the rational approach to change. Women's suffrage, on the other hand, would only add voters who were "led by tradition or self-interest or emotion, rather than by intelligent zeal for the welfare of the nation." The only valid basis for female suffrage lay in the claim that it would strengthen democratic constitutional government. Unfortunately, the mind of woman (like that of the "inferior races") delighted the demagogue because it was so easily manipulated by emotional persuasion; impulses could turn from constitutional to more revolutionary forms of government.[58] Echoing these fears, George F. Talbot, M.D., demanded a reappraisal of the feminist's political demands.

When by a heroic effort we lifted a million of ignorant and degraded slaves to the rank of citizens and electors, the immediate result was negro justices of the peace, negro judges of the courts, negro members of Congress, and in more than one State negro legislatures, which proceeded in a summary way to confiscate the property of the late masters by taxation, ostensibly expended in public works and largely wasted by private plunder. If the effect of raising to the grade of voters the whole mass of illiterate slaves was to give them the whole political control of several States, why will not this complete enfranchisement of women give them the political control in all the older States, where they will be in the numerical majority.[59]

Scientists observed that the fundamental difference between the sexes reduced ultimately to an essentially "disruptive diathesis" in the male and a "constructive diathesis" in the female.[60] Otto Charles Glaser of the University of Michigan as well as the Scottish biologists Patrick Geddes and J. Arthur Thomson used the distinction to defend women's rights. Nothing could be more fatal to the body politic, Glaser warned, than failing to recognize "that the natural endowments of the sexes are complementary, racially essential, and fortunately bred in the bone." Glaser regarded the enfranchisement of women as a conservative influence upon the body politic; and

58. *Ibid.*, 295–96.
59. George F. Talbot, "The Political Rights and Duties of Women," *Popular Science Monthly*, XLIX (1896), 84–85.
60. Otto C. Glaser, "The Constitutional Conservatism of Women," *Popular Science Monthly*, LXXIX (1911), 299.

in the light of male jingoism that periodically distorted the domestic and international scene with inflated prices and imperialistic wars, woman's conservative instincts would provide a healthy counterbalance to the male's disruptive political behavior.[61]

Despite the remarks by Glaser, however, medical scientists generally condemned the popular movement for women's rights as blatantly disregarding the findings of their research. Only through intelligent cooperation of the sexes would society avoid harmful ameliorative measures designed to change women's role in the political, educational, and legal framework of the nation. "The most devoted patron of woman's political and educational advancement," observed Iowa psychologist and philosopher George T. Patrick in 1895, "would hardly deny that the success and permanency of the reform will depend in the end upon the fact that there shall be no inherent contradiction between her duties and her natural physical and mental constitution." That science might find woman's present intellectual and physical constitution in a state of weakness would not justify, according to Patrick, the denial of her political and educational rights. Much would ultimately depend on whether her condition was the result of the "subordinate position which she has been compelled to hold," or whether it resulted from more fundamental peculiarities in her nature. If, on the basis of science, experts determined that woman might assume more rights, then these should be granted through a gradual process "in order that disaster to her cause might not follow the over-taxing of her strength."[62]

Opponents of the women's rights movement depicted the characteristics most peculiar to woman's nature—trust, charity, dependence, temperance, devotion, intuition, and fidelity—as infantile traits. Like the more primitive races, she tended toward conservatism, imitativeness, precocity, deceitfulness, emotionalism, fickleness, and religiosity rather than toward reason, analysis, and logic. The whole vasomotor system of the female

---

61. *Ibid.*, 302; Patrick Geddes and J. Arthur Thomson, *The Evolution of Sex* (London, 1897), 270–71.
62. Patrick, "The Psychology of Women," 209.

was far more excitable than that of the male, marking her with a tendency to greater tension, irritability, and emotionalism. Laughing, crying, blushing, and quickened heart beat were all marks of her peculiar mental state. She was more prone to hysteria, hypnotism, trances, superstitions, as well as pity, sympathy, and charity. Woman's most noted characteristic was her altruism; "in her altruistic life of love and self-sacrifice," wrote George Patrick, "woman shows herself the leader in the supreme virtue of Christian civilization." But to the extent that she excelled in altruism, she was deficient in truthfulness and veracity. "Deception and ruse in woman, far more than in man, have become a habit of thought and speech," Patrick added. The social, intellectual, and physiological condition of her makeup "have forced this habit upon her as a means of self-defense."[63] Woman's retarded or infantile evolution, according to the Iowa psychologist, was much more evident in her dress and adornment—her use of oils, perfumes, stones, colorful garments, ornaments, and mutilations (corset and high-heeled shoes). Although modern woman had evolved progressively from the adornment of earlier and more primitive centuries, she still partly reverted to those ancient customs.[64]

Antifeminists urged the enthusiasts for women's rights to consider their goals in the light of the female's supplemental role in society. The social reformer should "learn that woman's cause may suffer irretrievable damage if she plunged too suddenly into duties demanding the same strain and nervous expenditure that is safely borne by man." The reforms desired by feminists were far too extreme and basically unnatural to woman's nature. Would it not be better, they asked, if woman remained the conservator of humanity and carried forward traits of passivity, reserve, and calmness? Woman's responsibility in the history of the race was "too sacred to be jostled roughly in the struggle for existence"; she deserved exemption from the restless conflict.[65]

Some medical men saw the influx of feminist ideas as an

63. *Ibid.*, 220–21; Romanes, "Mental Differences between Men and Women," 658–59.

64. Patrick, "The Psychology of Women," 224–25.

65. *Ibid.*; Ely Van de Warker, "Sexual Cerebration," *Popular Science Monthly*, VII (1875), 289–92.

insidious incursion of foreign and atheistic thought into the mainstream of American life. For J. L. Ziegler, M.D., president of the Pennsylvania Medical Society, liberalism, evolution, communism, rationalism, equality of the sexes, and women's rights were the harbingers of darkness threatening the "Christian beacon" that had helped to guide the nation.

The doctrine of the equality of the sexes is one of these incorrect premises from which logical conclusions are deduced; many of those advocates are tainted with an impertinent rationalism, chilled by an icy unbelief imbued with the spirit of a devastating criticism that criticizes the Bible out of its covers and the title-page of the volume—degrading the holy bonds of matrimony into a mere civil contract to be dissolved by the caprice of either part—striking at the root of those divinely ordained principles upon which is built the superstructure of society. They assume as an axiom that the sexes are equal, and if this is admitted the logical conclusion will be irrefutable. . . . The pretensions of a class of political and social reformers based upon the idea of the equality of the sexes has given rise to many other delusions, advocated by men educated and prominent in science and literature, no regard being had for the ultimate effect upon the destiny of mankind. . . . It may be safely asserted that any doctrine or scheme of reform, no matter how plausible, which conflicts with the plain teachings of the revealed will of God, is ruinous to the present happiness and ultimate destiny of mankind.[66]

It was the "unerring light of Divine truth," he wrote, that placed the sexes in distinct but complementary relation to each other. While man could be heard in the "angry forum" or "directing the fury and rushing tide of battle," the woman's voice, lutelike and sweet, warmed the affections and sympathies of the world, helping to mold the minds of youth. Her responsibilities gave her a place of honor and respect far greater than the rough and tumble struggle of the fittest that so characterized man's destiny.[67]

As far as Ziegler was concerned, the feminist, like the atheist and evolutionist, was attempting to destroy the basic tenets of Christian faith. If it had been intended from the beginning that woman would occupy a position of equality with the male, he wrote, then Christ would have commissioned her to go out

66. J. L. Ziegler, "Address—Woman's Sphere," *Transactions,* Medical Society of the State of Pennsylvania, XIV (1882), 26–27.
67. *Ibid.,* 31.

and preach the gospel. Men such as John Stuart Mill and A. J. Ingersoll, whose book *In Health* (1884) argued that sex was a wholesome appetite and most of women's psychological problems stemmed from their fear of the sexual appetite, were conspiring with treasonous as well as heretical ideas. The problem was one which affected both the physical organization of woman and the fundamental doctrines of Christianity. He feared that in the age of steam and "electric speed," men had abandoned the principles of their forefathers and succumbed to the temptations of pernicious pleasure-seekers and false prophets.[68]

Nature's Nuns

In spite of the efforts of physicians to keep women safely in the home circle, by the end of the century, American society had begun to look benignly, if not approvingly, upon women in community and civil projects, in education, and, slowly, in the professions. The suffragette, the temperance leader, and the cyclist in her shortened dress and bloomers became common sights as the initial shock of women in public activity began to wear off. Vocal dissenters in the medical profession, however, remained wary of this newly "emancipated" woman and yearned for the rebirth of the nineteenth-century homebody. Their warning, sounded amid the cacaphony of other less euphemistic prose, suggested that the feminists had waged their crusade in blithe disregard of the intentions of creation. Blinded by their womanly sentiments and emotions, feminists believed that by stripping away the doctrinal deadwood of custom, prejudice, and archaic beliefs, they could erase the workings of God and evolution. Many doctors thought, however, that the feminist movement had grown out of an unholy alliance of unproven ideas, and its stubborn crusade would ultimately culminate in a macabre finale. The feminists had gambled recklessly with the laws of nature and lost, and those who had taken part in the naively contrived movement would suffer the ultimate barbarism—loss of femininity.

In 1895, physician and author James Weir, Jr. (1856–1906),

68. *Ibid.,* 37.

warned of the effects of female suffrage on posterity. A graduate of the University of Louisville Medical School, Weir brought his medical background to bear on subjects ranging from feminism to *Religion and Lust* (1897) and *The Psychical Correlation of Religious Emotion and Sexual Desire* (1905). According to Weir's medical and psychological analysis, the suffrage demands of the "new woman" threatened to weaken sexual restraints that had evolved over thousands of years of civilization-building by encouraging a return to polygamy and matriarchy. Evidence of this "psychic atavism," which attacked the weakest elements of civilization, was appearing in epidemic proportions among the feminists of the day, particularly those who were neurasthenic. According to his analysis, any woman who promoted equality of the sexes had "either given evidences of masculo-femininity (viraginity), or had shown, conclusively, that she was a victim of psycho-sexual aberrancy." This prognosis, first announced by Weir in 1893 in the *New York Medical Record*, attacked the feminist movement as an example of hermaphroditism. Searching history for proof of his theory, he listed similar traits in Joan of Arc ("victim of hystero-epilepsy"), Catherine the Great ("dipsomanic of inordinate sensuality"), Messalina ("Woman of . . . gross carnality"), and Queen Elizabeth ("a pronounced viragint, with a slight tendency toward megalomania"). Anticipating the worst, he predicted that American feminists would degenerate into either uninhibited libertines or an anomalous phalanx of barrel-chested women.[69]

In his efforts to identify the many insidious forms of viraginity in the feminine world of the nineteenth century, Weir noted the young tomboy inclination of girls who abandoned dolls for masculine sports, the "loud-talking, long-stepping, slang-using young woman," and the increasing problems of homosexuality and gynandry.[70] Those women who advocated equal rights and pursued a life-style fundamentally different from that which had evolved out of past race development

---

69. James Weir, Jr., "The Effects of Female Suffrage on Posterity," *American Naturalist*, XXIX (1895), 818–19.

70. *Ibid.*, 820; S. P. White, "Modern Mannish Maidens," *Blackwood Magazine*, CXLVII (1890), 252–60.

were clearly viragints and psychically abnormal. Because Weir assumed that the feminist movement was atavistic, he predicted that its efforts to reform the social and political system would inaugurate a revolution overthrowing the present form of government and establishing a matriarchy. While the effects of this phenomenon would emerge slowly, the inevitable change in woman's condition would nonetheless undermine the entire social and political fabric of the nation. The psychical inheritance of the ages which had produced the highest level of ethical purity in the modern woman would degenerate into sensuousness, moral decadence, and free love. "The right of suffrage," Weir predicted, "would . . . very materially change the environment of woman at the present time, and would entail new and most exhausting draughts on her nervous organism."[71] He compared what he believed to be the degenerates and psychical atavists of the Oneida community of John Humphrey Noyes to the coming society of perverted men and women in America who accepted equal rights for the sexes. The right of women to vote gave free reign to those tendencies which carried them "ever backward toward the abyss of immoral horrors so repugnant to our cultivated ethical tastes— the matriarchate."[72]

For medical science in the late nineteenth century, woman's place in nature rested ultimately on biological laws. The only method to achieve equality, wrote one physician, was to "unsex" the species, a process naturally repugnant and contrary to normal sexual instincts. The division of labor reflected centuries of evolutionary race development and corresponded accurately to the differentiation of physical and psychical structure. Just as woman's sphere was the home and family, so her psychological function was one of patience, kindness, and sacrifice to her offspring.[73] According to Marion Harland, author of a number of sex-in-life manuals for women, and a strong ad-

71. Weir, "The Effects of Female Suffrage on Posterity," 822–23; Mearkle, "The Woman Who Wants to Be a Man," 173–74.
72. Weir, "The Effects of Female Suffrage on Posterity," 824–25; Norman Bridge, "The Place of Women in the Modern Business World as Affecting Health and Morals," *Bulletin,* American Academy of Medicine, IX (1908), 348; A. A. Bulley, "Political Evolution of Women," *Westminster Review,* CXXXIV (1890), 1–8.
73. Pembrey, "Woman's Place in Nature," 134.

vocate of the home economics movement, a radical band of seditious women voicing demands for equal rights had formed an entente with "weak men who can not hold their own with their proper sex." Furthermore, by usurping the role of the male in society, these women became "sexless beings" replete with physical and psychological degeneration.[74] Believing that the medical profession had the unpleasant obligation of warning women of the consequences of their mannish pursuits, Otto Juettner, M.D., of Cincinnati predicted a tragic ending to their efforts.

Nature is a relentless task-maker. Inasmuch as function is dependent upon structure and perfection of structure is maintained by perfection of function, we see structure degenerate in the absence of proper function. This is true of every organ in the body, it holds good of the whole organism and the same law—*caeteris paribus*—applies in the life of the race. We, therefore, conclude that woman must degenerate structurally and functionally in proportion to her deviation from her fixed physiologic standard. When she invades the sphere of man in the modern business or political world, she departs from the sex-idea and becomes a sexless substitute for man. She destroys the physical and psychic elements of womanhood without, however, being able to create the things that are supposed to take her place. She descends from a higher to a lower physiological level and soon shows the evidence of biologic retrogression.[75]

Authors writing in the 1880s urged women to attend to the duties of the family circle before bringing upon themselves newer and graver responsibilities in the business world. Society, for all its wrongs, could only be cleansed of its "moral foulness" when women returned to the family and its needs. Women had no reason "to go forth into wider fields claiming to be therein the rightful and natural purifiers." If women maintained the proper moral purity of the home, then "the streams which flow therefrom will .sweeten and purify all the rest."[76] Medical men blamed the prevalence of prostitution on those emancipated women who, in leaving home and childbearing

74. Marion Harland, *Eve's Daughters; or, Common Sense for Maid, Wife, and Mother* (New York, 1882), 424–25; Searcy, "The Mental Characteristics of the Sexes," 555–57.

75. Otto Juettner, "The Place of Women in the Modern Business World as Affecting the Future of the Race," *Bulletin*, American Academy of Medicine, IX (1908), 351.

76. (Anony.), *Letters from a Chimney-Corner: A Plea for Pure Homes and Sincere Relations between Men and Women* (Chicago, 1886), 22.

duties, forced their husbands to seek liaisons among the diseased degenerates of the lower classes.[77] As builders in the spiritual realm, women had the responsibility of giving "bias to the brain cells and soul impulses of ante-natal and post-natal infantile life." They were the mothers and teachers of youth, whose purpose was to infuse civilization's children with "fine ennobling sentiments, the solid truths of social relations, and the sterling principles of rightness, honor, honesty, and fraternal love." Women were the "perfecting agency" for the character and ideals of civilization. The intuitive members in civilization's struggle for existence, women, like the Aeolian harp, should touch upon the "secret springs of life" and add direction as well as spiritual meaning to man's progress.[78]

It was a sad waste of time, wrote Henry Smith, M.D., in his book *Woman: Her Duties, Relations and Position* (1875), for woman to forsake her inherited responsibilities in the home. By thrusting herself into the whirlwind of public activity, she would inevitably become viragint in her attitude and manners. "Public matters will make her mannish," he warned, "and a mannish woman is of all women the most disagreeable and the most to be shunned."[79] In her own way, woman wielded unlimited power, but only when acting in the home circle. Her nature revolved around God and family, and woman without either of those essential elements was "an anomaly in nature."[80] "As between the power of the ballot and this moral force exerted by women there can not be an instant's doubt as to the choice," wrote an anonymous author in 1886. Woman could not wield both without a drastic and degenerative change in her nature. Her descent into the "coarse scramble for material power" alongside the aggressive male would destroy the dignity and womanly prerogatives that high civilization had bestowed upon her.[81]

77. Hutchinson, "The Economics of Prostitution," 975–76.
78. Lucinda B. Chandler, "The Woman Movement," *Arena*, IV (1891), 708–9; (Anony.), "Woman in Her Social Relations, Past and Present," *Journal of Psychological Medicine and Mental Pathology*, IX (1856), 521–44.
79. Henry Smith, *Woman: Her Duties, Relations and Position, a Medical and Social Work* (London, 1875), 8.
80. *Ibid.*, 59.
81. (Anony.), *Letters from a Chimney-Corner*, 24–25; Alexander Walker, *Beauty; Illustrated Chiefly by an Analysis and Classification of Beauty in*

In the opinion of Arabella Kenealy, a graduate of the London School of Medicine for Women, the feminist threatened irreparable damage to her health by indulging in the more brutish activities of man. Her competition in the marketplace as well as her excessive activity endangered not only her grace and charm, but also that mysterious essence that made woman so lovely and delicate. The lean, restless, hipless, breastless woman, Kenealy warned, harmed her sympathetic nervous system by directing the vital energies responsible for the graceful curves and wonderful evolvement of the woman's molded figure into coarser muscular development. Her militancy encouraged such moral and spiritual indifference in woman's proper activities that her complexion became strong and "her glance . . . unswerving and direct."

Where before her beauty was suggestive and elusive, now it is defined. . . . The haze, the elusiveness, the subtle suggestion of the face are gone; it is the landscape without atmosphere. . . . She inclines to be, and in another year will be, distinctly spare, the mechanism of movement is no longer veiled by a certain mystery of motion which gave her formerly an air of gliding rather than of striding from one place to another. In her evening gown she shows evidence of joints which had been adroitly hidden beneath tissues of soft flesh, and already her modesty has been put to the necessity of puffing and pleating, where Nature had planned the tenderest and most dainty of devices. Her movements are muscular and less womanly. Where they had been quiet and graceful, now they are abrupt and direct. Her voice is louder, her tones are assertive. She says everything—leaves nothing to the imagination.[82]

Instead of the charm of womanhood, the mannish maiden (for surely few would ever marry) became stout with marked lines of degenerative tissue and carelessly stacked muscles. It had been nature's plan, Kenealy wrote, to set special disabilities—added width and weight of hip—to the woman's activities. "Nature had other uses than merely muscular for this fine beautiful creature she had proudly evolved—moral, spiritualizing, tender, and dainty uses wherein muscular abilities have

Woman (London, 1836); Mearkle, "The Woman Who Wants to Be a Man," 173–74.
82. Quoted in T. P. W., "The Redundancy of Spinster Gentlewomen," *Scottish Review*, XXXVI (1895), 104–5; Arabella Kenealy, "Woman as Athlete," *Daily Telegraph*, June 17, 1899.

little portion." The muscular reformer, however, who saw woman's role as one which required the ability to do the same things man could do, transformed femininity into a "cult of masculinity." But Kenealy, whose writings were frequently intended as a challenge to feminist Olive Schreiner, felt that manliness in the woman was as improper as effeminacy in a man; both were degenerative aspects which rendered the sexes sterile. Thus the "new woman," if fortunate enough to marry, "passed through the human epochs of love-making, marriage, and motherhood with the most astounding insensibility."[83] No matter to what degree woman acquired masculine characteristics and aptitudes, she remained a creature of instinct; to overdevelop rationalism in her was to render her "prey of smouldering subconscious impulses which burst fitfully and mischievously into flame." Kenealy practiced medicine for only a short time, and then, after an attack of diphtheria, voluntarily retired from professional life. Taking her own advice seriously, she withdrew to the protection of the home circle where she spent a lifetime writing biographical defenses of her father (a poet and outspoken lawyer who had been disbarred), several novels, and assorted medical works such as *Feminism and Sex Extinction* (1920) intended to explain the generatrix of woman's life.[84]

Not all women lamented the "cult of masculinity." According to one feminist, nature, like religions, had nuns, and while they were a "race of physically passive and of mentally neutralized women," they were nonetheless indispensable contributors in the modern world. Like the bee and ant communities whose "neuters" performed many of the essential duties of the insect community, that same element among modern womanhood could perform similar functions of nursing, social-welfare activity, philanthropy, or general relief services.[85]

But the medical profession viewed "nature's nuns" with calamitous alarm, believing that women could not have the best of both worlds—they could hardly perform the functions

---

83. T. P. W., "The Redundancy of Spinster Gentlewomen," 106–7; B. F. Hatch, *The Constitution of Man, Physically, Morally, and Spiritually Considered: Or the Christian Philosopher* (New York, 1866), 304–5, 373.

84. Arabella Kenealy, *Feminism and Sex Extinction* (London, 1920), 105.

85. T. P. W., "The Redundancy of Spinster Gentlewomen," 92; Higginson, *Women and Men*, 41.

of motherhood and maintain a professional life outside the home circle at the same time. Unless women were willing to become sexless "neuters," they would have to avoid the technical and competitive skills. That which marred the scheme of nature and impaired the fitness of the woman to perform her cosmic functions in the home had to be relentlessly stamped out. Womanly functions and professional activities could not co-exist without a major compromise. Any attempt to erase those qualities which had been "built up by natural selection during the existence of innumerable generations [was], in truth, an effort to counteract the prime factor in organic evolution."[86] "Better fewer books, better less company, better less culture, better less almost everything," wrote Marcus P. Hatfield, M.D., in his *Physiology and Hygiene of the House in which We Live* (1887), "than to start into life such wretched apologies for womanhood as are too many of our high-school graduates." A professor at the Chicago Medical College from 1875 to 1896, Hatfield believed that the price women paid was too dear, despite the occasional Frances Willard or Jane Addams who seemed to survive the headaches, anemia, and neurasthenia that affected the educated woman. Unless women recognized their natural limitations and took measures to prevent nervous and physical degeneration as they approached womanhood, they would invariably become destined for the sofa, the shawl, and neuralgia.[87] Woman's greatest achievement, advised the purity author of *Manhood's Morning* (1896), lay behind the throne rather than on it. "The world's greatest and truest women have been the mothers of its noblest and best men. To become the mother of a Wesley or Wilberforce, a Webster or Washington, is greater than to be a Joan of Arc . . . or the Queen of Sheba. To rock the cradle and shape the destiny of Shakespeare, Milton, Bunyan, Luther . . . Morse or Edison is a greater work than to wield the sceptre of the world's fashion or wear a royal crown."[88]

86. Irwell, "The Competition of the Sexes and Its Results," 317; Wallace, "Women and Natural Selection in Marriage," 236–37.

87. Marcus P. Hatfield, *The Physiology and Hygiene of the House in Which We Live* (New York, 1887), 110–111.

88. Joseph A. Conwell, *Manhood's Morning; or "Go It While You're Young." A Book to Young Men between 14 and 28 Years of Age* (New Jersey, 1896), 163.

In an almost matter-of-fact manner, nineteenth-century physicians depicted in apocalyptic detail the perverted virago world of women's rights. Those women whose activities had taken them beyond the boundaries of polite society would inevitably degenerate into rooftop mehitabels with voracious sexual appetites or depersonalized neuters sublimating their natural instincts for those of a neurotic drone. Concealing their punitive moralism in the guise of medical prognosis, doctors maintained the facade of the disinterested professional when faced with the open discontent of the woman seeking to fulfill her potentialities as a human being. Having identified her as "a lesser man," they could only accept a passive, self-denigrating, and noncompetitive helpmate. Any effort on her part to deny or escape that role was considered an unnatural atavism that only reaffirmed her dependent and parasitic nature. Woman's efforts to escape from the home circle merely precipitated any number of newer medical theories to explain her actions.

According to Italian sociologist and historian Guglielmo Ferrero (1871–1942), whose research was published widely in the United States, evolutionary law determined that man must labor and struggle for his existence while woman should not. Only when the male sustained the female in the struggle for life was she able to accomplish those reproductive functions assigned her in the division of labor.[89] Ferrero suspected, however, that the women's rights phenomenon created pathological as well as sociological atavisms which threatened to overthrow the natural relation of the sexes. Like physicians Arabella Kenealy and James Weir, he feared that such atavisms would cause many women to grow ugly, coarse, bold, and masculine. For these reasons he considered it ridiculous as well as unnatural for woman to expend physical and mental forces "in laboring for what she may gain without any effort on her part."[90] Using the law of evolution in support of his argument,

89. G. Ferrero, "The Problem of Women from a Bio-Sociological Point of View," *Monist*, IV (1894), 262–63; Stephen Gwynn, "Bachelor Women," *Contemporary Review*, LXXIII (1898), 866–75.

90. Ferrero, "The Problem of Women from a Bio-Sociological Point of View," 269–70; E. F. Andrews, "Will the Coming Woman Lose Her Hair?," *Popular Science Monthly*, XLII (1892–93), 370–73; M. T. Runnels, "Physical Degeneracy of American Women," *Medical Era*, III (1886), 297–302.

Ferrero maintained that the American woman should see herself as a queen surrounded by homage, veneration, and love, whose husband bore the brunt of fatigue and suffering and the "daily scars that are gained in the deadly struggle for life." It was men, he wrote, who should object to the division of labor which removed women from the struggle for existence. The burden of struggle had caused an increasing number of "maimed and wounded" males to break down both in body and mind; and similar attempts by women to seek the same labor would turn into disaster. Ferrero could not understand why so many women were taking part in the feminist movement; he considered it a profitless activity which they did not need to undertake.[91] As civilization had progressed out of barbarism, man had endowed his mate "with all the benefits which have accrued therefrom, without her having to put forth any exertion." There was no advantage in woman's participation in the competition resulting from the survival of the fittest; she had only to wait until the man placed the fruit of his labor at her feet.[92]

Physicians who sensed the growing unrest of American womanhood during the first decades of the twentieth century blamed the women's rights movement for fomenting a large portion of the turmoil. Feminism had become a part of American literature and politics, and was even "beating frantically . . . against the barriers of political economy and social morality, whose fall would unsettle the very foundations of society." Looking back through the nineteenth century, they acknowledged that the American woman had made impressive achievements, but they earnestly hoped she would confine her future goals to those duties pertaining to the home circle. Since creation, the Deity had "not shown any decided intention of changing her mental qualities into replicas of the biped He created a short time previous, and called man." And surely, if

91. Ferrero, "The Problem of Women from a Bio-Sociological Point of View," 272–73; J. Oliver, "Women Physically and Ethically Considered," *Liverpool Medical-Chirurgical Journal,* IX (1899), 223–24.

92. Ferrero, "The Problem of Women from a Bio-Sociological Point of View," 274; J. S. Weatherly, "Woman; Her Rights and Her Wrongs," *Transactions,* Medical Association of Alabama (1872), 68; Talbot, "The Political Rights and Duties of Women," 87–89.

God had shown no such inclination, there was little justification for man's choosing to act differently.[93]

The comments of John R. Irwin, M.D., in the *Charlotte Medical Journal* in 1914 seemed to draw together the diverse attitudes expressed by medical prognosticators on the feminist revolt. Fearing that socialism and communism lurked on the horizon, he thought it important for the public to question seriously the viragint tendencies in American womanhood. "The most enduring element of our national strength," he wrote, "lies in the fact that our American life centers around the fireside." The bravery of American men and the purity and beauty of American women were the results of the qualities of the home. Pathological evidence had decreed that women "must respect and revere the divine mission of their sex, which is motherhood." The feminist movement not only distorted this divine mission, but presaged a tragedy of national importance as well. Because feminist unrest was upsetting the home and disrupting the politics of the nation, he urged a new renaissance in the home environment through the development of courses in home economics and domestic science, fostering newer techniques based on scientific methodology to simplify household chores. Although women should have the best education available, it should be directed toward the moral and spiritual side of their nature, based upon a strong biblical foundation and "not an expurgated woman's Bible." With this emphasis, American women would not only become the truest source of spirituality in morals and discipline but also the "temples of science" in their advanced use of civilization's achievements for improving the home circle.[94] If the female were educated with the full knowledge of the potentialities of the home, the "new woman" would eventually prize her dominion all the more, and the "complexities of her nature will find full play in the evolutions in the American home." There lay the answer to the nation's problems as well as the key to the nation's future. There lay also the rejuvenative source of the race—"woman's divinest opportunity, her su-

93. John R. Irwin, "Womanhood, from a Physician's Viewpoint," *Charlotte Medical Journal*, LXX (1914), 104.
94. *Ibid.*, 105–6.

premest obligation and her richest reward." Protected in the safety of the home circle she wielded a mighty force against the strifes and temptations of the world.[95]

95. *Ibid.*, 107.

Chapter III

BEHIND THE FIG LEAF

Few women understand at the outset, that in marrying, they have simply captured a wild animal, and staked their chances for future happiness on their capacity to tame him. He is beautiful physically very likely, of pleasing manners and many external graces, and often possessed of noble qualities of mind and heart; but at the core of his nature he cherishes still his original savagery, the taming of which is to be the life-work of the woman who has taken him in charge. It is a task which will require her utmost of Christian patience, fidelity, and love. The duty is imposed upon her by high heaven, to reduce all these grand, untamed life-forces to order—for it is not the man who has the strongest, but he who has the most ungoverned passions, who is dangerous to society— to make them subservient to the high behests of her nature, and to those vast undying interests which, to these two and to their posterity, center in the home.

[Anonymous], *Letters from a Chimney-Corner*, 1886

The same society which placed such great emphasis upon race progress, national improvement, and material prosperity could only see sexual promiscuity and the break up of the home circle as the most serious threat to the advance of civilization. For Victorian America, sexual promiscuity was an ominous indication of national decay, not a sign of progress or of women's liberation. It represented a pandering to the lower instincts, a lessening of family structure, and a serious weakening of society's order and stability. The "twilight talks" for men and women concealed in manuals of hygiene and ethics, religious pamphlets, medical articles, and etiquette books were thus calculated to impress their readers with sentiments of virtue and chastity, and offered the notion that physical love somehow interfered with the realization of society's greater objectives. Discussions of sex predisposed the Victorians to an assortment of inferences in which sexual urges were somehow at variance with the search for morality and the proper definition of virtue. Love, like nature, proceeded according to an established set of laws or principles which, when carefully observed, would prevent the sexes from yielding to the lower passions. Love had a certain order and harmony which manifested the infinite wisdom of the Deity and which, when platonic, appeared to express its most perfect form; only under the most stringent rules did the physical aspects of love include similar attributes of beauty and goodness. Though Victorians admitted the power and value of sex, they interpreted its use in terms of its function in the species' evolutionary advance. Just as race progress demanded a higher specialization of man's talents in both the arts and sciences, so the purpose of sex was less a means of personal enjoyment than a specialized function of race and national development. The same providence that watched over America in its victories and peace was similarly

A portion of this chapter has been previously published. See "From Maidenhood to Menopause: Sex Education for Women in Victorian America," *Journal of Popular Culture*, VI (1972), 49–68.

engaged in the management of the Victorians in their capacity as preservers of the species.

Sex as described in the manuals of Victorian America became middle class, with all the marks of sobriety, propriety, modesty, and conformity, and supplied for rural and working-class America much the same function it provided for urban America looking across the Atlantic for cues to correct behavior. From another point of view, the sex-in-life manuals were a carry over from the dabblers of the mid-nineteenth century society in the areas of pseudo-science, liberal Christianity, Transcendentalism, and perfectionist tendencies. With the sex manuals the clergy, who were declining in their function as moral advisors (possibly due to their involvement in the social gospel movement), and the physicians, who were attempting to widen their function as spiritual as well as physical healers, met to reform both medicine and morals. Strands of Thomsonianism, Swedenborgianism, homeopathy, phrenology, and animal magnetism converged to create a congenial atmosphere for reconciling the spiritual affections of middle-class morality with matters of the flesh. Deeply Augustinian in tone, with a strong undercurrent of Old Testament vengeance, the purity literature of the late nineteenth century portrayed sex as the most primitive human tendency (amativeness being located at the base of the brain and not among the higher convolutions), the aberrations of which were invariably detected and punished through disease and mental anguish.

Sexuality: From Pleasure to Prudery

The seventeenth- and eighteenth-century manuals of love and marriage contrasted sharply to those of the later Victorian period. The most obvious difference lay in their emphasis on "pleasure," since many earlier manuals were merely advertisements for patent and proprietary medicines to strengthen the sexual powers. An anonymous author in 1719 suggested, for example, that "when young persons are not early happy in their conjugal embraces as [they] may wish to be, and it is suspected from a coldness, and insufficiency upon that account on either side," the use of either Strengthening Electuary or Restorative Nervous Elixir would not fail "to render their intercourse prolific, as it actually removes the causes of impotency in one sex, and of sterility, or barrenness, in the other."[1] Another popular manual encouraged sexual pleasure by demanding that both sexes meet "with equal vigour" in the conjugal act. The woman's interest in sex as well as her ability to conceive depended entirely upon pleasurable reciprocity. The clitoris, which achieved an erection similar to the male penis ("yard" or "codpiece") as a result of stimulation, "both stirs up lust and gives delight in copulation, for without this, the fair sex neither desire mutual embrace, nor have pleasure in them, nor conceive by them."[2] Noted medical scientist John Hunter (1728–93) had identified the clitoris as the reciprocal organ of the male penis: "There is one part in common to both the male and female organs of generation, in all the animals that have the sexes distinct; in the one it is called the penis; in the other the clitoris. Its special use, in both, is to continue by its sensibility, the action excited in coition till the paroxysm alters the sensation."[3]

The most popular manuals of the seventeenth, eighteenth, and early nineteenth centuries were the "Aristotle" series, which first appeared anonymously in England in the mid-seventeenth century. Drawing from random selections of the writings of the Greek philosopher (indeed, often contradicting his teachings), literary pirates with a cursory knowledge of medicine incorporated legends, folklore, ancient medical practices, and mysticism of the sexual act into a compendium of information which quickly disseminated throughout England and the American colonies. In the absence of standard medical works on marriage relations, the Aristotle pamphlets provided

1. (Anony.), *Onanism Displayed: Being I. An Enquiry into the True Nature of Onan's Sin II. Of the Modern Onanists III. Of Self-Pollution, Its Causes, and Consequences; with Three Extraordinary Cases of Two Young Gentlemen and a Lady Who Were Very Much Addicted to This Crime IV. Of Nocturnal-Pollutions Natural and Forced V. The Great Sin of Self-Pollution with the Judgment of the Most Eminent Divines upon this Subject VI. A Dissertation Concerning Generation with a Curious Description of the Parts and of Their Proper Functions, etc.*, According to the Latest, and Most Approved Anatomical Discoveries (2nd ed.; London, 1719), 35.

2. Aristotle (pseud.), *Aristotle's Complete Master-Piece in Three Parts, Displaying the Secrets of Nature in the Generation of Man* (Worcester, 1795), 16, 35.

3. Quoted in Rufus W. Griswold, "Some Observations on the Physiology of Coitus from the Female Side of the Matter," *Clinical News*, I (1880), 447.

the major source of sex and gynecological knowledge to mass audiences. The first American edition appeared in 1766, and in the next eighty years more than 100 different editions were printed under varying titles and with changing texts. Usually titled *Aristotle's Master-Piece,* the *Last Legacy,* and the *Compleat and Experienced Midwife,* the pamphlets were a valuable source of erotic and medical lore. Gleaned from stray passages of Aristotle, the writings of Sylvius, the teachings of French physician Ambroise Paré (1510–90), and any number of Greek, Roman, and medieval myths, the manuals dealt with those problems of most concern to the populace—impotence, infertility, the marking of unborn children, and sexual malfunctions —as well as topics such as puberty, coition, conception, and the development of the fetus. The name Aristotle lent respectability, and the erotic nature of the poetic passages made the pamphlets appealing. With few doctors available in most areas of America in the eighteenth century and with their medical knowledge limited, the Aristotle pamphlets, although they had little actual medical standing, served an important function, and their widespread availability accounted for their popularity.[4]

Eighteenth-century manual writers regarded sex as a healthy passion governed by natural laws. The inclinations of virgins for marriage became evident soon after the flow of "natural purgations" at the age of fourteen or fifteen. Then the blood ceased to serve the development of their bodies and turned instead to "stir up their minds to venery." At puberty, the female body became heated by the additional eating of "sharp and salt things, and by spices, by which their desire of venereal embrace becomes very great, at some critical junctures almost insuperable." Although authors extolled the virtues of virginity, they nonetheless cautioned against making more of it than necessary. Virginity was the "boast and pride of the fair sex," but women must "honestly rid of it" without too great an emphasis as to its importance; "for if they keep it too long," wrote the author of an Aristotle pamphlet, "it grows useless, or at least loses much of its value, a stale virgin (if such a thing there be) being looked upon like an old almanak out of date."[5]

4. Otho T. Beal, Jr., "Aristotle's Master Piece in America: A Landmark in the Folklore of Medicine," *William and Mary Quarterly,* XX (1963), 207–222.

5. Aristotle (pseud.), *Aristotle's Complete Master-Piece,* 26, 29.

Manuals thus encouraged early marriages to prevent disorders resulting from the unnatural confinement of the "seed" in the male and female. Both sexes were "thrown into a deplorable Condition, which will find no absolute Cure, till the stagnating Seed is evacuated by Marriage."[6] In discussing the sexual act, the Aristotle love manuals gave the most glowing description.

> Now my fair bride, now will I storm the mint
> of love and joy and rifle all that's in't.
> Now, my enfranchis'd hand on ev'ry side,
> Shall o'er thy naked polish'd iv'ry slide:
> Freely shall now my longing eyes behold
> Thy barred snow, and thy upbraided gold.
> Nor curtains, now, tho' of transparent lawn,
> Shall be before thy virgin treasure drawn.
> I will enjoy thee, now, my fairest; come
> And fly with me to Love's Elysium.
> My rudder, with thy bold hand, like a try'd
> And Skilful pilot, thy shalt steer; and guide
> My bark in Love's dark channel, where it shall
> Dance, as the bounding waves do rise and fall,
> Whilst my tall Pinnace in the Cyprian strait,
> Bides safe at anchor, and unlades the freight,
> Having by these and other amorous acts (which love
> can better dictate than my pen) wound up your
> fancies to the highest ardour and desires,
> Perform these rites, nature and love requires,
> Till you have quenched each other's am'rous fires.[7]

With sexual congress completed, manuals advised the husband to refrain from withdrawing "too suddenly out of the field of love, lest he should, by so doing, make way for cold to strike into the womb, which might be of dangerous consequences." It was better for the husband to remain in "the great slit" until the "matrix" had time to close after receiving the "active principle." This would encourage the possibility of conception. While manual writers recommended a healthy accommodation to the passions of love, they nonetheless cautioned against excesses. As one author suggested, "women rather choose to have a thing done well, than have it often."[8]

6. (Anony.), *Onanism Displayed*, 97.
7. Aristotle (pseud.), *Aristotle's Complete Master-Piece*, 36–37.
8. *Ibid.*, 37; G. Archibald Douglas, *The Nature and Causes of Impotence*

Love manuals written during the first half of the nineteenth century treated women as potentially equal partners in the marriage bed, but they were not nearly as explicit in their discussion of sex as those of the previous century. For one thing, authors tended increasingly to limit the pleasurable aspect of sexuality. While encouraging healthy persons to exercise the sexual instinct, they cautioned against too frequent satiation of the senses.[9] Although there was to be a definite decorum in the privacy of the bedchamber, marriage manuals allowed that normal sexual relations could be enjoyed four or five times a week without difficulty, and the wife should experience orgasm along with the husband. "A modest female will be found always to possess . . . sufficient degree of effeminate decorum not to outstrip her sex, and play the harlot, even though her passions be strong," wrote one author in 1846, "but she ought not to be denied what a healthy husband ought to be able to give."[10] Part of the male's responsibility was to excite those sexual feelings which were thought to be comparatively dormant in the woman at marriage. "Almost any wife whose husband is not repugnant, can be persuaded to all the intensity of emotion necessary or desirable." The husband was to hold himself in readiness for the wife's invitation "which woman knows full well how to give, without the shadow of impropriety, and, in reality, leading while she seems to follow." On the other hand, the wife should "yield cheerfully," never prove remiss, but be always eager to comply.[11]

One of the first significant changes in marital advice came with the writings of Sylvester Graham (1794–1851), whose health crusade during the 1840s demanded certain rules re-

---

in Men, and Barrenness in Women, Explained. With the Methods by Which It May Be Known in Any Case and Whose Part the Imperfection Lies; and Instructions for the Prevention and Remedy (London, 1758), 15–27.

9. (A Physician), *Licentiousness and Its Effects upon Bodily and Mental Health* (New York, 1844), 30.

10. Robert J. Culverwell, *Professional Records. The Institutes of Marriage, Its Intent, Obligations, and Physical and Constitutional Disqualifications* (New York, 1846), 54.

11. Orson S. Fowler, *Love and Parentage, Applied to the Improvement of Offspring: Including Important Directions and Suggestions to Lovers and the Married concerning the Strongest Ties and the Most Sacred and Momentous Relations of Life* (New York, 1846), 126–27, 134.

garding the frequency of intercourse for married couples. Graham observed that American men were suffering from increased incidence of debility, skin and lung diseases, headaches, nervousness, and weakness of the brain—all of which he blamed on sexual excesses in marriage. Believing as so many others in his day that an ounce of semen equaled nearly forty ounces of blood, Graham concluded that sexual excesses lowered the life-force of the male by exposing his system to disease and premature death. Demanding that men radically change their diet to include such foods as unbolted wheat, rye meal, hominy, and Graham flour, he also hoped that healthy and robust husbands would limit their sexual indulgences to twelve times each year. More frequent intercourse would impair the male's constitutional powers, shorten life, and increase liability to disease and suffering. Graham's dietary rules and his views on intercourse eventually became common currency among physicians who saw in male abstinence a means not only of replenishing nervous energy, but also for radically changing the prevailing views of sexuality in the nineteenth century.[12]

The publication of William Acton's *Functions and Disorders of the Reproductive Organs* (1857) was responsible for much of the subsequent medical justification for the changing role of women in marriage. Speaking as a physician with countless hours of private consultation, Acton observed that women had little sexual feeling, and in fact, remained indifferent to the physical aspects of marriage. Only out of fear "that they would be deserted for courtesans if they did not waive their own inclinations," Acton wrote, did passionless women submit to their husbands' embraces. Woman's indifference to sex was naturally ordained to prevent the male's vital energies from being overly expended at any one time. For a century which was beginning to focus exclusively upon the male as the center of force and vitality, the role of woman in the personal sexual relationship could only be a supportive position, conserving male strength by matching the brassy edges of his ego with submissive femininity. According to Acton, since the sexual act

12. Sylvester Graham, *A Lecture to Young Men, on Chastity. Intended also for the Serious Consideration of Parents and Guardians* (Boston, 1839), 83; (Anony.), "Excessive Venery; Softening of the Brain," *New England Journal of Medicine*, XXXVI (1847), 41–42.

was such an enormous drain on the nervous system, the male should perform this function in as short a time as possible, preferably a few minutes. The female's lack of complementary satisfaction only helped to preserve the male's vital energies for other more serious responsibilities.[13] "I should say that the majority of women (happily for society) are not very much troubled with sexual feeling of any kind," he remarked. "What men are habitually, women are only exceptionally. . . . There can be no doubt that sexual feeling in the female is in the majority of cases in abeyance, and that it requires positive and considerable excitement to be roused at all: and even if roused (which in many instances it never can be) it is very moderate compared with that of the male."[14]

Young men falsely formed their ideas of women's sensuous nature as a result of their contact with "low and vulgar women." In every society there were certain females who, while not actually prostitutes, were nonetheless willing to "make a kind of trade of a pretty face." But such women, Acton observed, misrepresented the true feelings of the sex. "Many of the best mothers, wives, and managers of households," he pointed out, "know little of or are careless about sexual indulgences. Love of home, of children, and of domestic duties are the only passion they feel."[15] Similarly, George Napheys remarked in his *Transmission of Life* (1871) that only in rare instances did women experience a tenth of the sexual feelings familiar to most men. "Many of them are entirely frigid," he wrote, "and not even in marriage do they ever perceive any real desire."[16]

The attitude of the medical profession toward women's sexu-

13. William Acton, *The Functions and Disorders of the Reproductive Organs in Childhood, Youth, Adult Age, and Advanced Life Considered in Their Physiological, Social, and Moral Relations* (3rd. Am. ed.; Philadelphia, 1871), 135–40; C. B. Riggs, "Social Purity and Marriage," *New York Polyclinic Journal,* IX (1897), 77.

14. Acton, *The Functions and Disorders of the Reproductive Organs,* 163; William B. Carpenter, *Principles of Human Physiology* (London, 1842), 696.

15. Acton, *The Functions and Disorders of the Reproductive Organs,* 164.

16. Quoted in Griswold, "Some Observations on the Physiology of Coitus from the Female Side of the Matter," 445; George Henry Napheys, *The Transmission of Life. Counsels on the Nature and Hygiene of the Masculine Function* (Philadelphia, 1871); George Henry Napheys, *The Physical Life of a Woman: Advice to the Maiden, Wife, and Mother* (Cincinnati, 1873).

ality, however, was in no way monolithic. Although most manual writers alluded to woman's lack of sexual desire, physicians like Elizabeth Blackwell challenged Acton's thesis, maintaining that most female repugnance for sexual passion resulted from terror of pain, fear of injury from childbirth, and past experiences with awkward or brutal conjugal encounters. These women, for whom the sexual act was devoid of both romance and pleasure, and was, in fact, a source of discomfort, found sexual abstinence and frigidity an "easy virtue."[17] According to Frederick R. Sturgis, M.D., of New York, women were passive because they believed the sexual act to be simply for the pleasure and relief of the male's sexual needs. Consequently, the male attempted intercourse without any effort to excite the woman sexually. "Having gained entrance, he goes through the performance as rapidly as possible, and, the act being completed, he disengages long before she has had the opportunity of experiencing any sexual pleasure."

In other words, the act is begun, continued, and finished before the woman has hardly time to realize what is going on, and it is small wonder, under the circumstances, particularly, if this procedure be frequently repeated, that the woman comes to the conclusion that coitus has no pleasure for her, and that if she yields herself to the embraces of her husband it is only because she feels it to be her wifely duty, and perhaps because she wishes to please him. . . . Of course, I need not tell my readers that in most women the orgasm takes a long time for its advent, and is separate and distinct from the secretion of the glands, which are first provoked into action by the titillation by the male organ. If, now, the male forgets his partner in the act, her feelings are naturally hurt; I do not mean her physical, but her mental feelings, and she regards herself simply as a passive instrument for the gratification of the man's animal passions, and she often feels resentment and anger against the man who thus treats her merely as a machine.[18]

Some nineteenth-century doctors even suspected that the female's capacity for sexual satisfaction was more intense and prolonged than the male's. Clearly, medical science did not

17. Elizabeth Blackwell, *The Human Element in Sex: Being a Medical Enquiry into the Relation of Sexual Physiology to Christian Morality* (London, 1884), 45; Thomas W. Galloway, *Love and Marriage; Normal Sex Relations* (New York, 1924), 62.

18. Frederick R. Sturgis, "Sexual Incompetence: Causes and Treatment," *Medical Council,* XII (1907), 62.

fully understand the physiology of coitus, but they felt that Acton and others like him had erred in their impression that the vaginal canal and not the clitoris was the reciprocal organ for sexual satisfaction in the woman. As a result, only one woman in four knew she had a clitoris because it remained dormant without sufficient titillation, and even in coitus was not usually touched.[19] The editors of the *Alkaloidal Clinic,* writing in 1899, blamed this ignorance on woman's education, which had taught her to think that sexual feeling was indecent, immoral, and silly—that it was "morally wrong to indulge in sexual pleasures even with the husband." The result was "a race of sexless creatures, married nuns," for whom the clitoris had only ordinary sensation, and who experienced no pleasurable feeling in the vagina during intercourse.[20]

Unfortunately, the views of Acton remained dominant among physicians who were unwilling to make the connection between the clitoris and the woman's feeling for excitement. "There is an ingrained and inborn prudery prevailing," wrote one distraught physician, "which stifles the few and hesitant endeavors of medical men who occasionally feel impelled to speak of this subject."[21] By the 1870s, purity authors had begun to monopolize marriage manuals and extolled frigidity in the female "as a virtue to be cultivated, and sexual coldness as a condition to be desired."[22] As one manual suggested in 1876, women had "more of the motherly nature than the conjugal about them. . . . Their husbands are to them only children of larger growth, to be loved and cared for very much in the same way as their real children. It is the motherly element which is the hope, and is to be the salvation of the world. The higher a woman rises in moral and intellectual culture, the more is the sensual refined away from her nature, and the more pure and perfect and predominating becomes her motherhood. The real woman regards all men, be they older or younger than

19. Griswold, "Some Observations on the Physiology of Coitus from the Female Side of the Matter," 447.

20. (Anony.), "Sexual Hygiene," *Alkaloidal Clinic,* VI (1899), 646.

21. Samuel S. Wallian, "The Physiological, Pathological and Psychological Bearings of Sex," *Transactions,* Medical Society of the State of New York (1890), 255.

22. Griswold, "Some Observations on the Physiology of Coitus from the Female Side of the Matter," 448.

herself, not as possible lovers, but as a sort of step-sons, towards whom her heart goes out in motherly tenderness."[23]

To restrain the aggressive nature of the male, purity authors advised women to remain cold, passive, and indifferent to the husband's sexual impulses. Careless and amative acts destroyed the "innate dignity" of the wifely role and led to the misuse of the sexual function in immodest responses in the male.[24] It was part of nature's plan, wrote Mary Wood-Allen, M.D. (1841–1908), national superintendent of the Purity Department of the Woman's Christian Temperance Union, for women to "have comparatively little sexual passion." Though women loved, and while they gladly embraced their husbands, they did so "without a particle of sex desire." For Wood-Allen, the most genuine sort of love between man and wife existed in the lofty sphere of platonic embrace.[25] As a passive creature, the wife was to endure the attention of her husband in a negative sense, if only to deter the greater weakening of his "vital forces." Late nineteenth-century moralists likened the sexual role of women to that of the flower—motionless, insentient, passive, and inanimate. Women must follow nature, and like the flower, lie "motionless on [the] stalk, sheltering in a dazzling tabernacle the reproductive organs of the plant."[26] In contrast to the writers of the eighteenth- and early nineteenth-century love manuals, purity authors agreed that the experience of "any spasmodic convulsion" in coition would interfere with conception—the primary function of the marriage act. "Voluptuous spasms" in the woman, wrote one author, caused a weakness and relaxation which tended to make her barren.[27]

The common stereotype of a Victorian marriage in which

23. Eliza B. Duffey, *The Relations of the Sexes* (New York, 1876), 219.

24. Emma F. (Angell) Drake, *What a Young Wife Ought to Know* (Philadelphia, 1908), 85.

25. Mary Wood-Allen, *Marriage; Its Duties and Privileges* (Chicago, 1901), 194.

26. Margaret Cleaves quoting from Maurice Maeterlinck, "The Intelligence of Flowers," *Harper's Monthly*, CXIV (1907), in her "Education in Sexual Physiology and Hygiene," *Woman's Medical Journal*, XVIII (1908), 223.

27. Alexander Walker, *Intermarriage: Or the Mode in Which and the Causes Why Beauty, Health, and Intellect Result from Certain Unions, and Deformity, Disease, and Insanity from Others* (New York, 1839), 256; William M. Capp, *The Daughter: Her Health, Education and Wedlock* (Philadelphia, 1891), 94.

the wife's sexuality was realized completely in the breeding of legitimate heirs was all too real for many women. While American wives struggled successfully to redefine their legal status within marriage in order to overcome their distinction as chattels of their husbands, attempts to liberalize the personal relationships of the marriage bed resulted in a moral code that severely restricted sexuality. With minor exceptions, women were not only willing to maintain their circumscribed sexuality, but actually regarded the marriage stereotype as a convenient excuse for salvaging a sort of dignity within marriage. Although ostensibly giving preference to the self-centered hedonism of the Victorian male, the purity literature and its theories on female passivity allowed women to sidestep the popular concept which held the man as master of his wife by establishing the limits within which they would act as a sex object. In a certain masochistic sense, Victorian women used the purity literature of the late nineteenth century as a vehicle in their efforts to obtain greater freedom of person. Disappointed in their role as sex objects, and unwilling or unable to break from the confines of an inherited moral code, they sought to reject sexual pleasure completely through assorted fantasies. Women attempted greater personal freedom not by enjoying sex but by relegating it to the narrow procreative role. The prevailing public strictures against artificial birth control, the fear of conception, and the problems attending childbirth, tended to confine women's revolt to a policy of nonsexuality. The century's purity literature became a double-edged tool: while it allowed the woman to maintain a propriety necessary to her station in the home circle, it also circumscribed her sexuality to the extent that she often suffered psychologically. Not understanding their need or capacity for sexual fulfillment, many wives remained frigid in marriage, resulting in part in their high incidence of hysteria and sexual neurasthenia.

From Maidenhood to Wifehood

Nearly all purity literature condemned the romantic novel as responsible for the increase in sexual neurasthenia, hysteria, and generally poor health among American women. Not only did sentimental novels tempt them to impurity, but the emotional stimulation that accompanied novel reading tended "to develop the passions prematurely, and to turn the thoughts into a channel which led in the direction of the formation of vicious habits."[28] Whatever stimulated emotions in the young girl caused a corresponding development in her sexual organs. Overindulgence in romantic stories produced a flow of blood to certain body organs causing "excessive excitement" and finally disease.[29] For this reason, children's parties, staying up late, puppy love, hot drinks, "boarding-school fooleries," loose conversation, "the drama of the ballroom," and talk of beaux, love, or marriage were contributing causes to unnatural sexual development.[30] The physician's duty was to oppose novel reading as "one of the greatest causes of uterine disease in young women." There was little doubt that such reading habits injured not only the mind, but the sexual organs and their functions as well. "Reading of a character to stimulate the emotions and rouse the passions may produce or increase a tendency to uterine congestion, which may in turn give rise to a great variety of maladies, including all the different forms of [womb] displacement, the presence of which is indicated by weak backs, painful menstruation, and leukorrhea."[31] Thousands of women who had in their youth "intently por[ed] over the vulgar poems of Chaucer or the amorous ditties of Burns or Byron" were subsequently forced "to wage a painful warfare for years

28. John H. Kellogg, *Ladies Guide in Health and Disease. Girlhood, Maidenhood, Wifehood, Motherhood* (Des Moines, Iowa, 1883), 208–9.

29. Catherine Ester Beecher, *Letters to the People on Health and Happiness* (New York, 1855), 45; Joseph H. Greer, *Woman Know Thyself; Female Diseases, Their Prevention and Cure: A Home Book of Tokology, Hygiene and Education for Maidens, Wives and Mothers. A Clean and Clear Exposition of Nature's Laws and Mysteries* (Chicago, 1902), 90–92.

30. Orson S. Fowler, *Maternity; or the Bearing and Nursing of Children including Female Education and Beauty* (New York, 1856), 16; Anna M. Galbraith, *The Four Epochs of Woman's Life; a Study in Hygiene* (Philadelphia, 1904), 28; Helen Maria (Fiske) Hunt Jackson, *Bits of Talk about Home Matters* (Boston, 1873), 184–88.

31. Kellogg, *Ladies Guide in Health and Disease*, 208–9; Orson S. Fowler, *Creative and Sexual Science: Or Manhood, Womanhood, and Their Mutual Interrelations: Love, Its Laws, Power, etc., Selection, or Mutual Adaption; Courtship, Married Life, and Perfect Children; Their Generation, Endowment, Paternity, Maternity, Bearing, Nursing, and Rearing; Together with Puberty, Boyhood, Girlhood, etc.; Sexual Impairments Restored, Male Vigor and Female Health and Beauty Perpetuated and Augmented, etc., as Taught by Phrenology and Physiology* (Cincinnati, 1870), 891.

to banish from their minds the impure imagery generated by the perusal of books of this character." Most complications during pregnancy and menopause were traced to this source.[32] Thus, writers cautioned parents to examine carefully every piece of literature placed in their daughters' hands, even to the extent of editing prurient Sunday-school books.[33]

Doctors advised parents to prevent "silly letter-writing" between boys and girls in their early school years. "We have known of several instances," warned John Harvey Kellogg, M.D., in his *Ladies Guide in Health and Disease* (1883), "in which the minds of pure girls became contaminated through this channel." Kellogg, famous for his health foods (he helped to found the W. K. Kellogg cereal company) and rest homes for the century's neurasthenics, campaigned for "eternal vigilance" and enjoined parents to guard the chastity of daughters in all their relations. This vigilance included the prohibition of tea and coffee until they were at least eighteen years of age. These "comforting properties" were addictive and sometimes led the young woman to seek stronger tonics to satisfy her craving for stimulants.[34]

Like novels and letter-writing, dancing was another source of impurity. Kellogg, for example, claimed that the dance had caused the ruin of three-fourths of the degenerate women in New York City.[35] One young lady confessed that the waltz had awakened a "strange pleasure" in her constitution—her pulse fluttered, her cheeks glowed with the approach of her partner, and she "could not look him in the eye with the same frank gayety as before." According to Sylvanus Stall, author of a sex-

32. Kellogg, *Ladies Guide in Health and Disease*, 209–10; George M. Beard, *American Nervousness, Its Causes and Consequences* (New York, 1881), 111; George F. Comfort and Anna M. Comfort, *Woman's Education and Woman's Health; Chiefly in Reply to "Sex in Education"* (Syracuse, 1874), 116; William A. Alcott, *The Young Husband, or Duties of Man in the Marriage Relation* (Boston, 1839), 206, 209.

33. Kellogg, *Ladies Guide in Health and Disease*, 157–58; Gordon Stables, *The Girl's Own Book on Health and Beauty* (London, 1891), 191–92.

34. Kellogg, *Ladies Guide in Health and Disease*, 160; Richard W. Schwarz, "Dr. John Harvey Kellogg as a Social Gospel Practitioner," *Journal*, Illinois State Historical Society, LVII (1964), 5–22; Marion Harland, *Eve's Daughters; or Common Sense for Maid, Wife, and Mother* (New York, 1882), 116; Stables, *The Girl's Own Book of Health and Beauty*, 49, 139.

35. Kellogg, *Ladies Guide in Health and Disease*, 214.

in-life series in 1897 which sold more than a million copies and was translated into a dozen or more foreign languages, the male transferred his physical emotions to the woman through animal magnetism. Not the dance itself, nor even the intentions of the male dance partner, caused the woman pleasure; rather, the female absorbed the male's more domineering and passionate nature through magnetic contact. Thus, wrote a ruined and repentant girl, "I became abnormally developed in my lowest nature."[36]

The proper training of girls, their personal hygiene, their relations with other children, their reading habits, and the embarrassing problem of masturbation (variously called the "solitary vice," "self-pollution," "self-abuse," or the "soul-and-body-destroyer") dominated a major portion of the sex manuals of the day. Manual writers cautioned girls never to handle their sexual organs, for, while it gave temporary pleasure, the habit left "its mark upon the face so that those who are wise may know what the girl is doing."[37] The misuse of the sexual organs brought inevitable disease and severe complications in later life. "The infliction of the penalty may be somewhat delayed," wrote one physician, "but it will surely come, sooner or later."[38] The young girl who practiced the solitary vice would never escape the consequences of her indiscretion. She would become subject to a multitude of disorders such as backaches, tenderness of the spine, nervousness, indolence, pale cheeks, hollow eyes, and a generally "languid manner." Her attitude, once pure and innocent, would turn peevish, irritable, morose, and disobedient; furthermore, she would suffer loss of memory, appear "bold in her manner instead of being modest," and manifest unnatural appetites for mustard, pepper, cloves, clay, salt,

36. Sylvanus Stall, *What a Young Husband Ought to Know* (Philadelphia, 1897), 244–45; Sylvanus Stall, *What a Young Man Ought to Know* (Philadelphia, 1897), 243; Beecher, *Letters to the People on Health and Happiness*, 18–19; Fowler, *Maternity*, 130–32.

37. Mary Wood-Allen, *What a Young Girl Ought to Know* (Philadelphia, 1897), 106; Samuel B. Woodward, *Hints for the Young in Relation to the Health of Body and Mind* (Boston, 1856); Edith B. Lowry, *Herself; Talks with Women concerning Themselves* (Chicago, 1911), 137–48.

38. Kellogg, *Ladies Guide in Health and Disease*, 146–47, 154; Beecher, *Letters to the People on Health and Happiness*, 12–13; Walker, *Intermarriage*, 35.

chalk, and charcoal.[39] Seeing a connection between sexual perversity and certain foods, Kellogg and other late nineteenth-century purity writers departed radically from the eighteenth-century belief that these food cravings were signs of a young woman's sexual development, and preached a moral and ethical system which borrowed heavily from the health crusades of Sylvester Graham and William Andrus Alcott of the American Physiological Society. Other writers conjectured that a girl's eyes became dull, with bluish rings, that she would experience difficulty in concentration and in study, and that blindness, stupidity, and even idiocy could occur. All through life, "the penalty of unlawful transgression [would] be visited upon her," and when she became a wife and mother, her earlier abuse would make the perils of pregnancy and menopause much more dangerous. Actually, these latter ideas appear to have been first suggested in an anonymous pamphlet, *Onania; or, the Heinous Sin of Self-Pollution, and All Its Frightful Consequences, in Both Sexes Considered,* published in London in 1737, which most nineteenth-century manuals accepted without question and elaborated upon with great skill. Masturbation left such obvious marks on the face and personality that a careful parent could know the habits of a son or daughter and guard them from "polluted" friends.[40]

The manuals passed hurriedly over another nasty habit—the display of unnatural affections of girls for other girls. The custom of holding each other's hands, of kissing and caressing "should be kept for . . . hours of privacy, and never indulged in before gentlemen." The reasons for this admonition "readily

39. Wood-Allen, *What a Young Girl Ought to Know,* 106–7; Kellogg, *Ladies Guide in Health and Disease,* 152; Lowry, *Herself; Talks with Women concerning Themselves,* 140–41; Goss and Co., *Hygeiana, a Non-Medical Analysis of the Complaints Incidental to Females* (London, 1823), 30–31; Samuel Gregory, *Facts and Important Information for Young Women on the Self-Indulgence of the Sexual Appetite* (Boston, 1857).

40. Henry S. Cunningham, *Lectures on the Physiological Laws of Life, Hygiene and a General Outline of Diseases Peculiar to Females, Embracing a Revival of the Rights and Wrongs of Women, and a Treatise on Disease in General, with Explicit Directions How to Nurse, Nourish and Administer Remedies to the Sick* (Indianapolis, 1882), 98; R. H. McDonald, "The Frightful Consequences of Onanism; Notes on the History of a Delusion," *Journal of the History of Ideas,* XXVIII (1967), 423–31.

suggest themselves," and there were other motives, wrote one purity writer, "known to those well acquainted with the world."[41] Perhaps women sought to compensate for the masculine attentions that Victorian strictures forbade, and turned to feminine intimacy to supply this lack; perhaps they sought to fulfill a deeper desire. In a masculine-feminine relationship, the woman could only be a passive object, whereas in a feminine-feminine relationship she could be the subject as well as the object. In these friendships a latent lesbianism might have lurked, for here the woman could assuage the loss of prerogatives bestowed on the male by his sex, and undertake, in a slight and subtle way, to step outside the limits imposed on her by her gender.[42]

The mistaken notion of delicacy left many girls unprepared for the physiological changes at puberty. One doctor remarked that nearly a fourth of his female patients were ignorant of the significance of bodily changes, and many of them were "frightened, screamed, or went into hysterical fits."[43] However, part of the problem was surely due to the manuals themselves, which touched ever so gently on the subject of menstruation. Jules Michelet, in *Love* (1859), for example, explained that for a period of fifteen or twenty days out of twenty-eight, the woman was "not only an invalid, but a wounded one." It was woman's plight, he wrote, to ceaselessly suffer "love's eternal wound."[44] Second only to the ignorance surrounding the "periodical ordeal" was the mistaken notion of delicacy that the "calls of Nature" were inconvenient as well as unfeminine. Thus, constipation seemed to dominate many of the century's manuals. "I have known girls, and matrons old enough to be grandmothers," wrote Marion Harland in *Eve's Daughters; or, Common Sense for Maid, Wife, and Mother* (1883), "who pushed ignorant complacency to the fatuity of boasting that

41. Mrs. John Farrar, *The Young Lady's Friend* (New York, 1860), 241–42; Wood-Allen, *What a Young Girl Ought to Know*, 173.

42. Simone de Beauvoir, *The Second Sex* (New York, 1952), 404–24.

43. Edward J. Tilt, *On the Preservation of the Health of Women at the Critical Periods of Life* (London, 1851), 20.

44. Jules Michelet, *Love* (New York, 1859), 48.

the calls of Nature upon them averaged but one or two demands per week."[45]

In one of her most important functions, the young lady was to provide a constant source of idealism to her brothers. "So many temptations beset young men of which young women know nothing," wrote the author of *The Young Lady's Friend* (1860), that it was of utmost concern that the sister tend to her brothers' needs. Her evenings should be devoted to their happiness, encouraging them to spend more time at home, and to make their friends her own friends; furthermore, she should encourage "innocent amusements" within the family circle for their benefit. In this manner, brothers could pass "unharmed through the temptations of youth," and would owe their purity to the "intimate companionship of affectionate and pure-minded sisters." Once having enjoyed the influence of the "home engagement," brothers would refrain from "mixing with the unpure." Because of the loving attentions of sisters, many brothers would lay aside the wine cup and even stronger tonics "because they would not profane with their fumes the holy kiss, with which they were accustomed to bid their sisters goodnight."[46]

In their relations with males, purity authors constantly advised girls to play a passive role. "The safest and happiest way for women," wrote one author, was "to leave the matter [of courtship] entirely in his hands." Though matrimony was a great and noble vocation, it was "an incident in life, which, if it comes at all, must come without any contrivance of [the woman]."[47] And in all relations with the wooer, the girl was to maintain a strict modesty in order to guard against personal familiarity. She was never to participate in any "rude plays" that would make her vulnerable to a kiss. She was not to permit men to squeeze or hold her hand "without showing that it displeased [her], by instantly withdrawing it." Accept no unnecessary assistance, one author cautioned, "sit not with another in a place that is too narrow; read not out of the same

45. Harland, *Eve's Daughters; or, Common Sense for Maid, Wife, and Mother*, 81.

46. Farrar, *The Young Lady's Friend*, 201–4; WCTU, *Physiology for Young People* (New York, 1884), 13–17.

47. Farrar, *The Young Lady's Friend*, 258–59.

book; let not your eagerness to see anything induce you to place your head close to another person's."[48]

Girls were to carefully guard themselves from strangers. More important, they should have little confidence in men whose intentions were not yet known. "Watch them, and be ever on your guard," wrote Henry S. Cunningham in his *Lectures on the Physiological Laws of Life* (1882), "never give them ANY chance to abuse your confidence."[49] According to H. N. Guernsey, M.D., author of *Plain Talks on Avoided Subjects* (1882), young women should have no "sexual propensity, or amorous thoughts or feelings." Guernsey's admonitions were reinforced in nearly all the purity manuals of the era and reflected the influence of Acton, whose *Functions and Disorders of the Reproductive Organs* expressly limited the emotions of the modest woman to love of home and domestic duties. If properly educated, Guernsey observed, women would live through the years before marriage "perfect strangers to any such sensations" and would develop these feelings only when a suitable gentleman proclaimed his intentions. "After this acquaintance has ripened into love, and when she has become convinced of the purity of his heart [the woman] enjoys being with him, in sitting by his side, and is unhappy in his absence. When betrothed, owing to her great and pure love for him, she takes pleasure in receiving such marks of affection from him as are shown by a tender father or brother, but nothing more. After marriage, she feels that she is really his and that he has become a part of herself—that they are no more twain but one flesh. All this has transpired without her hardly suspecting such a quality in herself as an amorous affection."[50]

Manuals cautioned the woman to passively await the male's declaration of matrimonial intentions before expressing the slightest evidence of reciprocating love. To allow herself even a "partially animal basis" during courtship was to fall prey to the evils of blighted love which weakened not only her modesty but also her most important organs. Trifling with love was

48. *Ibid.*, 263.

49. Cunningham, *Lectures on the Physiological Laws of Life,* 100–101.

50. Henry N. Guernsey, *Plain Talks on Avoided Subjects* (Philadelphia, 1882), 78–79; Steven Marcus, *The Other Victorians: A Study of Sexuality and Pornography in Mid-Nineteenth Century England* (New York, 1964), chap. 1.

immoral as well as damaging to the physical and mental balance of the woman's delicate structure. When a gentleman engaged the affections of the woman, his amorous attentions caused those special organs of her sex (bosom and reproductive organs) to quicken in their development. Love not only enhanced charm and virtue, but also brought womanly functions to sexual fruition. One writer described the woman in love as one whose breasts "rise and fall with every breath, and gently quiver at every step." But when the male suitor broke off the relationship (usually as a result of the woman's immodest actions), he destroyed her charm and attractiveness, and because of the "perfect reciprocity which exists between the mental and physical sexuality," he crippled the physical organs of her sex, causing deterioration as well as disease.[51] As a member of the Social Purity League wrote in 1896, society held the woman more accountable to breaches of sexual morality than the male, for the woman's infidelity was both conserved and transmitted in the family circle while the male's offense was not. "In her person, society itself is defiled by the offense, and is compelled in self-defense to visit upon her a penalty which does not fall upon her partner."[52]

Young girls were also to avoid the hazards of early marriage. Premature love robbed the nerve and brain of their natural needs and blighted the organs of sex. It was consummate folly, wrote one author, for girls to "rush into the hymeneal embrace" since it would only exhaust the love powers, and precipitate disease and an early grave. To prevent this, young women were to place themselves on "high ground" apart from "gushing affections," holding their love as the "choicest treasure," not conferring even the smallest degree of affection to the male wooer. This etiquette would promote in the male a higher understanding of love, as he expressed "upon the bended

51. Fowler, *Maternity*, 75–79; Lowry, *Herself; Talks with Women concerning Themselves,* 157–62; Fowler, *Creative and Sexual Science,* 923.
52. S. D. McConnell, "Sexual Purity," *Medical and Surgical Reporter,* LXXIV (1896), 130; George Z. Gray, *Husband and Wife; or, the Theory of Marriage and Its Consequences* (Boston, 1885), 87–88; Benjamin F. Hatch, *The Constitution of Man, Physically, Morally, and Spiritually Considered* (New York, 1866), 404–6.

knees of confession and solicitation" only the purest form of veneration.[53]

While it was not the purpose of nineteenth-century purity manuals to make the woman unaware of the differences between male and female, they did little to inform her, in other than the most restrictive terms, of the physical aspects of married life. A large number of women entered marriage ignorant of sex; indeed, one writer remarked that there were some women "into whose minds the thought of coition has never once entered."[54] The honeymoon, therefore, was the focus of much of the marriage counselor's attention. Many marriages which would normally have developed into lasting relationships, wrote Emma Drake, professor of obstetrics at the Denver Homeopathic Medical School and Hospital, were ruined in the first days of married life by the male's thoughtless passions. "Frightened and timid, and filled with a vague unrest at the mysteries of marriage which await their revelation," innocent brides not too infrequently put their lives in the possession of husbands who "thought that every right is theirs immediately." This "rapacious passion" wrecked whatever love and honor the young bride had developed for her husband. Manuals advised young brides to avoid these problems by introducing, through the intervention of a friend, such books as the bridegroom might wisely read for the good of the marriage. The ignorance of the young bride concerning the physical aspects of marriage could hardly produce harmony; the woman particularly suffered, because her necessary chastity could not allow her to betray any knowledge or understanding of the sex act.[55]

Reflecting the efforts of the urban middle class to imitate Britain's Victorian mood, the sex-in-life manuals were almost unanimous in pointing out that the English had the most reasonable understanding of marriage relations. It was the custom in English homes, they wrote, for the husband and

53. Fowler, *Maternity*, 78–79; Lowry, *Herself; Talks with Women concerning Themselves*, 155.

54. Stall, *What a Young Husband Ought to Know*, 126.

55. Drake, *What a Young Wife Ought to Know*, 54; John Cowan, *The Science of a New Life* (New York, 1871), 105.

wife to have separate bedrooms. Though "freedom-loving Americans might think it a rather cold custom," separate bedrooms provided the perfect environment when "proper self-control seems difficult" and when too much freedom "degenerates into license."[56] According to Wood-Allen in her *Marriage: Its Duties and Privileges* (1901), if the husband found sleeping with his wife a source of great temptation, then, for the sake of chastity, he must take a bed to himself.[57] While the doors separating the two rooms should "seldom be shut," nonetheless, the custom relieved the married couple of temptation and "prevented the familiarity, which even in married life, breeds contempt."[58] Furthermore, undressing in one another's presence caused excessive emotion that harmed lasting marital relations. "If the husband cannot properly control his amorous propensities," wrote another author, the couple "had better by all means occupy separate beds and different apartments, with a lock on the communicating door, the key in the wife's possession."[59] The male body, argued Sylvanus Stall in *What a Young Man Ought to Know*, is "like a cage that encloses a beast, an angel and a devil, and no young man can afford to arouse the beast."[60] The pseudo-scientific reasoning behind separate beds, as with dancing, grew out of speculation regarding animal magnetism and the belief that the vital forces of both the husband and wife would change from too frequent intimacy—the wife becoming masculine in her cravings and the husband showing signs of effeminacy. "There is nothing that will so derange the nervous system of a person who is eliminative in nervous force as to lie all night in bed with another who is absorbent in nervous force," wrote Edward Foote in 1888. "The absorber will go to sleep and rest all night, while the eliminator will be tumbling and tossing, restless and nervous, and wake up in the morning fretful, peevish, fault-finding, and discouraged."[61]

56. Drake, *What a Young Wife Ought to Know*, 85; Greer, *Woman Know Thyself; Female Diseases, Their Prevention and Cure*, 67.
57. Wood-Allen, *Marriage; Its Duties and Privileges*, 49.
58. Drake, *What a Young Wife Ought to Know*, 85.
59. Stall, *What a Young Husband Ought to Know*, 94–96.
60. Stall, *What a Young Man Ought to Know*, 241.
61. Gustavus Cohen, *Helps and Hints to Mothers and Young Wives* (London, 1880), 88; Edward B. Foote, *Plain Home Talk about the Human System*

The separate bedroom theory was prominent in late nine-teenth-century purity literature, and represented a major effort to contain the passionate nature of the male's appetite. The double bed, wrote J. H. Greer, M.D., was a relic of a more primi-tive age. "No matter who else may sleep together," he de-clared, "husband and wife should not."[62] According to Dio Lewis, M.D., the bed "is the most ingenious of all possible de-vices to stimulate and inflame the carnal passion. No bed is large enough for two persons. If brides only knew the great risk they run of losing the most precious of all earthly posses-sions—the love of their husbands—they would struggle as resolutely to secure extreme temperance after marriage as they do to maintain complete abstinence before the ceremony. The best means to this end is the separate bed."[63] Since the hus-band was seldom strong-willed enough to master his appetites, added homeopath Emma Drake, the custom of separate beds encouraged him to subordinate the bestial nature, and allow his thoughts to "soar above the earth, even unto the region of the heavens."[64]

Contraception

Englishman Robert Malthus (1766–1834), whose alarming thesis of population growth in a geometric progression while the means of subsistence increased at only an arithmetical pro-gression, precipitated much of the discussion concerning birth control in the nineteenth century. He found willing ears among those seeking to change the prevailing strictures concerning women, the married state, and conjugal relations by suggesting that the population could be kept within bounds by preventive measures. While Malthus himself merely recommended ab-stinence ("moral restraint") from sexual intercourse as a solution to the crisis, later Neo-Malthusians like Francis Place were willing to support more direct application of contraceptive

—the Habits of Men and Women—the Causes and Prevention of Disease—Our Sexual Relations and Social Natures (New York, 1888), 867–68.

62. Greer, Woman Know Thyself; Female Diseases, Their Prevention and Cure, 186.
63. Dio Lewis quoted in Stall, What a Young Husband Ought to Know, 95; Dio Lewis, Our Girls (New York, 1871).
64. Drake, What a Young Wife Ought to Know, 86.

theories. Extensive dissemination of these latter ideas, however, came only after the founding of the Malthusian League
in 1877, which included John Stuart Mill, Charles Drysdale,
Charles Knowlton, Annie Besant, and Charles Bradlaugh.
Knowlton encouraged birth-control techniques for those men
and women who normally would have postponed marriage for
business and educational reasons. Believing that late marriages
resulted in poorly formed and weak children, and that furthermore, a man or woman's happiness need not be restricted to
the celibacy rules of the Shakers, he advised the use of coitus
interruptus, the baudruche ("French secret"), vaginal "tents"
(diaphragms), vaginal douches after intercourse with alum,
pearlash, white vitriol (sulphate of zinc), infusions of white oak,
bark, red rose leaves, nutgalls, or simple water.[65]

Although physicians were divided on the question of birth
control, the majority of those who published books or pamphlets on the subject took a strict view of conjugal pleasures and
remained publicly opposed to the use of contraceptives. Doctors wrote of weak, scrofulous, and even monstrous children
born of parents who had brought the devices of the street
prostitute into their homes, of husbands who were despondent
and subject to impotency or involuntary losses of semen as a
result of their fraudulent efforts, and of women whose fear of
pregnancy led to horrible disorders of the uterus.[66] Not without
reason, then, medical practitioners were particularly critical of
coitus interruptus ("pull back" or "withdrawal") and referred
continually to men and women who suffered physically and
psychologically from the practice. Specifically, the male's withdrawal the moment before ejaculation caused the sexual act to
stop before the vas deferens completely emptied of semen.
Enough of the fluid remained "to tease his organs and to
kindle in him desires too importunate to tolerate any self-
control." Thus men indulged in repeated venereal excesses
to satisfy unfulfilled desires, leading to a constant drain on the
"life-giving fluid" and a continual expenditure of the "nerve-

65. Charles Knowlton, *The Fruits of Philosophy. A Treatise on the Population Question* (Chicago, n.d.), 8, 39–41.
66. Culverwell, *Professional Records*, 185–86; C. Bigelow, *Sexual Pathology*
(Chicago, 1875), 75–80; S. G. Moses, "Marital Masturbation," *St. Louis
Courier of Medicine*, VIII (1882), 168–73.

forces." And for the wife, conjugal onanism, or what the French called a "coup de piston," prevented the "bathing" action of the semen upon the uterus.[67] For many years, the medical profession was almost unanimous in its belief that measures taken to prevent the comingling of the male and female fluids resulted in tumors, uterine colics, neuroses, polypi, and even cancer.[68] Wives were known to become hysterical because their wombs had not been "refreshed and soothed" by a teaspoonful of seminal secretion. In the 1870s, however, Bertillion, in his *Hygiene Matrimoniale,* argued that there were no scientific grounds for the assertion that the spermatic fluid vitalized the membranes of the uterus. Similarly, Ely Van de Warker, one of the foremost gynecologists of the century, published "A Gynecological Study of the Oneida Community" in the *American Journal of Obstetrics* demonstrating that the nonejaculation of the male in no way hindered the health of the woman. The women of the Oneida community, some of whom had sexual relations oftener than seven times a week without the discharge of semen into the vagina, did not suffer from uterine disease.[69]

Besides withdrawal, probably the most common contraceptive other than a woman's headache, was the condom, which Madame de Stael once described as "a breast plate against pleasure and a cobweb against danger." Doctors condemned the device as deterring sexual enjoyment, and most doubted its effectiveness. One physician remarked that "at any moment it is liable to rupture and place the wearer in the position of the virtuous swain, who used an eel-skin as a prophylactic and

67. William Goodell, "Clinical Lecture on Conjugal Onanism and Kindred Sins," *Philadelphia Medical Times,* II (1872), 163; L. B. Bangs, "Some of the Effects of Withdrawal," *Transactions,* New York Academy of Medicine, LX (1893), 119–24; Culverwell, *Professional Records,* 103–4; Bigelow, *Sexual Pathology,* 92–93. The term onanism was used to describe both coitus interruptus and masturbation. The word derives from Genesis 38:9 "And it came to pass, when he [Onan] went in unto his brother's wife, that he spilled it on the ground, lest that he should give seed to his brother. And the thing which he did displeased the Lord; wherefore he slew him."

68. Wallian, "The Physiological, Pathological, and Psychological Bearings of Sex," 255; Fowler, *Creative and Sexual Science,* 672; T. E. McArdle, "The Physical Evils Resulting from the Prevention of Contraception," *Transactions,* Washington Obstetrical and Gynecological Society, II (1887–89), 162.

69. (Anony.), "Does Male Copulation without Emission Injure Female Health?," *Medical News,* XLV (1884), 240–41.

neglected to sew up the eye holes."[70] "Male continence" was yet another form of contraception in vogue during the late nineteenth century, and although its main adherents were the members of the Oneida community, medical journals as well as some marriage manuals discussed its applicability. The founder of the Oneida community, John Humphrey Noyes, had divided the sexual act into three stages: the presence of the male organ in the vagina, the series of reciprocal motions, and last, the ejaculation of semen. Since the only uncontrollable portion of the sexual act was the final orgasm, he claimed that with sufficient mental control, the male could voluntarily govern the first two stages, prolonging the motions of sex so that mutual satisfaction could be obtained without orgasm. Certain members of the medical profession looked enviously on the ability of the Oneida communitarians to prolong carnal pleasures, but most agreed that the mental discipline was far too demanding for the ordinary man, and that its effectiveness would probably be obvious to those who practiced the technique in nine months. In addition, doctors suspected that prolonging the sexual act without proper ejaculation induced discomfort, atrophy, urethritis, insomnia, impotency, melancholia, and severe spermatorrhea. The only result of Noyes's sexual experimentation, claimed one skeptic, was the substitution of "wet dreams" for natural ejaculation.[71]

Since complete intercourse was thought to expend a large amount of vital force, J. H. Greer, M.D., in his *Woman Know Thyself* (1902), suggested an alternative to Noyes's technique of "male continence" called Zugassent's Discovery. The husband and wife united as in intercourse but refrained from orgasm, achieving "magnetic harmony" through the exchange of vital magnetic currents.[72] Similarly, Ida C. Craddock, the

70. F. W. Abbott, "Limitation of the Family," *Massachusetts Medical Journal*, X (1890), 341.

71. Cowan, *The Science of a New Life*, 109–10; John Humphrey Noyes, *Male Continence* (New York, 1872), 7–12.

72. Greer, *Woman Know Thyself; Female Diseases, Their Prevention and Cure*, 188–89; Albert Ellis and Albert Abarbanel (eds.), *The Encyclopedia of Sexual Behavior* (2 vols.; New York, 1961), I, 289; R. A. Parker, *A Yankee Saint. John Humphrey Noyes and the Oneida Community* (New York, 1935); Hubbard Eastman, *Noyesism Unveiled: A History of the Sect Self-Styled Perfectionists* (Brattleboro, 1849); Maren Lockwood Carden, *Oneida: Utopian Community to Modern Corporation* (Baltimore, 1969), 49–65.

author of *Right Marital Living* (1899), divided the sexual organs into "love organs" and those intended for procreation. With proper control, she wrote, the husband could achieve orgasm without ejaculation of semen, thus reabsorbing the semen into the system and conserving male vitality. Craddock's book was condemned by Anthony Comstock as "the science of seduction" and although she claimed to have the endorsement of several members of the WCTU, she was found guilty of obscenity and committed suicide to escape legal penalty.[73]

During the first half of the nineteenth century, druggists reported more purchases of abortive drugs than contraceptive devices and germicides. Women sought to induce "accidental miscarriages" by using ergot, prussic acid, iodine, strychnine, cotton root, savin, or oil of tansy. Southern women frequently resorted to cotton-seed tea to induce abortion. In addition, there were a host of patent and proprietary medicines which claimed to correct "female problems," and while many gullible wives purchased the nostrums in the hope of inducing abortion, there were repeated cases of women who were poisoned or maimed by their use. When these agents failed, women sometimes purchased uterine probes and catheters containing spring stylets to produce abortion. For five dollars, a woman could buy a silver probe, and for three dollars more, receive special instructions for relieving her "female complaint."[74] In *My Life and Loves*, nineteenth-century literary critic Frank Harris wrote: "We make a pointed pencil of certain ingredients which swell with the heat of the body. This pencil would be introduced slowly and carefully into the neck of the womb; as soon as it began to swell, the abortion was begun: nature then made its own effort and got rid of the intruding semen."[75] By the 1870s, however, the trade changed to contraceptive devices

73. (Anony.), "Sexual Hygiene," 649; Theodore Schroeder, "Censorship of Sex Literature," *Medical Council*, XIV (1909), 95–96.

74. Sidney Ditzion, *Marriage, Morals and Sex in America; a History of Ideas* (New York, 1953), 317–53; Beryl Suitters, "Contraception in Ancient and Modern Society," *Journal*, Royal Society for the Promotion of Health, LXXXVIII (1968), 9–11; F. R. Bruner, "Is Onanism Justifiable," *Medical Register*, III (1888), 79; Wesley Grindle, *New Medical Revelations, Being a Popular Work on the Reproductive System, Its Debility and Disease* (Philadelphia, 1857), 180–87, 212–13; Norman E. Himes, *Medical History of Contraception* (Baltimore, 1936).

75. Frank Harris, *My Life and Loves* (New York, 1963), 907–8.

such as the pessarium occlusivum, which Annie Besant advertised in private circulars to women. Besant's "womb veil" or
"tent" consisted of a small rubber cap surrounded at the rim by
a flexible ring.[76] Women sometimes used vaginal injections of
carbolic acid to prevent conception and avoid venereal contagion, a solution popular in many houses of prostitution.[77] Other
contraceptive douches consisted of injections of cold or warm
water, solutions of bicarbonate of soda, borax, bichloride of
mercury (which, improperly used, caused mercurial poisoning),
potassium bitartrate, alum, dilute vinegar, lysol, creolin, and
other agents to remove or sterilize the sperm. Tampons of
sponge, cotton, and other substances were retained in the
vagina for as long as twenty-four hours after intercourse to
prevent conception. Physicians who recommended "prevention"
sometimes prepared vaginal suppositories of cocoa butter and
boric acid to be applied before intercourse to act as a germi-
cide. Tannic acid and bichloride of mercury were also used in
place of boric acid, while olive oil or glycerin were substitutes
for the cocoa butter. Another contraceptive device consisted
of borated cotton pledgets which were attached to a piece of
string and pushed into the vagina against the cervix. Women
who were less knowledgeable employed handkerchiefs to
cleanse the vagina after intercourse, and one physician recalled
a patient who was accustomed to wiping out her uterus with a
crochet needle around which she attached a piece of cloth.[78]
One popular belief was that if a woman engaged in vigorous
exercise (usually dancing or horseback-riding) after intercourse,
she would avoid conception.[79]

The advocates of Neo-Malthusianism were by no means
monolithic in their attempts to curb the swelling population.
Some abstained from intercourse except during the "agenetic"
period. However, complete confusion within medical circles

76. John C. King, "Ethics and Methods of Preventing Conception," *Southern California Practitioner*, XIV (1899), 272; William P. Chunn, "The Prevention of Conception; Its Practicability and Justifiability," *Maryland Medical Journal*, XXXII (1895), 304–5.

77. Webb J. Kelly, "One of the Abuses of Carbolic Acid," *Columbus Medical Journal*, I (1883), 433–36.

78. Abbott, "Limitation of the Family," 343.

79. Harris, *My Life and Loves*, 907; Martin Larmont, *Medical Advisor and Marriage Guide* (New York, 1859), 88.

concerning the fertile and infertile periods of the woman's monthly cycle meant most nineteenth-century men and women relied on an assortment of medical guesses. Carl Capellmann, in his *Pastoral Medicine* (1879), for example, recommended "moral restraint" from intercourse for fourteen days after the woman's menstrual period and then for three to four days before the period in the belief that it was during those two times that women were most susceptible to fecundation.[80] Others preached abstinence during the months of May and June, when they believed women were most easily impregnated. Another popular theory of contraception dictated that women remain passive in intercourse. It was believed that the passionless submission of the female in the marital act, whether from personal repulsion or fear of impregnation, would render the act less fertile. Legal arguments were sometimes made in cases of rape which resulted in pregnancy that the woman's fertile condition was grounds for defense against the charge. The idea originated from the earlier Aristotle love manuals which suggested that the "want of love in the persons copulating, may also hinder conception as is apparent from those women deflowered against their will: No conception following any forced copulation."[81] Women thus concluded that by remaining passive to their husband's embraces, they might avoid pregnancy. Although the theory was widely held among women, and surely contributed toward their lack of response during coitus, it was easily refuted by those who pointed out that "loose" women who abandoned themselves to voluptuous sensations in the venereal act were least capable of conceiving, while those who were vulgarly called "cold women" were impregnated with ease.[82]

To be sure, there were more exotic forms of contraception. Karl Buttenstedt in *Happiness in Marriage* (1904) and Richard E. Funcke in *A New Revelation of Nature* (1906) maintained

80. Carl Capellmann, *Pastoral Medicine* (New York, 1879), 54; Carl Capellmann, *Facultative Sterility, without Offense to Moral Laws* (Aachen, 1883).

81. Aristotle (pseud.), *Aristotle's Complete Master-Piece*, 50; Augustus K. Gardner, *The Causes and Curative Treatment of Sterility, with a Preliminary Statement of the Physiology of Generation* (New York, 1856), 49; James Matthews Duncan, *On Sterility in Women* (Philadelphia, 1884), 96.

82. Abbott, "Limitation of the Family," 340.

that if a husband continued to suck his wife's breasts after a child was weaned, natural contraception would be continued, and give "everlasting life for humanity."[83] The woman's milk was an "elixir of life" for the male partner as well as a contraceptive. As Funcke wrote: "Thou shalt not leave thy vital force unutilized; thou shalt not menstruate unless thou hast the firm will and desire to become pregnant; thou shalt allow thy vital force in the form of milk to flow from thy breasts for the benefit and enjoyment of other human beings."[84]

Advocates of animal magnetism held that the friction generated by the mixture of the alkaline fluid in the female vagina and the acid fluid secreted by the male penis produced chemical electricity; the pubes, considered a nonconductor, confined the electrical energy generated and exchanged during the act by insulating the sexual organs from the rest of the body.[85] Any number of variations of this theory were advanced by individuals seeking to utilize animal magnetism for contraceptive purposes. Dianism, a form of magnetic contraception proposed in an anonymous pamphlet in 1882, referred to the man and woman as sexual batteries of positive and negative electricity, who during "sexual companionship or contact, [caused] a radiation or conduction which reduces the polarity, and restores the equilibrium." Believing that friction of the sexual parts during intercourse led "to the gradual accumulating attraction, which suddenly reaches the point of explosion of instant discharge; [at which] the two bodies becoming identical in polarity, repel each other," the author sought to discover a way of reducing the electrical polarity. Unlike other advocates of animal magnetism, Dianists thought it important for husband and wife to sleep together "with some degree of nude contact" in order to prevent sexual polarity from becoming excessive. Sleeping together tended to diminish the passions and bring couples to "sexual equilibrium." Hence, the practice indirectly led to marital continence by dissipating the strong

83. Iwan Bloch, *The Sexual Life of Our Time in Its Relations to Modern Civilization* (London, 1909), 700; Karl Buttenstedt, *Happiness in Marriage (Revelation in Women): A Nature Study* (Friedrichshagen, 1904).

84. Richard E. Funcke, *A New Revelation of Nature; a Secret of Sexual Life. No More Prostitution* (Hanover, 1906), 70.

85. Foote, *Plain Home Talk about the Human System,* 628, 630.

passionate attractions stimulated by sexual polarity. "When men and their wives can learn to be together, seeing each other, and embracing each other without the intervention of clothing, and to enjoy such caresses disassociated from passional feelings, there will be little danger that there will ever be such sexual excess between them as to endanger the perpetuity of their mutual attraction." The author dedicated the doctrine of "Dianism" to the principle of "continence except for procreation" achieved through sexual satisfaction and sexual contact. The contact, however, was accomplished by sexual "equilibration" (a word borrowed from Herbert Spencer's theory of evolution, referring to the progressive integration of matter, accompanied by dissipation of motion) of minds and bodies through physical nude contact.[86] Those who supported magnetism as a means of limiting family size believed that coition was merely one form of magnetic exchange between the electrical batteries of the sexes. "There is no difference in kind, but only in degree," wrote one Dianist, "between the pleasures of the dance, of a kiss, or even of the mere presence of a person of the opposite sex, and the most exciting feeling of sexual orgasm." Many married couples lived happily together and limited the size of their family through these alternative forms of magnetic exchange.[87]

Most Protestant church leaders ignored the question of contraception altogether. While condemning feticide, they seldom dealt with the problem of prevention, preferring to leave the matter to private conscience. As one Presbyterian minister wrote in 1899, "the sin [of prevention], if sin existed, must be a purely physiological one, and in physiological matters the clergy must sit at the physicians' feet as learners." The Catholic clergy, on the other hand, was united in its condemnation, despite the fact that its laity represented a significant percentage of patients requesting prevention information. Although

---

86. (Anony.) *Diana: A Psycho-Fyziological Essay on Sexual Relations for Married Men and Women* (New York, 1882), 22, 29, 42; Hatch, *The Constitution of Man, Physically, Morally, and Spiritually Considered*, 337–58; Edward B. Foote, *Dr. Foote's Reply to the Alphiles, Giving Some Cogent Reasons for Believing that Sexual Continence Is Not Good for the Health* (New York, 1882).

87. Albert Chavannes, *Vital Force and Magnetic Exchange, Their Relation to Each Other and to Life and Happiness* (Knoxville, Tenn., 1888), 16.

many medical men agreed with the church's position, they seldom expressed public support because of medical repugnance to the church's cast-iron position against craniotomy, which had for decades antagonized the moral sense of doctors who favored the life of the mother over the life of the fetus.[88]

The medical profession touched very gingerly on the question of contraception in its journals. The *Medical and Surgical Reporter* in 1888 described several contraceptive methods considered simple and harmless compared with the dangers of too frequent pregnancies. Although not openly advising contraception, doctors began to speak of select cases in which health demanded that women avoid pregnancy. "The vicious and immoral do not ask for or need this advice," wrote Ernest C. Helm, M.D., "for they have plenty of devices of their own; but as physicians, as humanitarians, should we withhold it from those who seem to need it very much, and denounce the prevention of conception as a crime second only to criminal abortion?"[89] A supporter of Malthus's theories, Texan physician Thomas A. Pope feared that the time would come when the world population would become so dense that mere existence would entail struggle. He rejoiced in the decisions of Congress to restrict Chinese immigration and to deport diseased European immigrants. This policy constituted "the beginning of a struggle for the survival of the fittest that henceforth will not cease as long as mankind shall continue to multiply and replenish the earth."[90] Another practitioner, disgusted with the arguments calling contraception a form of homicide, suggested that such men should "doubtless go into mourning after an erotic dream."[91] Physician W. R. D. Blackwood reminded the medical profession that certain circumstances imperatively demanded preventive devices.

If prostitution—a gigantic evil—is ever to be eradicated, it can only be

88. King, "Ethics and Methods of Preventing Conception," 273.
89. Ernest C. Helm, "The Prevention of Conception," *Medical and Surgical Reporter*, LIX (1888), 646.
90. T. A. Pope, "Prevention of Conception," *Medical and Surgical Reporter*, LIX (1888), 523.
91. (Anony.), "The Prevention of Conception," *Cincinnati Medical News*, n.s., XIX (1890), 307.

done by encouraging judicious marriage relations; and as law and custom have recognized or prescribed monogamy as the proper form of married life with us; and as it is a fact that the male is ever ready and generally solicitous for intercourse during his prime, whilst the female is only so at periodical intervals when at all, at which time she is more exposed to conception than in the interim, it is evident that unrestrained indulgence must lead to rapidly recurring pregnancies in women during the child-bearing period provided they are not sterile. This being so the question is reduced to this—Is it proper, is it humane, is it desirable that the lot of a married female should be a continual round of impregnation, delivery and lactation? Would such conduce to the happiness of the home; to the welfare of the family; to the sturdiness of the progeny thus generated? I do not hesitate for an instant to say NO! and I look with more than suspicion on the fulminations of those who, assuming superior virtue, condemn any and all attempts to control conception—I don't believe what they say! . . . To me the matter reduces itself to a choice between foeticide and prevention. The one is an indefensible crime—the other a necessity.[92]

Most doctors, however, continued to feel that contraceptive information would only encourage prostitution, fewer marriages, and more disease among women. Part of their opposition grew from the fear that the "woman question" might possibly turn in this direction as the woman claimed the right to her body. They hoped that higher education would not result in learning how to prevent fecundation. "Her elevation in the social state," wrote T. M. Dolan, M.D., in a paper read before the Ninth International Medical Congress held in Washington in 1887, "should not be purchased by degradation personal to herself."[93] Though there were individual cases in which the threat of disease, death, or abortion made prevention a necessity, most physicians were at a loss to explain the best means to solve the dilemma. "Let it become generally known that the medical profession countenances a preventive even in a few cases," remarked one concerned practitioner, "and there is reason to fear this will be stretched to a license which will work much mischief to women who are already experimenting

92. W. R. D. Blackwood, "The Prevention of Conception," *Medical and Surgical Reporter,* LIX (1888), 396.

93. T. M. Dolan, "On the Evils of Artificial Methods of Preventing Fecundation, and on Abortion-Production in Modern Times," *Medical Register,* II (1887), 395; Goodell, "Clinical Lecture on Conjugal Onanism and Kindred Sins," 163.

in this direction."[94] Rather than face the problem, doctors preferred to preach abstinence to the laity. "If the world to-day is suffering from an over-population of human beings," wrote one doctor, "let us endeavor to teach men and women to bridle their passions instead of trying to place in their hands a thing that will eventually prove disastrous and will at the same time lead to an excess of sexual indulgence."[95]

Marital Continence

Most American Victorians were aware of contraceptive devices but, for a variety of reasons, clung to the rigid sexual mores of the day. Women authors of purity manuals were even more vocally opposed to birth-control practices. While there were, of course, feminists like Annie Besant and later Margaret Sanger who sought greater sexual freedom through birth-control techniques, most sex-in-life authors chose the route of "marital continence," which they hoped would lessen women's role as sex objects. Marital continence meant the "voluntary and entire absence from sexual indulgence in any form, and having complete control over the passions by one who knows their power, and who, but for his pure life and steady will, not only could, but would indulge them."[96] Women reared under the influence of the WCTU and other purity-minded organizations felt that artificial birth control would destroy the sanctity of the home circle by bringing into it the tools of the street prostitute, and within the framework of nineteenth-century male guardianship would perpetuate in a most licentious manner women's continuing role as sex objects. Moreover, manual writers shied from talk of birth-control techniques after the legislative successes of purity fanatic Anthony Comstock, secretary of the New York Society for the Suppression of Vice, and the subsequent passage of anticontraceptive laws in

94. Isaac Pierce, "The Prevention of Conception," *Medical and Surgical Reporter*, LIX (1888), 616.

95. L. Huber, "The Prevention of Conception," *Medical and Surgical Reporter*, LIX (1888), 580–81; C. E. Swift, "Conception: The Fallacy and Evil of Attempted Prophylaxis," *Medical Summary*, XIX (1897–98), 13; Louis F. E. Bergeret, *The Preventive Obstacle; or, Conjugal Onanism. The Danger and Inconveniences to the Individual, to the Family, and to Society, of Frauds in the Accomplishment of the Generative Functions* (New York, 1870).

96. Cowan, *The Science of a New Life*, 114–15.

some twenty-four states after 1879. The American attitude toward the discussion of sex (which George Bernard Shaw called "Comstockery") forced manual writers to broach the subject in only the vaguest language, for public morality judged such practices as unnatural and illegal. For these reasons, most married couples either avoided the issue completely by leaving the problem to chance or practiced variations of marital continence.[97]

In reply to those Malthusians who advocated limitation of families without contraceptive devices, women responded with the demand for total abstinence, prohibiting coition except when there was a desire for parenthood. "No pandering to sexual indulgence" or "gratification of the lower nature" was permitted as long as the slightest unwillingness for parenthood existed. Those not wishing to have children had to have a "proper manly and womanly Christian temperance in those things." Too many marriages were nothing more than licensed prostitution in which the lower natures of both man and wife were "petted and indulged at the expense of the higher."[98] Since the sexual act caused an expenditure of vital force in the male body, any release of seminal fluid "prostituted to the simple gratification of fleshy desire" weakened the husband and endangered the well-being of his physical and mental state. He should conserve his seminal fluid for limited coition only— the implication being that the vital energy not expended in the sexual act would then be diverted to the "mental and moral force of the man." According to purity advocates, the conservation of sperm illuminated the mind and soul through its assimilation by the brain, where it was expended in thought.[99]

The obsession with misuse of the passions appears in part to have been borrowed from the earlier humoral pathology of the body. If the body had a certain natural order and temperament, excess of passion would not only injure the tranquillity

97. C. F. Brooks, "The Early History of the Anti-Contraceptive Laws in Massachusetts and Connecticut," *American Quarterly,* XVIII (1966), 2–23; Mary Ware Dennett, *Birth Control Laws* (New York, 1926); Denslow Lewis, "The Control of the Sexual Instinct," *Medical Examiner and General Practitioner,* XIX (1908), 105–9.

98. Drake, *What a Young Wife Ought to Know,* 87–88.

99. *Ibid.,* 88–89; Greer, *Woman Know Thyself; Female· Diseases, Their Prevention and Cure,* 110–13, 153–54.

of the mind but precipitate a change in the solid and fluid balance in the system as well. Every disposition of the mind was intimately connected with the peculiar temperament of the body. Thus, when the body indulged in one of the passions, it induced "a consentaneous temperament of the body," and similarly, when the body formed a particular habit, a corresponding disposition of the mind followed. A cogent remark from Henry Rose's *Dissertation on the Effects of the Passions upon the Body* (1794) illustrates this thinking.

But when [love] becomes deeper seated, it disturbs the serenity of the mind, and the general economy of the body—the countenance then becomes hung over with languor, the eyes indicate some remarkable desire; the breast rises and falls like the disturbed waters of the ocean, with deep and languishing sighs. The body becomes effeminated, and it unlocks every manly power of the soul. The afflicted person is particularly agitated when in presence of the beloved object. The heart leaps, and its Systole and Dyastole is repeated with increased rapidity; the pulse performs an inordinate action; the countenance at first is suffused with redness and then suddenly becomes pale. In proportion to the vehemence of the passion, these symptoms are increased, and when violently excited, fever attended with great heat, palpitation of the heart, and a sense of burning through the whole circulatory system, have been the consequences. Sometimes the breathing is laborious, the eyes are veiled with a cloud of mist, and the body is covered with a cold sweat. No passion so imperceptibly undermines the constitution as the one now under consideration; debility, the predisposing cause and mother of almost every disease, to which the human species is liable, inevitably follows: that pleasant languor, which at first was so welcome to the body, at length proves to be its destroyer. From the beginning the induced debility and effeminacy, the various perturbations, which immediately follow, cannot be sustained without the greatest agitation of both body and mind.[100]

According to many of the purity writers of the century, love had gone through a process of natural selection, attaining its most spiritual form among the higher civilizations. As Jennie G. Drennan, M.D., reminded the readers of the *New York Medical Journal* in 1901, however, Western civilization had reached a precarious point in its evolution where the backsliding nature of man's passions and instincts threatened to delay higher spiritual attainment. The chief obstacle to man-

100. Henry Rose, *An Inaugural Dissertation on the Effects of the Passions upon the Body* (Philadelphia, 1794), 16, 26.

kind's evolutionary ascent was sexual intercourse as a means of pleasure. "As long as mankind marries in order to indulge in a licensed sexual intercourse," she pointed out, "it will seek happiness in vain. No purely animal pleasure can satisfy its nature, which is striving Godward."[101] As the lower races evolved to the lordly Caucasian, sexual relations underwent a similar evolution. Reason began to encroach more on the instincts. "If neither intellect nor instinct guide the primitive man to well-regulated marital relations," wrote Henry T. Finck in his book *Romantic Love and Personal Beauty* (1887), "so again his emotional life is too rude and limited to allow any scope for the domestic affections."[102] Finck believed that the "inferior races" along with the working classes of the urban cities knew only certain levels of conjugal attachment, and that romantic love existed solely in the refined sensitivities of the advanced peoples of the world, in particular, the urban middle class. To Finck, however, the American Negro presented an anomaly. "It is a very interesting question how far the negroes transplanted to America, who have adopted so many of the habits and ways of thinking of their white neighbours, are capable of forming a true romantic attachment," he wrote. "I have not been able to find any conclusive evidence on this head, and should any readers of this book positively know any cases, I should be greatly obliged if they would forward a detailed account of them to me, in care of the publisher." Only those educated men and women in the upper strata of society, whose minds had sufficient time to comprehend and feel the complex emotions which constituted personal relationships, could attain the qualities of romantic love. As for the "great unwashed," they plodded a frightfully narrow path between an awareness of purity and the backsliding character of their instincts.[103]

Purity manuals expressed hope that married couples would

101. Jennie G. Drennan, "Sexual Intemperance: Some Explanation of What Is Meant by the Term," *New York Medical Journal*, LIV (1901), 70; Jennie G. Drennan, "Sexual Intemperance," *International Record of Medicine*, LXXXIII (1901), 19–20.

102. Henry T. Finck, *Romantic Love and Personal Beauty; Their Development, Causal Relations, Historic and National Peculiarities* (New York, 1887), 55.

103. *Ibid.*, 66.

accept strict continence as a standard in marital relations. If parents would assure their children that sexual powers in the human species were properly used only for reproduction, "the whole veil of mystery would be blown away and the subject would then be presented in a beautiful and ennobling light." There would be no further necessity for prostitution, no need for governmental regulation of vice, no white slave traffic, nor further reason for the degradation of women. The world would be safe from the greatest social evil of life, and men and women would meet "upon the basis of intellectual congeniality" without the perplexing issue of sex, and, for the first time, "the delight of friendship, now practically unknown, could be enjoyed to the fullest extent." If sexual continence prevailed in marriage, the husband and wife would not have to live as "comparative strangers" in separate bedrooms, in constant fear of inflammatory desires. "If the human body were always held in thought as a sacred temple," wrote Wood-Allen, "its outlines would be suggestive of nothing but the purest and holiest feelings." Woman's figure would cease to inflame the passions of men and there would result a "social mingling of men and women without a thought of sex in their minds." Marital continence, she urged, would become a valid and proper substitute for physical pleasure, and eliminate forever the thought that woman was "the means of gratifying desire."[104]

Nineteenth-century purity manuals quoted extensively from ministers on the subject of sexual relations; both Emma Drake and Mary Terhune (Marion Harland), writers of popular manuals for Victorian society, were married to ministers. "I firmly believe," remarked a minister in Wood-Allen's book, "that the purpose of the Creator in the institution of the marital relation can be fulfilled only when the two parties in the relation are agreed to *make no provision for the flesh* in thought, desire, or practice." There was a loss of dignity to both husband and wife if either thought of the other as a "sexual being." In spite of "pet names" given to the sexual appetite, it was lust of the basest sort. Any use of the sexual act other than for procreation was "a waste of vital energy," deteriorating the conservation of necessary forces in the body and depriving the

104. Wood-Allen, *Marriage; Its Duties and Privileges,* 196–97, 208–9.

system of its legitimate needs. Perfect continence in marriage did not mean mere moderation in sexual relations; moderation was a casuist rationalization for the gratification of the physical appetites.[105]

Delos F. Wilcox dedicated his *Ethical Marriage* (1900) to youths and maidens "who do what they think they ought to do, admitting no ideal that is impractical, and omitting no duty that is seen." Using a Spencerian formula, he, like Henry Finck, argued that the institution had undergone an evolution from brute savagery to nomadic marriage, and finally to ethical marriage. The new ethical family was founded on the principles of love, intelligence, and duty, and would perpetuate only those traits which it considered of "superior social value."[106] Evolutionary law ruled that sexual intercourse "should be had at long intervals and during a limited portion of adult life." Any nonprocreative sexual union was contrary to nature's laws. In practice, this meant that married couples ought to be "loyally affectionate" until they chose to have children, at which time they "should have a single complete sexual congress. . . . Time should then be given to ascertain whether or not conception has taken place. Normally menstruation ceases during pregnancy. If the menses are not interrupted, the probabilities are strong that conception has not taken place, and then another copulation will be necessary. Intercourse may take place once a month until there is reason to believe that the woman is pregnant, or until the season favorable to reproduction has passed. After impregnation has been secured there should be no more intercourse until another child is desired."[107]

Wilcox, whose ideas reflected a confusing mixture of eugenics, the perfectionist tendencies of Shaker Mother Ann Lee, and the crusading vengeance of Anthony Comstock, believed that continence was a practical answer to the sexual passions in marriage. Speaking from his own experience, however, he

105. *Ibid.*, 201–3.
106. Delos F. Wilcox, *Ethical Marriage* (Michigan, 1900), 56–57.
107. *Ibid.*, 82–84. Because the child's character was influenced by the intentions of the parents at the moment of conception, physician J. H. Greer advised intercourse in the morning when "the best qualities of each parent . . . have been refreshed by rest." See Greer, *Woman Know Thyself; Female Diseases, Their Prevention and Cure,* 194.

argued that the mere desire for sexual continence was not enough; married couples needed to take specific steps to prevent the unleashing of their unhealthy passions. These steps included an understanding that marriage "should make no more immediate difference in their lives than the taking of a roommate does to a student," avoiding a honeymoon, the use of separate beds or sleeping quarters, abstaining from stimulants, encouraging exercise, and finally, the proper education of children to prevent sexual curiosity or abnormal habits.[108] Similarly, Gustavus Cohen wrote in his *Helps and Hints to Mothers and Young Wives,* that "principle should be the controlling power of every thought and action." Continence was one of the more important principles that governed every relationship. A horrible blight to the marriage contract could be removed if woman had the right "to deny all approaches, save and only when she desired maternity."[109] Wilcox predicted that the benefits from marital continence would become self-evident—cessation of habits that encouraged passion, the conservation of vital energies in the male, increased love and respect, and fewer doctors' bills.[110] Women would be freed from the "taxes of lust," they would develop a higher sense of social responsibility; marriage "would no longer . . . be the bartering of [their] freedom for a mess of pottage," and they could enjoy a far greater freedom in dress. Indeed, if men accepted continence, women could wear shorter skirts "without the sensuous desires of men being aroused." Women, whose clothes had been styled in order to prevent the "prurient curiosity of men" from creating a sense of shame in the virtuous woman, could now cast off the oppressive garments of defensive purity.[111]

The majority of purity manuals for women certainly sanctioned continence as the ideal marriage relationship in the late nineteenth century. Manuals for men also suggested strict continence in married life. Few of them, however, were as adamant in their proposal as the authors of women's manuals.

108. Wilcox, *Ethical Marriage,* 124–25.
109. Cohen, *Helps and Hints to Mothers and Young Wives,* 83; Greer, *Woman Know Thyself; Female Diseases, Their Prevention and Cure,* 206–8.
110. Wilcox, *Ethical Marriage,* 133–34.
111. *Ibid.,* 137–39.

Sylvanus Stall's book, *What a Young Husband Ought to Know*, showed that many married couples who had chosen strict continence secured "not only greater strength and better health, but greater happiness also."[112] The passions, "the controlling organ of which lies at the very bottom and lowest part of the brain," degraded both the mind and the morals of the individual.[113] Some writers, of course, were content to accept a moderate sexual indulgence. Acton, for example, recommended coitus every seven or ten days; those men whose sexual impulses were excessively strong could have intercourse twice on the same night provided they allowed the body a period of ten days for repair.[114] Other practitioners, while not specifying exact time periods, indicated that long abstinences ("hymeneal postponement") were not beneficial to male vitality.[115] According to Mrs. E. B. Duffey in her *Relations of the Sexes* (1876), too many writers advocated "sexual starvation" theories. Although women were never troubled with the lascivious dreams that affected the male, and their passions seldom developed until after marriage, women nonetheless were able and willing to enjoy their rights in intercourse. Attempting to reach a compromise somewhere between absolute continence and promiscuity, Duffey suggested coition once every month, with the decision in the hands of the woman. To encourage this, she counseled separate beds, avoiding bodily contact, and "no robing or disrobing in each other's presence." Only by showing the husband that he was injuring himself with his frequent enjoyment of pleasure could the wife make him conscious of his lustful sins. "All the train of evils which follow masturbation," she wrote, "attend, only in a lesser degree, the too lustful marriage bed."[116]

Responsibilities of Motherhood

Nearly all manuals restricted sexual relations during pregnancy. The very fundamentals of Victorian science and mo-

---

112. Stall, *What a Young Husband Ought to Know*, 81.
113. *Ibid.*, 93–94.
114. Acton, *Functions and Disorders of the Reproductive Organs*, 145; Bigelow, *Sexual Pathology*, 85.
115. Fowler, *Creative and Sexual Science*, 697.
116. Duffey, *The Relations of the Sexes*, 206, 221–22, 224.

rality ruled against this practice. "The submission of an unwilling wife or the sexual irritability that may be engendered through the mother who gives herself up to the indulgences of desire" would jeopardize the physical and moral future of the child. The upheaval of the child's embryonic home "through gusts of passion" left an indelible mark on his character.[117] Coition during pregnancy, according to one physician, predisposed children to epilepsy. "The natural excitement of the nervous system in the mother by such a cause," he wrote, "cannot operate otherwise than inflicting injury upon the tender germ in the womb." Kellogg believed that the mental and nervous sensations of the mother molded the brain of the fetus, and when the mother indulged in sexual relations, she increased the chances of the child's developing an abnormal sexual instinct. "Here is the key to the origin of much of the sexual precocity and depravity which curse humanity," wrote Kellogg.[118] "Every pang of grief [or passion] you feel," added Orson S. Fowler in his book on maternity, "will leave its painful scar on the forming disk of their soul."[119]

The child's future depended upon his mother's conduct during pregnancy, a conduct that concerned not only her diet, but also her reading material, relations with her husband, and her most private thoughts. Martin Luther Holbrook, M.D., in his book *Stirpiculture*, explained why some children were more virtuous and beautiful than others. A Darwinian who crusaded for healthy marriages on the basis of community-controlled eugenics and high ethical behavior, he pointed out that the child's character, morals, and even physical appearance depended on how the parents conducted themselves during the pregnancy. "In my early married life," confessed one mother, "my husband and I learned how to live in holy relations, after God's ordinance. My husband lovingly consented to let me live apart from him during the time I carried his little daughter under my heart, and also while I was nursing her." These were the happiest days in her life. "My husband and I were

117. Wood-Allen, *Marriage; Its Duties and Privileges*, 207.

118. Stall, *What a Young Husband Ought to Know*, 200–201; Kellogg, *Ladies Guide in Health and Disease*, 425–26.

119. Fowler, *Maternity*, 16, 124; Aimée Raymond Schroeder, *Health Notes for Young Wives* (New York, 1895), 31.

never so tenderly, so harmoniously, or so happily related to each other," she exclaimed, "and I never loved him more deeply than during these blessed months." As a result of the parents' relationship, the child born at this time was beautifully formed, and grew to be virtuous, healthy, and extremely happy. Several years later, wrote Holbrook, the same mother became pregnant with a second child, but during that period, her husband "had become contaminated with the popular idea that even more frequent relations were permissible during pregnancy." Yielding to her husband's rapacious demands, the wife became "nervous and almost despairing." The child was born sickly and nervous, and after five years of constant difficulty, died "leaving them sadder and wiser."[120]

A woman during her pregnancy was a "soul-gardener." The beauty and virtue of her children depended ultimately upon the manner in which she acted during the nine months of pregnancy. Since she had to provide the "good soil" in which the child grew during its prenatal life, the pregnant woman was to direct herself to the goal of creating the best possible child. She must change her dress, allowing no weight to hang around her hips; "the union suit of underclothing, the union skirt and waist combined, and the gown," wrote Emma Drake, "are all that should be worn throughout the entire period."[121] Most important, however, the expectant mother should cultivate her mind with only the highest thoughts. Mind engendered physiological and psychological character upon the unborn child. Italian children bore "a striking resemblance to the pictures of the child Jesus, from the veneration which the mothers give to the Madonnas." From this, Drake concluded that "we not only become like we most love, and think most about, but . . . we may transmit this likeness to our little ones." In order to ensure beautiful and vigorous children, the woman was to study beautiful pictures and statuary, yet "for-

120. Holbrook quoted in Drake, *What a Young Wife Ought to Know,* 91–93; Greer, *Woman Know Thyself; Female Diseases, Their Prevention and Cure,* 182–83; John Humphrey Noyes, *Essay on Scientific Propagation* (New York, n.d.); (A Physician and Sanitarian), *Marriage and Parentage and the Sanitary and Physiological Laws for the Production of Children of Finer Health and Greater Ability* (New York, 1882), 142–43, 158–59.

121. Drake, *What a Young Wife Ought to Know,* 101–2; Kellogg, *Ladies Guide in Health and Disease,* 294–95.

bid as far as possible the contemplation of unsightly and imperfect models."[122] In particular, she was warned to avoid the alcoholic and tobacco breath of her husband. Many wives suffered from ill health "directly traceable to the inhaling, night after night, of the breath of the husband, poisoned with nicotine. Many a little one is wailing through its infancy, and if it have strength sufficient, inherited from its remote ancestors, to pull it through, yet will it all its life suffer from its antenatal and postnatal poisoning; and the chances are that as soon as it is old enough it will take up the habit which is already acquired, to pass down along the line a more enfeebled heritage."[123]

Just as the mother's emotions during pregnancy went into the making of the child's emotional system, so the nursing period was extremely important to the child's mental development. For this reason, sexual intercourse was also restricted during lactation. There was no doubt in Kellogg's mind, for example, that the gratification of passions during the nursing period would cause "the transmission of libidinous tendencies to the child."[124] For the same reasons, mothers were continually warned not to employ wet nurses with bad habits—women who drank or carried on affairs in secret. Invariably, the examples listed in the manuals were Irish wet nurses. The child suffered irreparable harm because the low mentality as well as the emotional excesses of the wet nurse transferred to him in feeding.[125] Physician Gustavus Cohen believed that mothers who neglected this important function would invite disease and any number of constitutional disorders. The failure of women to nurse their own babies, he wrote, caused eventual barrenness, premature aging, and even early death.[126]

Purity writers advised endlessly on the dangers of meno-

---

122. Drake, *What a Young Wife Ought to Know*, 105–9; Lowry, *Herself; Talks with Women concerning Themselves*, 98–100.

123. Drake, *What a Young Wife Ought to Know*, 119; Kellogg, *Ladies Guide in Health and Disease*, 309.

124. Kellogg, *Ladies Guide in Health and Disease*, 425–26; Cowan, *The Science of a New Life*, 116, 119.

125. Harland, *Eve's Daughters; or, Common Sense for Maid, Wife, and Mother*, 23–35.

126. Cohen, *Helps and Hints to Mothers and Young Wives*, 57; Cowan, *The Science of a New Life*, 117.

pause. Physicians invariably characterized it as the "Rubicon" in a woman's life, and they measured the extent of discomfort and disease by the degree of abuse she had inflicted on her constitution. In typically Calvinistic terms, manuals blamed the frequency and seriousness of disease during this period upon the "indiscretions" of earlier life. Excesses of any kind, whether in sexual passion, dress, reckless use of stimulating foods, prurient reading, contraception, or solitary vice, accentuated the hardships of this period of change. The woman who transgressed nature's laws, remarked Kellogg, "will find this period a veritable Pandora's box of ills, and may well look forward to it with apprehension and foreboding."[127] "Many things that have been laid to our ancestors remotely distant," observed Emma Drake, "are really the result of wrong-doing and living in the first decade and a half of our lives."[128] Charles Meigs, M.D., in his *Females and Their Diseases* (1848), a book which was extensively quoted in manuals of the day, described a young woman's efforts to prevent her monthly period in order that she might go to a ball. To achieve this, she accepted the advice of her "confidential servant" and took a hip bath in cold water. Although she succeeded in stopping the flow, she suffered an attack of "brain fever" and in her later years "felt the effects of the dereliction of duty." As a result of that single breach of nature's law, her life "was rendered a scene of bitterness, of vapours, of caprices."[129] Nature, remarked Drake "rebels and compels the payment of her violated laws." Usually nature accomplished this through malignant disease, or "failing in this, a slow and dangerous change is likely to be experienced, followed by years of discomfort or invalidism."[130]

The Victorian era has pictured itself to later generations in terms of stereotypes, sometimes conflicting, often grossly overdrawn. In many cases, however, the gap between the stereotypes handed down to twentieth-century America and life in

127. Kellogg, *Ladies Guide in Health and Disease*, 372–73.
128. Emma F. (Angell) Drake, *What a Woman of Forty-Five Ought to Know* (Philadelphia, 1902), 39, 137.
129. Meigs quoted in Cohen, *Helps and Hints to Mothers and Young Wives*, 6; Edward H. Dixon, *Woman and Her Diseases, from the Cradle to the Grave* (Philadelphia, 1860), 156.
130. Drake, *What the Woman of Forty-Five Ought to Know*, 55; Guernsey, *Plain Talks on Avoided Subjects*, 104–5.

Victorian society only reflects the disparity between the pretensions of a middle-class society and the reality it often chose to ignore. In one sense, there seems to be a certain status-suffix evident in its aspiring view of the role of sex. The sex-in-life manuals were an arena for imaginative writing in nineteenth-century society, and appear at times to shroud the urban middle class in a romantic arcadia set apart from the lusty vernacular of urban immigrants and city slums. The manuals were caricatures of subjective prejudices and assumptions concerning middle-class values and behavior. The romanticization of family and marriage portrayed in the manuals was not so much a plea for reshaping the marriage relationship as it was a technique for explaining the incongruity that existed between middle-class "principles" and reality. The middle class measured its greatness not only by its achievements but also by its principles—a situation which allowed it to blame any discrepancy upon a gallery of villains. Manual writers stalked the victims of sexual deviation in the empirical reality of the "lower races" and working classes, where disease, poverty, and depravity seemed to spawn the world's problems.

As moral pronouncements of society, the sex-in-life manuals became documentaries of middle-class myths seeking both to justify the prevailing social and moral fabric of Victorian America and to explain, without a sense of personal guilt, the survival of a less imaginative reality. The history of the century's manuals of love and marriage reveals an effort to interpret and grapple with the lack of tradition in urban life, and to reach for an understanding of sexual relationships in a way that would give added relevance to the class consciousness of middle-class America. A sense of pretension, along with a very real sense of educational, ethical, and economic superiority to the rawness of working-class America, combined to create a thinly concealed romantic moral code, steeped in fictitious parables and impossible ideals, struggling to assert a new and imaginative perspective for the American class structure. The aspirations of the middle class form a vital link in a proper understanding of sexual attitudes of the nineteenth century. It was this group in America which, in the absence of a hereditary class system, sought to create a moral and ethical barrier between themselves and the working class. And it was perhaps the rising expectations of the working class which allowed such pretensions to go unchallenged in spite of an obvious discrepancy between pretensions and reality.

Chapter IV

BODY RELIGION

Heredity may not be able to shoulder all of the sins of mankind, but, at least, it must bear its share. The coming woman must not only be well-born, she must be bred in more hygienic methods. She must not only possess inherited vigor, she must also be educated nearer to Nature. The genuine child of nature is not a morbidly emotional child. The girl who lives in the open air, who knows every bird and flower and brook in the neighborhood, has neither time nor inclination to spend in reading the sentimental histories of departed child-saints, and takes small delight in morbid conversation.

Mary T. Bissell, M.D., *Popular Science Monthly*, 1887

The Victorian woman cultivated beauty in the same manner that she attended to her private thoughts. With her sexuality circumscribed by society's harsh moral incantations, she turned for relief toward narcissism. Unable to find rewarding pleasures in either her projects or objectives, the woman, as Simone de Beauvoir has pointed out, was "forced to find her reality in the immanence of her person," a reality which existed precariously between the extremes of modesty and exhibitionism. "Ineffective, isolated, woman can neither find her place nor take her own measure," Beauvoir added, "she gives herself supreme importance because no object of importance is accessible to her."[1] But here, again, the physician was in chronic demand, bringing advice and moral suasion to bear on her dress and personal habits. Beauty was a moral concern that required the most dedicated zeal. Complexion, cleanliness, and stature had to express a harmony of form. Unsightly warts, sunburn, freckles, or a "gymnastic face" not only destroyed the harmony of form but also suggested that the moral character of the woman had undergone a modification for the worse. While it was the duty of every woman to look as beautiful as she possibly could, she was taught to cultivate beauty without giving the impression of having worked too assiduously in the process. Governed by moderation in both her toilet and her passions, and observing scrupulously the rule that cleanliness was akin to godliness, she was to employ only the most gentle effort in cultivating the "house of her soul." By preserving and enhancing personal beauty through proper hygiene, the woman was approaching "that Celestial Beauty, which is so closely allied to the Good and the True."[2]

As in so many other aspects of the woman's private and public life, nineteenth-century doctors considered themselves notably responsible for bringing their medical training and moral

1. Simone de Beauvoir, *The Second Sex* (New York, 1952), 630.
2. Daniel G. Brinton and George H. Napheys, *Laws of Health in Relation to the Human Form* (Springfield, Mass., 1870), 323.

authority to bear on questions of hygiene. Dominated by their promptings to a wider ministry, they proved themselves equal to the task of applying their proselytizing methods to the problems of cleanliness, exercise, and personal beauty. Here again, health depended upon not only a judicious management of bodily powers, but also a careful application of moral force. Archibald Hunter's description of women's hygiene as a "body religion" in his *Health, Happiness and Longevity* (1885) meant, for all practical purposes, that hygiene demanded all the care and ritualism of a vestal virgin. Poor health, ugliness, constipation, "American dyspepsia," and lack of cleanliness had all the attributes of sin and intimated indiscretions of the basest sort.

Beauty Hints

When writing about beauty and general body hygiene, doctors offered helpful hints on everything from crooked noses to red ears and wrinkles. Included were diets for "female Falstaffs," suggestions as to the proper size of the neck, breasts ("the distance from nipple to the lower edge of the collarbone of the same side should equal that from one nipple to the other, which, in turn, should be precisely one-fourth of the circumference of the chest at their level"), hints on cosmetics, cleanliness, and the maintenance of a whitened complexion. As for those "symbols of maternal love and fruitfulness," Daniel G. Brinton, M.D., the assistant editor of the *Medical and Surgical Reporter,* and George H. Napheys, M.D., recommended in their book *Laws of Health in Relation to the Human Form* (1870) that women who wished to "create a figure" should avoid the use of hair or cotton pads because they only flattened or distorted the breasts. Instead they suggested hollow India-rubber hemispheres or woven wire which were both firm and elastic and would exert little pressure. For pendulous breasts, they recommended cadmium or iodine ointment as well as internal doses of iodide of potassium; in addition, bandages of adhesive plaster were to be firmly applied to the breasts. The authors also advised the use of a vacuum cup to promote the health and shapely beauty of the breasts. The vacuum cup consisted of a glass bowl to which was fitted a stopcock. The woman placed the cup over each breast and then exhausted the air by means of an air syringe. The procedure, which was based on the widespread use of "dry cups" to draw blood from the internal organs to the surface, caused a flow of blood into the breasts. "It is highly likely that this device would be of considerable service," wrote the authors, "and that the breasts would be rendered much more shapely, and better adapted to fulfill their functions. The theory of the instrument is philosophical, and if used regularly for a sufficient time must certainly restore the organs in a great measure to their proper shape, size, and function."[3]

Because women went to extremes to preserve their complexions, doctors offered a number of suggestions to maintain a white, wrinkle-free countenance. First, they advised against too much laughing as it destroyed the contour of the face, making it far more difficult to maintain the "classic repose."[4] They also deplored the widespread habit of drinking vinegar or arsenic (*poudre rajeunissante*) to obtain the frail, gossamer appearance. The medical world first learned of the phenomenon of arsenic-eating around 1855 when Dr. Von Tschudi announced that peasants living in the areas of lower Austria and Styria were literally thriving on the mineral. According to Tschudi, whose original discussion of the habit became popularized in James F. W. Johnston's *The Chemistry of Common Life* (1855) and a number of English and American journals, the Styrian peasant woman saw in arsenic-eating a "lovemaker," a "harbinger of happiness," which through its effects upon the complexion soothed her "ardent longings" and bestowed "contentment and peace" upon her and her lover. "Stirred by an unconsciously growing attachment," wrote Johnston, "confiding scarcely to herself her secret feeling and taking counsel of her inherited wisdom only," she found that arsenic-eating added to "the natural graces of her filling and rounding form," and imparted "a new and winning lustre to her sparkling eye." News of the habit spread quickly, and following the example of the Styrian peasants, Victorian women be-

---

3. *Ibid.*, 60–63; George H. Napheys, *The Physical Life of a Woman: Advice to Maiden, Wife and Mother* (Cincinnati, 1873).
4. Henry T. Finck, *Romantic Love and Personal Beauty; Their Development, Causal Relations, Historic and National Peculiarities* (New York, 1887), 421.

gan to drink Fowler's Solution (potassium arsenite) and a variety of patent medicines which contained arsenic for their complexion, using them as a cosmetic wash.[5]

Brinton and Napheys accepted moderate arsenic-eating, but they believed that the recent popularity of wallpaper in homes, which were colored with arsenical dyes (Paris or Scheele's green), had threatened to poison the woman beyond her tolerance level. Although long use of arsenic had rendered many women immune to the mineral, their husbands occasionally came to untimely ends as a result of a romantic embrace.[6] As an alternative, some physicians prescribed two teaspoonsful of flowers of sulfur in a cup of boiled milk which the woman was to drink an hour or so before breakfast.[7] Others recommended wash solutions of borax and rain water, aqua ammonia and hot water, cucumber juice, or horse-radish root and buttermilk. In addition, women could apply solutions of benzoin and alcohol ("virgin's milk"), or bismuth ("pearl powder"). There was an unfortunate problem with bismuth, however. Women who might be wearing a "bismutine creame" in a room where improper management of the coal furnace had allowed sulfurous gases to penetrate would discover with embarrassment that their bismuth complexion changed to a dirty ash color.[8]

Women were to keep their hands soft and white by wearing "tight cosmetic gloves" filled with cold cream or glycerin at night. If the glycerin disagreed with the skin, they were to substitute dry oatmeal. Upon waking, they were urged to rub a mixture of oatmeal and water on their hands, or a preparation made from the white of an egg and a grain of alum. Still others preferred to use an acid solution.[9] Doctors were cautious

5. W. B. Kesteven, "On Arsenic-Eating," *Association Medical Journal*, IV (1856), 721; James F. W. Johnston, *The Chemistry of Common Life* (2 vols.; London, 1855), II, 202–4, 207; Craig McLagan, "On the Arsenic-Eaters of Styria," *Edinburgh Medical Journal*, X (1864,) 201.

6. Brinton and Napheys, *Laws of Health in Relation to the Human Form*, 239–40.

7. Anna Kingsford, *Health, Beauty, and the Toilet. Letters to Ladies from a Lady Doctor* (New York, 1886), 25.

8. Brinton and Napheys, *Laws of Health in Relation to the Human Form*, 208–9; Finck, *Romantic Love and Personal Beauty*, 460–61; Marion Harland, *Eve's Daughters; or Common Sense for Maid, Wife, and Mother* (New York, 1882), 109.

9. Finck, *Romantic Love and Personal Beauty*, 404, 407; E. Marguerite Lindley, *Health in the Home* (New York, 1896), 344, 350, 357.

in prescribing cosmetic face masks. Too many husbands, they felt, became irritated with the habit and it was a genuine cause of many "domestic infelicities." Brinton and Napheys thought that the husband's opinion of the cosmetic face mask had been best expressed in a choice comment by Henry IV, who, attempting to find his wife Margaret of Navarre behind her mask, allegedly said: "Madam, with that confounded black mask on, you look so much like the devil that I am always tempted to make the sign of the cross and drive you away."[10]

Since cleanliness was next to godliness, the Victorian woman was continually advised to keep herself spotless. Ironically, however, many doctors opposed the recent invention of the bathtub. "That zinc coffin," wrote Dio Lewis, M.D., "in which you lie down, put your head upon a strap at one end, and keep yourself from drowning and then balance yourself for a while in a sort of floating condition, is simply a stupid absurdity." Believing that the rubber or oil-cloth bathing mat which the woman placed on the floor of her bedroom was the most hygienic, he explained the bath procedure for the woman.

Of course you must have a wash-bowl with two or three quarts of water. Next a pair of bathing mittens,—simple bags,—loosely fitting your hands. These are made of the ends of a worn out crass or Turkish towel, though any thick linen will do. Now with a piece of good soap,—matters little what kind,—you are ready. You have removed your night-dress, you are standing upon the centre of your bathing mat, with your mittens or bags upon your hands. Seize the soap, make abundant soap-suds, and go over every part of the skin. Rub the soap several times, that every portion of the skin may be thoroughly covered with soap-suds. Now, dipping your hands into the water, rinse off the soap, although if it is winter, and the free use of water chills you, you may apply very little water, and wipe the soap-suds from your skin. Indeed, with many persons, it is an excellent practice to leave a certain portion of the soap on the skin. It will continue the process of neutralizing the oil.[11]

Brinton and Napheys suggested that the woman might mitigate the problem of weak eyes, without resorting to spectacles, by wiping the brow of the eye and temple with a solution of red peppers or ginger root in alcohol. Another remedy was for

10. Brinton and Napheys, *Laws of Health in Relation to the Human Form*, 199.

11. Dio Lewis, *Our Girls* (New York, 1871), 276; Titus M. Coan, *Ounces of Prevention* (New York, 1885), 52.

the woman to immerse her eyes in a solution of salt water. This latter procedure, they wrote, was a good remedy for redness or inflammation of the eyes.[12] If the woman was going to a ball and desired to have her eyes glittering and sparkling, they urged her to carry a handkerchief doused slightly in a pungent perfume of oil of thyme and the oil of bitter almonds (containing prussic acid) which could be held before the face several times during the evening.[13] Brinton and Napheys ruled out musk, bergamot, and patchouli perfumes for the "cultured woman" since they were considered to be aphrodisiacs. These scents, they wrote, were popular "in our large American cities [and] especially among the lower and immoral classes of women, which is reason enough why they should be avoided by a lady."[14]

"Corsetitis": The Harnessed Woman and Her Diseases

The widely divergent viewpoints held by the feminists on the one hand and the conservative medical profession on the other converged in a common opposition to the corset. Although their reasons for disliking the harness were so dissimilar as to be almost conflicting, each operated within its own sphere to attempt to destroy the custom of tight-lacing. A relationship existed in the nineteenth century between the women's rights movement and efforts to improve upon women's dress. The bloomers of the 1840s, a skirt worn to six inches below the knee over wide pantaloons, were seized upon by advocates of women's equality such as Susan B. Anthony and Elizabeth Cady Stanton, who quickly appreciated that freedom of movement was an important step toward freedom of women. However, they soon reluctantly abandoned their liberating costume, for it provided an all-too-easy target for the derision of their audiences, and when the issues for which they spoke were lost in the laughter over their dress, they wisely forsook this innovative fashion in fear that it would harm their cause. But while women's rights advocates capitulated in their demands for ex-

12. Brinton and Napheys, *Laws of Health in Relation to the Human Form*, 90.
13. *Ibid.*, 93.
14. *Ibid.*, 112.

terior dress reform, they nonetheless continued to speak out against the corset which they depicted as the real villain in their struggle for freedom. Frances Willard, president of the WCTU, bitingly remarked that "niggardly waists and niggardly brains go together." A female physician in 1890 noted that the emancipated woman must first be free from the thralldom of her dress before undertaking greater tasks. "Woman has certain inalienable rights," she wrote, "and first and foremost among them is the right to occupy as much room in space as nature intended she would."[15]

Physicians adamantly opposed the corset in language almost as strong as that used by the feminists. However, they did not espouse the feminists' cry for freedom of movement; rather, physicians descried the corset's restricting features as harmful to the health of future mothers. Their argument against the harness was that it made childbearing more difficult, indeed, almost impossible in many cases. The medical profession thus favored a less restricting underpinning, but one which would nonetheless keep the woman hygienically—and modestly—confined. Perhaps in their rhetoric one can find a fear that the woman, suffocated inside her corsets, would be unable to maintain even her role as a sex object whose function was not to create or enjoy pleasure, but to bear children. And when fashion dangerously threatened this role, the physician was roused to speak out. Blaming the contraption for everything from hepatitis, split livers, cancer, and consumption, to red noses, soured tempers, wrinkles, clumsiness, apathy, and even stupidity, doctors waged a full-scale attack against the practice of tight-lacing.[16]

But though the medical profession expressed itself in copious ridicule and invective, the habit of tight-lacing seemed ines-

15. Theoda Wilkins, "Pelvic Congestion from Moderate Compression of the Waist," *Southern California Practitioner*, V (1890), 134.

16. Joseph H. Greer, *Woman Know Thyself; Female Diseases, Their Prevention and Cure. A Home Book of Tokology, Hygiene and Education for Maidens, Wives and Mothers. A Clean and Clear Exposition of Nature's Laws and Mysteries* (Chicago, 1902), 44; George R. West, "The Corset, as a Factor in Pelvic Diseases," *Transactions*, Tennessee State Medical Society (1892), 209; J. H. Kellogg, *Ladies Guide in Health and Disease. Girlhood, Maidenhood, Wifehood, Motherhood* (Des Moines, Iowa, 1883), 256; Anna M. Galbraith, *The Four Epochs of Woman's Life; a Study in Hygiene* (Philadelphia, 1904), 34–35.

capably compelling to the majority of middle-class women. There seemed to be a symbolic interplay between their willingness to suffer in its contorted shapes and the complicated ritual of fashion which conditioned them to look with virtuous indignation at those women who shunned the infernal device or, moreover, those who could not afford it. Perched like a gilded hourglass before an adulating crowd of urban businessmen, the corseted woman provided the aesthetic touch for many of the false values of the time. She was a sculptured vessel who sustained not only the misplaced piety of the age, but also the impulse toward mawkish sentimentality. Women seemed to act out a tortured drama with themselves over the mechanized horrors of the corset, and whether they cried loudly against the brutality of the device or viewed it with quiet contempt, they nonetheless were stubbornly addicted to its serpentine charms, its sophisticated Old World pretensions, and its defiantly antiproletariat look.[17]

There was a certain stateliness implicit in the image of the corseted woman. Her figure imparted just the right touch to an otherwise old-fashioned personality. Built into the stays and busk were notions of aristocratic leisure which prevented her from bending, from picking things off the ground, and from exercising. At best, she could stand or sit, and even then she must be catered in all her needs. The corset inspired a sense of responsibility (if only to avoid stooping or exercising), and an obsession for absolute mastery of the most simple movement; it tantalizingly suggested a sense of romance and shrewdly dressed the woman in a moral gown fit to face posterity. Despite the burdensome ordeal of concealing behind false fronts what at times must have been a colossal mismanagement of the flesh, the Victorian lady presented herself as the finest example of America's urban class, plumped out above and below, piously exposing a narrow waist. Cramped, but otherwise unruffled and unharried, she epitomized a deft blend of middle-class temperament and tolerance. As one fashion magazine of the 1870s put it, the corset "is an ever present monitor, indirectly bidding its wearer to express self-restraint; it is evidence of a

17. Thorstein Veblen, "The Economic Theory of Women's Dress," *Popular Science Monthly*, LV (1894), 198–205.

well-disciplined mind and regulated values."[18] Greedy for the products and riches of the new industrial society, yet repressing those yearnings in a kind of self-imposed purgatory, the urban woman concealed within her rigid frame all the marks of self-delusion, phallic sublimation, inflated emotions, and crude romanticism.

According to Sauveur Bouvier's *Etudes historiques et medicales sur l'usage des corsets* (1853), women began to shape their forms "as soon as men were sufficiently elevated above the beast to admire [them]." Corsets were used by the early Greeks and Romans, but seemed to disappear during the so-called Dark Ages, only to reappear again in the sixteenth century. Catherine de Medici and Queen Elizabeth, with their "corps" or corset and their "terrible engines" of rigid and unyielding metal busks, inaugurated the era of the small waist and, incidentally, the earliest known medical warning published in 1602 by Felix Plater. Before long, designers were constructing corsets to carry the female from cradle to grave. "Any mother would have laid herself open to the charge of gross indifference to her children's welfare," wrote Bouvier, had she neglected to corset her daughters. "These early cares," he maintained, were thought to be "indispensible to any regular formation of body."[19] By the time of the French Revolution, women had substituted a steel or hickory busk for the older iron, bone, and wooden busks of the seventeenth and eighteenth centuries, and also introduced a more pliable corset made of cloth. The busk or front piece was pushed into a sheath in the front part of the corset extending the length of the breast bone. The purpose of the busk was to "keep the body from bending forward in the center, and to prevent the dress and corset from 'hooping up,' as it was called."[20] In 1793,

18. An 1873 fashion magazine quoted in Cecil W. Cunnington and Phillis Cunnington, *Handbook on English Costume in the Nineteenth Century* (London, 1959), 499.
19. Quoted in Robert L. Dickinson, "The Corset: Questions of Pressure and Displacement," *New York Medical Journal*, XLVI (1887), 507; Felix Plater, *Praxis Medica* (Basileae, 1602); Sauveur Henri Victor Bouvier, *Etudes historiques et medicales sur l'usage des corsets* (Paris, 1853).
20. F. D. Godman, "Injurious Effects of Tight Lacing on the Organs and Functions of Respiration, Digestion, Circulation, etc.," *Boston Medical and Surgical Journal*, II (1829), 482.

Samuel T. Sömmerring wrote his *Über die Wirkungen der Schnürbrüste* on the injurious effects of the corset, and after that time physicians contributed hundreds if not thousands of warnings on the practice. Sömmerring listed over ninety seventeenth- and eighteenth-century works calling attention to the evil, including writings by the famed Peter Camper, Albricht von Haller, John George Zimmerman, John George Frider, Joseph Claudius Rougemont, John Henry Müller, Paul Mascagni, and John Frider Pierer.[21]

With the developments of the industrial age, the corset made even tighter advances on the woman's waist. Ingeniously contrived on mechanical principles, it became one of the finest examples of nineteenth-century technology. While the lacing on the back of the corset involved the age-old principle of the pulley, the "metallic age" provided strong steel catches for the front which were attached at intervals along two steel bands. Provided that the woman met with some success in applying the pulley principle, she then utilized the principle of the lever, "the first fastening affording sufficient fulcrum for drawing the gaping sides into apposition." With the battlements thus in place, she obtained "a form forbidden by God's workmanship but approved by society's dictum," and, assuring herself that the corset was quite safe, she forced her conscience to acquiesce to the squeeze as a mark of the lady's "emergence into womanhood."[22]

While naturalists found the curling nails and cramped feet of the Chinese women a mark of cultural degeneracy, and while they could point to the Australian savage practice of transfixing the nasal septum with six inches of bone, tortoise shells hanging from the chins and lips of the natives of the Corn Islands in Central America, and weights and dilators in the lips, nose, ears, and chin of African tribes, they needed to go no further than their own wives' dressing rooms for confirmation of yet another curious custom. There amid the droop-

21. Samuel Thomas Sömmerring, *Über die Wirkungen der Schnürbrüste* (Berlin, 1793), 79–84; Johnston Symington, "Notes on the Effects of Tight Lacing upon the Position of the Abdominal Viscera," *Edinburgh Medical Journal*, XXXVII (1891–92), 616–17.
22. W. Wilberforce Smith, "Corset-Wearing and Its Pathology," *Sanitary Record*, n.s., X (1888), 201–2.

ing ferns, petticoated lampshades, featherwork and embroidery of their dressing rooms, nineteenth-century women indulged in the agony of drawing their corsets "as tightly about the soft upper parts of the abdomen as silken and hempen strings could pull them." Many lacked the strength to lace themselves properly and depended in a certain demonic way upon the services of their serving maid who cordoned their bodies "with a power of muscle that would have insured a Saratoga trunk against the most energetic baggage-smasher." If they were the independent or shy type who performed such delicacies in private, they still required the aid of a bedpost to act as a "belaying-pin." With a loop of the lace around the bedpost, they strained away from it "until the creaking construction of buckrum and bone closely banded the waist as in a vice." Thus clothed in respectability and self-righteousness, with breasts forced almost up to the collarbone and the ribs compressed to the point of overlapping, they presented a sleek demure figure that instilled terror in physicians, created a chasm between themselves and the working classes, and forced upon themselves an image of boredom and a deathly pale complexion. Suffering in the close air of their own social ionosphere, they walked about breathless and half-swooning. They fainted by the score in crowded rooms and gallant males rushed to their rescue with trusty pocketknives which they used with almost surgical precision to cut corset strings as the quickest remedy for collapsed lungs.[23]

Physicians were hampered in their crusade for corset reform by the polemics of corset designers who took up their pens to attack the products of their competitors while writing paeons to the health and beauty preserved by their own patented brand. Madame Roxey A. Caplin's *Health and Beauty: Or, Corsets and Clothing Constructed in Accordance with the Physiological Laws of the Human Body* (1856) was an example. While Madame Caplin issued a doomsday warning of the horrible consequences of using her competitors' corsets, she nonetheless advertised the hygienic attributes of her own brand of harness. The purpose of the corset, she wrote, was to support

23. Harland, *Eve's Daughters; or Common Sense for Maid, Wife, and Mother*, 350–51.

the woman's bones as they developed through life, but without harming or obstructing the corresponding development of muscles. The true artist of corsets could "anticipate every requirement through life, and adapt her contrivances to the ever varying want of the body."[24] Anticipating these needs, Madame Caplin designed some twenty-three corsets which included the Hygienic Corset, a Self-Regulating Gestation Corset "calculated to answer all the phases of pregnancy," the Corporiform for "corpulent ladies," a Young Lady's Riding Belt, the Juvenile Hygienic Corset "for young ladies growing too rapidly," the Riverso-Tractor Hygienic Corset "for preventing children standing on one leg," and the Contracting Belt used by women during their confinement.[25] She even designed an Umbilical Band for infants which would provide "sufficient umbilical pressure, and [allow] all the great organs of life to perform their natural function."[26]

Similarly, Rebecca Mills, an elastic corsetmaker of the 1840s, advertised her own patented corset while criticizing the accursed tight-lacing that injured so many women. According to her, there were any number of reasons for the development of the corset, one of which stemmed from the smaller stomach of the woman. Her appetite for food was comparatively less than the male, and she could also abstain from food for a longer period of time. "These facts as to the subordination and delicacy of the preparatory vital organs," she wrote, "in some measure originate the taste for tight stays, and insure their consequences." Furthermore, the woman, unlike the man, was subject to any number of "crises" in her life which threatened the health of her organs. "Exposed to great shocks, to alternate extensions, compressions and reductions," the cellular structure of her tissue became unduly "lax and yielding." While nature provided woman with aids in neutralizing the shocks to her system, elastic harnesses adjusted to conform to the "general suppleness of the different organs" and immeasurably added

24. Roxey A. Caplin, *Health and Beauty; or, Corsets and Clothing Constructed in Accordance with the Physiological Laws of the Human Body* (London, 1856), 39.
25. *Ibid.*, 46–47.
26. *Ibid.*, 7.

to the life of the tissue by supporting its weakened state.[27] The proper object of the corset, she wrote, should be to provide gentle support for the figure "without diminishing the freedom of motion, and to conceal the size of the abdomen when it becomes disproportionately large, either from corpulence or from accidents which naturally occur."[28]

Miss Lydia Becker, one of the outspoken defenders of the corset in the 1880s, informed her readers that the instrument provided a "firm foundation" for the garments of the woman, and while giving firmness and support to the waist, it also offered warmth "which no loosely-fitting bodice can afford."[29] She observed that the corset should be chosen to adapt to the particular needs and habits of the wearer, and under no circumstances be laced "like a good old-fashioned family fire-grate." Those critics of the corset who looked to the beautiful models of Greek statuary for woman's real figure failed to realize, she added, that they were simply expressions of a sculptor's ideal and did not portray actual figures of women. The real model for woman's figure was not the form of Venus de Milo, but the women of Noah's Ark; and unlike the graceful lines depicted in the ancient statuary, the figures of the biblical women were far less beautiful. Indeed, the art of fashion exhausted all possible variations in order that women's figures might pass the test of time. Since only those fashions persisted which survived the law of evolution and survival of the fittest, Miss Becker argued that the corset was a natural product of woman's evolution. As an admirer of Herbert Spencer, she could not help but feel that women's fashions, particularly the corset, were included in the supra-organic social-Darwinian world.[30]

Lydia Becker also pointed out that women, because of gestation, breathed naturally from the upper part of the lungs, or "costal breathing" as she termed it, and that one purpose of the corset was to insure against the possibility of their breathing

27. Rebecca Mills, *The Influence of Well-Made Stays on the Health and Beauty of Women, and the Great Injuries Which Ill-Made Ones Inflict* (London, 1841), 4–5.

28. *Ibid.*, 82–83.

29. Lydia E. Becker, "On Stays and Dress Reform," *Sanitary Record*, X (1888), 149.

30. *Ibid.*, 151.

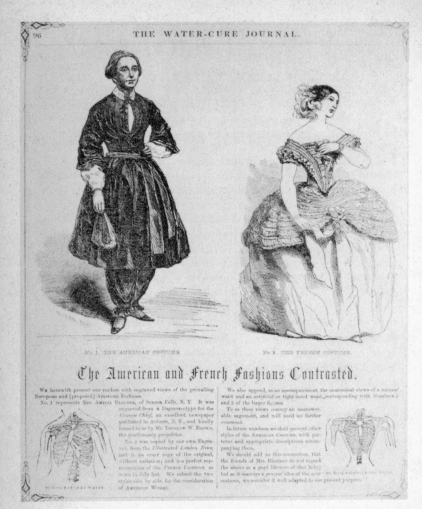

No. 1. THE AMERICAN COSTUME.

No. 2. THE FRENCH COSTUME.

The American and French Fashions Contrasted.

We herewith present our readers with engraved views of the prevailing European and [proposed] American Fashions.

No. 1 represents Mrs. AMELIA BLOOMER, of Seneca Falls, N. Y. It was engraved from a Daguerreotype for the *Cayuga Chief*, an excellent newspaper published in Auburn, N. Y., and kindly loaned to us by Mr. THURLOW W. BROWN, the gentlemanly proprietor.

No. 2 was copied by our own Engraver, from the *Illustrated London News*, and is an exact copy of the original, without variation; and is a perfect representation of the FRENCH FASHIONS, as worn in July last. We submit the two styles side by side, for the consideration of AMERICAN WOMEN.

We also append, as an accompaniment, the anatomical views of a natural waist and an artificial or tight-laced waist, corresponding with Numbers 1 and 2 of the larger figures.

To us these views convey an unanswerable argument, and will need no farther comment.

In future numbers we shall present other styles of the AMERICAN COSTUME, with patterns and appropriate descriptions accompanying them.

We should add in this connection, that the friends of Mrs. Bloomer do not regard the above as a good likeness of that lady; but as it conveys a general idea of the new costume, we consider it well adapted to our present purpose.

No. 3. NATURAL WAIST.

No. 4. TIGHT-LACED WAIST.

A wood engraving from *The Water Cure Journal*, 1851. National Library of Medicine, Bethesda.

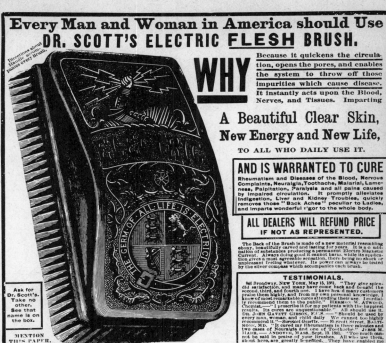

An advertisement from *Harper's Weekly*, October 29, 1881. National Library of Medicine, Bethesda.

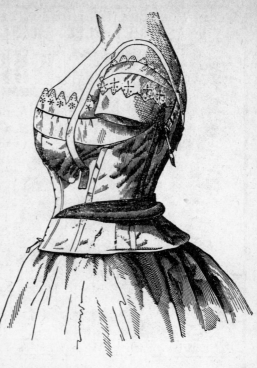

An advertisement from *The Water Cure Journal,* 1857. National Library of Medicine, Bethesda.

VIEWS *of* FOUR VARIETIES *of* MR. AMESBURY'S "PATENT BODY SUPPORT," *as they are used in various Conditions of the Body in the Single and Married State.*

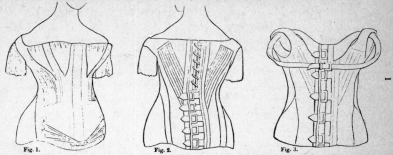

Fig. 1.   Fig. 2.   Fig. 3.

Fig. 1. Front View of the "PATENT SIMPLE SUPPORT," showing the Front Parts closed with Systems of Laces.—*Fig.* 2. Back View of the "PATENT SIMPLE SUPPORT," represented as having the Back Parts closed partly with Buckles and Straps and partly with a Lace.—*Fig.* 3. Back View of *either* of the other varieties of the Patent Support, shown as used to assist in correcting mal-position of the Shoulders.

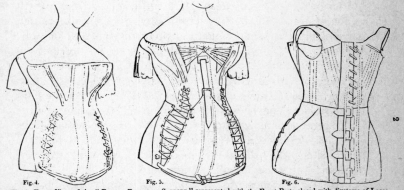

Fig. 4.   Fig. 5.   Fig. 6.

Fig. 4. Front View of the " PATENT REDUCING SUPPORT," represented with the Front Parts closed with Systems of Laces. —*Fig.* 5. Front View of the " PATENT ADJUSTABLE SUPPORT," shown with the Front Parts closed with Systems of Laces, and with the *Patent Adjustable Busk* partly extended.—*Fig.* 6. Back View of the " PATENT ADJUSTABLE SUPPORT, with the Back Parts partly closed with Buckles and Straps, and partly with a Lace.

N.B. *The Front and Back Parts of the Supports are frequently closed, partly with Buckles and Straps, and partly with Systems of Laces, and sometimes with Buckles and Straps only.*

AGENTS *are instructed to obtain the Supports from the Factory, closed in that manner most suited to the bodily condition of the Purchaser.*

An illustration from Joseph Amesbury, *Substitutes for Stays and Corsets, Patent Body Supports,* 1840.

abdominally like the male.[31] Her spirited heterodoxy caused an immediate furor in medical circles and evoked investigations by numerous physicians to prove the contrary. Writing in *Century Magazine* in 1893, Thomas Mays, M.D., of Philadelphia showed through his investigation of some eighty-one Indian girls that abdominal breathing was the natural form of respiration for both sexes, and that the clavicular, or costal, respiration occurred only with civilized women who artificially constricted themselves by garments that supported the abdomen.[32] In all cases, he wrote, Indian women, who knew nothing of corsets, busks, or stays and who had always worn loose clothing, breathed in an abdominal manner. Costal respiration was not due to the influence of gestation as Miss Becker had indicated, but due to the complex attitudes of fashion, figure, and civilization.[33] A superintendent and surgeon of the Battle Creek Sanitarium, John Harvey Kellogg, made similar inquiries on the matter of respiration and confirmed the investigation of Mays. He also suspected that costal breathing caused uterine difficulties and unnatural pressures that not only affected the abdominal cavity but also changed the voice of the female.[34]

Physicians continually warned women of the dress habits. Because their costume exhibited a total disregard for the laws of physiology, and because it was worn for display more than for comfort, urban women were threatening the natural laws governing their health. Corseted, and stuffed into tight high-heeled shoes, they threw their body axes forward to the point of destroying the "natural equilibrium of the body." They forced their carriages into "new positions" and subjected nearly all their body organs to "tension."[35] If men would not encourage the extravagance in women's dress, wrote one doctor, then women who continually sought the approving eye of men would enter a more healthful state. "If men would refuse to

31. Cited in Viscountess Harberton, "On Dress Reform and Stays," *Sanitary Record*, X (1888), 263.

32. Cited in Eugene Lee Crutchfield, "Some Ill Effects of the Corset," *Gaillard's Medical Journal*, LXVII (1897), 1.

33. Dickinson, "The Corset: Questions of Pressure and Displacement," 511.

34. West, "The Corset, as a Factor in Pelvic Diseases," 212.

35. M. T. Runnels, "Physical Degeneracy of American Women," *Medical Era*, III (1886), 298–99.

marry women who wear corsets," wrote M. T. Runnels, M.D., of Kansas City, "how long would it be before corsets would be 'out of fashion'?" Lamenting the fashion plates of *Harper's Bazaar, New York Fashion Bazaar, Young Ladies' Journal, Godey's Lady's Book,* and others, Runnels believed that modern culture had transformed urban women into neurasthenic wasps "wholly disqualified for marriage and maternity." The fact that more than 10,000 gross of nursing bottles were sold annually in the country pointed to a very fundamental constitutional degeneracy in urban mothers. "There can be no doubt whatever," he went on, "that the true and essential function of these glands at the present day is ornamental and aesthetic. Their noblest opportunities are not in the 'milky way,' but in the line of high art and realistic delineation."[36]

While most physicians of the nineteenth century agreed that the corset was designed to enlarge the pelvis and mammary region of the body, the phrenologist and medical quack, Orson Squier Fowler (1804–87), speculated even further in his philosophical critique on marriage. The enlarged pelvis, he wrote, represented an instinctive desire on the part of the female and indicated a very basic philosophy which women either consciously or unconsciously strove to maintain. In his book *Maternity* (1856), he maintained that fashion, despite its aberrations, was entirely philosophical. "In all their variations and mutations," he wrote, woman's costumes "PUFF OUT AND ADORN THE PELVIC REGION." Just as in Queen Anne's time when hoops were used to make dresses flare out ("because pregnancy does the same"), so the modern costume similarly filled out the skirts with the use of the bustle, corset, and extra skirts.[37] Though he admitted that tight-lacing was the "most accursed of all fashions, which has slain more women in a score of years than the sword has men in a century—stifled more children than the Ganges," it nonetheless had the rationale of giving the pelvic region a greater size by contrast to the small waist. "Mark the fact," he wrote, "that this lacing has always extended down

36. *Ibid.*, 300–301.

37. Orson S. Fowler, *Maternity* (New York, 1856), 60; Peter Camper, *The Works of the Late Professor Camper* (London, 1794); Crutchfield, "Some Ill Effects of the Corset," 10–11.

just to the very point which the early stage of child-bearing distends." The bodice waist had the same intent, since it filled out the pelvic area. It adorned the woman with added beauty by making that portion of her anatomy "seem large and fair, which when large and full indicates an excellent child-bearer."[38]

Unfortunately, according to Fowler, tight-lacing excited the husband's love, but it did little to retain that love. While the corset enabled the woman to deceive her husband into believing that she had "something where she is nothing," the deception lasted only until the husband saw the "naked truth" before him. "If he is green enough to be caught in her snares," Fowler warned, "his first introduction to her as his wife will show him, that what he thought was food for love was only cotton above and hemp below." "Seeing no charms on which love can feast," and piqued at having been outwitted, the angered husband now "hated where he would have loved if he had found what he had a right to expect."[39]

The same was true of the bustle. It seemed to one physician that the entire motive behind the bustle was to exaggerate the procreative functions of the woman. Since the male saw in woman the means of carrying on the species, woman instinctively aided that male desire by exaggerating those inclinations in her clothes. By compressing her waist she exaggerated both the mammal and pelvic development and thus "brought into lustful prominence the capacity of women for easy reproduction and subsequent plentiful lactation." She transformed the simple act of respiration into a perverted act of "subclavicular enticement."[40]

Maternity enlarges the pelvis, fills out around the hips, and throws the lower part of the spine out backward, while it causes its middle portion to bend inward—the very shape produced by childbearing. Now the entire paraphernalia of bustling, extra skirts, sacking, and all that, is to imitate, as nearly as may be, the form of a woman while carrying a child; and the entire philosophy of this hip-dressing, is to render the wearer INTERESTING, by making her appear as if actually in an "interesting situation." This is what gives to this apparent abdominal enlargement all its beauty. Woman knows by instinct that man loves to view a fullness of this

38. Fowler, *Maternity*, 61.
39. *Ibid.*, 71–72.
40. Crutchfield, "Some Ill Effects of the Corset," 11.

region—and he does so, because he instinctively admires whatever resembles or promotes child-bearing—and, therefore, puffs out these parts by cotton, bran, hemp, skirts, and surplus petticoats by the half-dozen, simply to excite this male passion.[41]

According to Dio Lewis, M.D., author of *Our Girls* (1871), there were psychological reasons why men preferred the wasp-waisted woman to the healthy maid. The reasons stemmed from ethnological evidence that women were once slaves to men's passions. While the gentlemen of the "better classes" had risen above that barbaric relationship, they had nonetheless made the women into "pets," thus perpetuating indirectly the older relationship. Just as the age had valued its pets in proportion to their almost toylike frailty, so husbands selected their wives as they would have selected a black-and-tan. Corseted tightly in gowns that were decorated in an assortment of laces, silks, trinkets, and rings, they sat in parlors receiving visitors, re-dressed several times during the day, and patiently awaited their husbands' return from the hectic business world.[42] The whole style of the woman's dress denoted her function in life. As Simone de Beauvoir has noted, "the significance of woman's attire is evident: it is decoration, and to be decorated means to be offered." In a society in which a man's wealth was gauged by the manner in which his wife was clothed, her "decoration" was important, and as the woman was the chief object in a home full of other objects, she had literally to dress her part.[43]

Picturing corsets as one of the decadent imitations from an even more decadent Europe, physicians implored Christian America to discard "the costumes devised by the dissolute capitals of Europe" and embark on a crusade for a more pure and free womanhood.[44] The languid, sickly women who read romantic novels and promenaded in tight-fitting gowns were poor models for the American girl to imitate. Such refined invalids masked extreme cases of physical, mental, and moral

41. *Ibid.*, 10.
42. Lewis, *Our Girls*, 86–87; George M. Beard, *American Nervousness, Its Causes and Consequences* (New York, 1881), 73–74; Louise Fiske-Bryson, "Women and Nature," *New York Medical Journal*, XLVI (1887), 627.
43. de Beauvoir, *The Second Sex*, 422.
44. Lewis, *Our Girls*, 55.

exhaustion. Their organs were jammed upward into the chest and throat and downward into the pelvis, resulting in chronic suffering from weak backs, delicate nervous systems, and severe invalidism.[45] Besides restraining the chest and arm movements, and hampering respiration and digestion, the corset heated the pelvic region to the point of "disturbing the circulation and inducing inflammatory troubles."[46] One physician remarked that the mind of physically exhausted women frequently weakened to the degree that the "exquisite sensibilities of the soul became weak and blunt." No physician of experience, he added, would fail to see instances in which physical exhaustion led to subsequent loss of modesty.[47]

According to Orson Fowler, the mental temperament of the woman decidedly altered with the application of corset pressure. In his book, *Tight-Lacing, Founded on Physiology and Phrenology; or, the Evils Inflicted on Mind and Body by Compressing the Organs of Animal Life, thereby Retarding and Enfeebling the Vital Functions* (1846), he argued that the woman's blood, hindered from its natural circulation, tended to flow to the head, inflaming the nervous system and causing an unnatural change in her personality. But even more disastrous to the corseted female was a situation which he reluctantly alluded to, admitting facetiously that in so doing, he would injure the popularity of his book.

I introduce it because it ought to go in—it ought to be KNOWN that it may be guarded against. Who does not know that the compression of any part produces inflammation? Who does not know that, therefore, tight-lacing around the waist keeps the blood from returning freely to the heart, and retains it in the bowels and neighboring organs, and thereby *inflames all the organs of the abdomen,* which thereby EXCITES AMATIVE DESIRES? Away goes this book into the fire! "Shame! shame on the man who writes this!" exclaims Miss Fastidious Small-Waist. "The man who wrote that, ought to be tarred and feathered." Granted; and then what shall be done to the woman who laces tight? If it be improper for a man to allude to this effect of lacing, what is it for a woman to cause and experience it? Let me tell you, Miss Fastidious, that the less you say about this, the better; because I have TRUTH on my side, and because it

45. *Ibid.,* 193.
46. George F. Comfort and Anna M. Comfort, *Woman's Education and Woman's Health; Chiefly in Reply to "Sex in Education"* (Syracuse, 1874), 105.
47. Lewis, *Our Girls,* 66–67.

is high time that men who wish virtuous wives knew it, so that they may avoid those who have inflamed and exhausted this element of their nature. It is also high time that virtuous woman should blush for very shame to be seen laced tight, just as she should blush to be caught indulging impure desires.[48]

Fowler prided himself on the fact that his earlier remarks on the subject had led to the formation of Anti-Lacing Societies, with their motto of "Natural waists or no wives."[49] He even went so far as to blame the corseted women for weakening or killing their children during pregnancy. "Yes, and that even by Christian mothers—by the daughters of Zion, the followers of the Lamb," he wrote. "Yea, more. These infanticides, with their corsets actually on, are admitted into the sanctuary of the Most High God, and even to the communion-table of the saints!"[50] The corset, stays, and tight-lacing must disappear from women's clothing altogether, added another physician in a pamphlet entitled *The Great Evil of the Age, a Medical Warning*, or the American woman's ability to bear healthy and well-developed children would decrease at a disastrous rate.[51]

The mischief of tight-lacing remained a popular topic in medical circles throughout the nineteenth century. Physicians attempted in many instances to shame the woman into abandoning the corset by picturing all sorts of diseases, and caricaturing the graceful "gait" of the corseted body. "From the shoulders down, as stiffly inflexible as the parlor tongs," wrote one practitioner, the corseted woman could walk only by a "sideling shuffle of the feet."[52]

Instead of the easy graceful inclination of a flexible form, we have an awkward ungainly attempt to balance the body on the limbs; the shoulders stiffened backwards, as if shackled with iron; the chest girded in, till breath can scarcely be drawn; and the trunk of the body as rigid as if carved in wood—the figure looking like a caricature upon nature, ease, and grace! When ladies in this trim enter a room, especially after

48. O. S. Fowler, *Tight-Lacing, Founded on Physiology and Phrenology; or, the Evils Inflicted on Mind and Body by Compressing the Organs of Animal Life, Thereby Retarding and Enfeebling the Vital Functions* (New York, 1846), 10–11.
49. *Ibid.*, 1.
50. *Ibid.*, 12–13.
51. John Ellis, *The Great Evil of the Age, a Medical Warning* (n.p., n.d.), 2.
52. Godman, "Injurious Effects of Tight Lacing on the Organs and Functions of Respiration, Digestion, Circulation, etc.," 487.

walking, they can scarcely speak for several minutes, and their bosoms heave with an unnatural agitation. If the busk be of the *fashionable* length, it is impossible for them to sit comfortably in a chair; they must perch on its outer edge, to prevent the busk from being pushed toward the chin, etc. All this torture, uneasiness, and inconvenience, is patiently endured, and for what? because it is fashionable! Grace, ease, elegance, and comfort, are alike immolated to this Miloch, who spares none who pretend to the rank of fashionable.[53]

According to another critic, too many women were willing to endure the corset, endless petticoats, and seemingly miles of material for the sake of fashion and a hopelessly narcissistic attitude of themselves. They were willing to accept even the constricted movement of the legs in walking in the belief that it was the most natural gait for the proper lady. Romantic and fashionable women of the time saw no reason to deprecate the artificially shortened step; rather, the fashionable lady indulged in an exciting life of the imagination. Exhausted but stubborn, she continued to implement the naively contrived pretensions of the urban class. Indeed, wrote one female, "the resisting weight of petticoats in walking, especially if there is the slightest wind, has been likened by some writers to the pleasant process of eternally walking through a field of long grass."[54] There were few women in the urban areas of the nation, remarked J. H. Kellogg, M.D., in his *Ladies Guide in Health and Disease,* who could walk in the natural step given them by the Creator. Stays, corsets, and the abominable "French heels" had created a "stiff, unnatural, mincing gait of the fashionable young lady [that] is not so much an affection as a necessity with her." "She struts or wriggles and minces along in the most ridiculous fashion," he added, "not because she desires to do so, but because it is impossible for her to walk in any other way."[55]

One physician observed, in an article written for the *Boston Medical and Surgical Journal,* that the corset was confined principally to countries with a common moral and religious code, and that the various harnessing contrivances devised were essentially "designed to *conceal,* as far as possible, the

53. *Ibid.,* 497.
54. Harberton, "On Dress Reform and Stays," 264.
55. Kellogg, *Ladies Guide in Health and Disease,* 132–33.

consequences of levity and imprudence." The argument that the corset improved the figure was "a mere excuse to cover the *real* object for which they were worn." Though women excused themselves from criticism with the argument that the corset was used only for the purpose of "support," more often than not their real desire was to "make" a figure. In reality, the woman's "horror of rotundity" led her to seek a flat bosom with the aid of cord and busk. Some women even attempted to conceal the evidence of pregnancy. "With all the mawkishness of false delicacy," they maintained a "fashionable appearance" at the expense of their unborn children.[56] According to a doctor writing in the *Southern Medical and Surgical Journal* in 1846, tight-lacing interrupted the "sympathetic communication between the uterus and mammae" causing constitutional problems in the fetus and inability of the mother to nourish her child after birth. It was his belief that tight-lacing not only deprived the woman of the maternal pleasure of nursing her own children, but also, because of the subsequent dependence upon artificial nourishment, was an indirect cause of colic, diarrhea, and gastric and intestinal problems that not too infrequently brought death to the infant.[57] In addition to destroying the joys of maternity, doctors suspected that the corset had "rendered the conjugal condition one of unceasing disappointment and gloomy solitude."[58] "I should not like to acknowledge that I ever got my arm around the waist of a woman," remarked one bachelor physician, "but these young men who have been there say that when they try that scheme with one of these young ladies whose waists are compressed to the highest degree there is no more pleasure in it than there would be in putting their arms around a lamp-post."[59] One female physician blamed the corset for the irritable personality of so many women. She also indicated that the corset was indirectly responsible for a good deal of the immorality of the age.

56. Godman, "Injurious Effects of Tight Lacing on the Organs and Functions of Respiration, Digestion, Circulation, etc.," 499.
57. Thomas W. Carter, "The Morbid Effects of Tight-Lacing," *Southern Medical and Surgical Journal*, II (1846), 409.
58. Godman, "Injurious Effects of Tight Lacing on the Organs and Functions of Respiration, Digestion, Circulation, etc.," 499.
59. Quoted in West, "The Corset, as a Factor in Pelvic Diseases," 221–22.

Husbands, she pointed out, were quicker to seek pleasure out-side the home dominated by the vile temper of a tight-laced wife.[60]

Because of the reluctance of fashionable women to part with the corset, physicians chose the circuitous route of noblesse oblige to attack the device. Reluctantly admitting that the "properly educated" lady might be well aware of the dangers of tight-lacing, and thus minimize her own discomfort with judicious use, doctors realized that there were nonetheless thousands of "females of the lower ranks of life" who imitated the better sort in matters of dress and manners without the proper knowledge of the cause and consequence of their ac-tions. The attempts by busty maids cramped into wasp-waists to carry out the normal household duties of sweeping, cleaning, cooking, mending, and serving, brought them to the brink of disease, disfiguration, exhaustion, and even death. It was not strange for such fashionable imitators to suffer from dyspepsia, chronic vomiting, fainting, and anemia in their voluntary im-prisonment. Unable to stoop without harming their respiratory systems and causing stresses on the abdominal cavity, they be-came chronic sufferers of "female diseases." According to one medical critic, it was a common occurrence for such women to "consult physicians for various supposed diseases, which are the immediate results of their preposterous attempts to make themselves fine figures." A good number of them, he added, wore their corsets and busks even in sleep, tightening them a bit more when they lay down, and then even more when they got up in the morning. On one occasion, he recalled, he noticed one of these "imitators of high life" laced in the fashionable manner of the day and occupied in sweeping the gutter outside her mistress's home. Nothing would have made the scene any more ludicrous than had one of the exquisitely dressed "gem-men" of the town shaded her with an umbrella while she dis-charged a chamberpot of "liquid-sweets."[61]

The so-called "high art" of fashion was a continual bane to

60. Wilkins, "Pelvic Congestion from Moderate Compression of the Waist," 139.

61. Godman, "Injurious Effects of Tight Lacing on the Organs and Func-tions of Respiration, Digestion, Circulation, etc.," 498.

the practitioner of the nineteenth century, who could point to the "tight-laced liver" as its only significant memorabilia to the fashionable lady. It was harmful enough to the upper classes "but it is a more grievous thing to reflect that the servile imitators of these women in the lowest orders shall be made to suffer also."[62] By splitting a subtle hair, doctors distinguished between the better sort of women who understood (or ought to) the nature of the instrument, its probable dangers, and the hygienic limits to constriction, and the inexperienced imitator who bought her corsets with little understanding of their mischief, who laced them too tight, and who wore them in working situations which made her grimaces absurd, and her contortions the bread and butter of itinerant quacks, patent medicine manufacturers, and concerned physicians. F. D. Godman, M.D., once recalled an incident at a boarding house in Philadelphia in which a young female housekeeper, whose duty it was to place a tea kettle over the kitchen hearth, was unable to do so because of the stooping it required. When her mistress inquired why the tea had not been placed on the fire to boil, the maid confessed to wearing a "long busk," and said she was laced so tight that she "could not possibly stoop to put on the kettle." The common disposition of the lower classes to imitate meant that both "elegant and innocent women fell into a fashion which promised improvement to the personal charms, while in reality, it was productive of their destruction."[63]

Doctors hoped that society women would dress "with greater plainness and economy" in order to impress the working class with a sense of decency and thrifty habits. Otherwise, society would be deluged with the vulgar caricatures of "pinchbeck and shams which women in humbler life affect in ridiculous imitation of their betters."[64] Since poorer classes used the corset as an article of warmth as well as support, and because they adopted it usually at the time of puberty, working girls would accustom themselves to the device at a time

62. Dyce Duckworth, "On Tight-Lacing," *Practitioner*, XXIV (1880), 11.
63. Godman, "Injurious Effects of Tight Lacing on the Organs and Functions of Respiration, Digestion, Circulation, etc.," 498–99.
64. S. C. Young, "The Evils Arising from Tight Lacing," *Journal*, Louisiana State Medical Society, XVIII (1860), 311.

when the organs of reproduction should have unrestricted development.[65] The upper classes, wrote one doctor, had the weighty responsibility for demanding not only gracefulness in woman's dress, but at the same time proper respect for the physiologists' views. "In matters of dress," he added, "beneficial influences proceeding from them must rapidly descend the social scale. It is much to be desired that women of high social rank should feel the importance of exercising their power aright."[66]

Physician Robert L. Dickinson, lecturer on obstetrics in the Long Island College Hospital, used a manometer in 1887 to determine the pressure of the corset on the woman's body. He discovered in his tests on over fifty women that the average amount of pressure from the corset was twenty-one pounds, while the greatest measured eighty-eight pounds. He also noted a distinct change in the pressure during the first twenty seconds after the women hooked their corsets. He believed that the change was due to "the displacement of organs and the expulsion of blood from the liver and abdomen and of air from the lungs." He also discovered that the contraction in the waist measured from two and one-half inches to six inches.[67] Another clinician, making use of a spirometer to test the cubic inches of air a woman could expel from her lungs after her deepest inhalation, found that the average for the uncorseted woman was 163 cubic inches, while the corseted woman, whose waist was two and one-half inches smaller, averaged a capacity of thirty cubic inches less.[68]

In their concern for the urban woman, doctors frequently bemoaned the increasing difficulty in childbearing. The abnormal attitude of the body axis caused by high heels, along with the constricted frame of the woman's body, produced a displacement of the uterus and other vital reproductive organs. But even more frightening to doctors was their belief that while corsets were making the pelvises of women smaller,

65. Duckworth, "On Tight-Lacing," 12–13.
66. W. Wilberforce Smith, "Corset-Wearing and Its Pathology," *Sanitary Record*, n.s., X (1888), 328.
67. Dickinson, "The Corset: Questions of Pressure and Displacement," 508.
68. *Ibid.*, 511; V. H. Taliaferro, "The Corset in Its Relations to Uterine Diseases," *Atlanta Medical and Surgical Journal*, X (1873), 683–85.

civilization was making the heads of children larger, due to the greater demands of brain force in the urban worker. In the struggle for existence, wrote one practitioner, the "man with the big head, and not the one with the strong arms, wins the battle of life." As the children of the civilized nations inherited the qualities of their parents, so too they were born with larger heads and cranial mass than their parents. The situation made the role of motherhood intolerable for many cultured women. Left to nature, it seemed to some that the woman with the small pelvis would "probably perish in her first confinement, so that the breed of women would at once die out." But the invention of forceps in child delivery had not only permitted women with small pelvises to give birth, but also to have a hereditary significance on the size of pelvises of their daughters. One physician even believed that because the tendency toward smaller and narrower pelvises was reaching a critical stage, only the removal of the uterus "would put a stop to such vicious breeding."[69]

In a speech before the International Medical College in Rome in 1894, Charles Cannaday, M.D., of Virginia suggested that the practice of tight-lacing, usually begun at the period of greatest uterine development in the female, interfered with the nutrition of the pelvic region, and, more seriously, the generative functions. Pelvic diseases were rare among those races which did not resort to the practice, and pregnancy was likewise relatively free of pain and complications. Besides race differences, there were remarkable differences between women living in rural districts where the practice of tight-lacing was rare and those in the urban areas who seemed to be addicted to the practice. Gynecology, he wrote, was a postcorset medical specialization which flourished in the urban areas. Cannaday further reminded the profession that the increased sterility prominent among the upper classes in American society could be blamed on the practice of tight-lacing. In applying Darwin's theory of natural selection to women, he predicted that "we may in the future expect our fair sex to have waists as slim as

69. Quoted in A. L. Smith, "What Civilization Is Doing for the Human Female," *Transactions,* Southern Surgical and Gynecological Association, II (1890), 358–59.

wasps, and generative organs incapable of performing physiological functions."[70] He even believed that cancer, which he thought was a disease common to the civilized nations, could be linked in some manner to the peculiar custom of lacing.[71]

The most common complaint of physicians dealing with women who practiced tight-lacing was the development of the "chicken-breast." Because her ribs turned inward and overlapped due to the continual pressure of the corset, the chicken-breasted woman suffered from insufficient respiration, fractured ribs, and injuries to the sternum and clavicle. The lungs, in the parts most compressed, atrophied and collapsed. One doctor writing in the 1860s blamed the corset for the high incidence of consumption in women, and, because their lungs were forced to perform under conditions injurious to wholesome breathing, he likened their problem to what he called the "heaves" in horses. He also suspected that the tendency of the corset to displace the liver from its natural position explained the high incidence of hepatitis among the fashionable ladies.[72] Another doctor recalled an incident in which the use of the corset had caused the "outraged" blood, forced from its legitimate channels, to retreat "vengefully" to the woman's nose, where it remained "a source of keenest mortification." In desperation she applied leeches to the inside of her nostrils but the "sullen red held the fort obstinately."[73]

In a paper read before the New York Homeopathic Medical Society in 1880, Walter Y. Cowl, M.D., remarked that tight-lacing was a primary cause of neurasthenia in the urban woman. The lessened respiration and impaired digestion and circulation, added to the lack of proper exercise, acted as catalysts upon her weak nervous system.[74] Samuel Weir Mitchell's treatment for the neurasthenic woman was designed specifi-

70. Charles Graham Cannaday, "The Relation of Tight Lacing to Uterine Development and Abdominal and Pelvic Disease," *American Gynecological and Obstetrical Journal,* V (1894), 636.

71. *Ibid.,* 638.

72. Young, "The Evils Arising from Tight Lacing," 310–12.

73. Harland, *Eve's Daughters; or, Common Sense for Maid, Wife, and Mother,* 349.

74. Walter Y. Cowl, "On Tight Lacing as Cause of Disease," *Homeopathic Journal of Obstetrics,* III (1881–82), 38; Smith, "Corset-Wearing and Its Pathology," 324–25.

cally to alleviate the effects of tight-lacing. Besides massage, rest, and forced feeding, he used faradic currents to strengthen the thoracic and abdominal walls, reduce intestinal constriction, and encourage circulation in the constricted woman. Physicians Peaslee and Emmett of New York City pointed out the frequency of uterine congestion, leukorrhea, menorrhagia, dysmenorrhea, and ulceration of the cervix, hemorrhoids, and constipation which resulted from the use of the corset. According to Cowl, the fact that the corset had replaced the function of the abdominal muscles was in a large part responsible for the frequent need to bandage women after their confinement in order to support their "pendulous belly." The difficulties of labor were directly related to weakness of the abdominal muscles. Surely, one of the direct results of the corset, according to R. L. Dickinson, M.D., was the need for instruments during childbirth, a need which seemed primarily urban in nature and principally for the fashionable woman and her children.[75]

One of the most dreaded difficulties resulting from the corset was prolapsus uteri, or the falling of the womb. When prolapsus uteri occurred, the womb tended to slide down the vagina until it sometimes projected out of the body. "In some cases," wrote A. M. Mauriceau, "it absolutely protrudes entirely without the parts."[76] Treatment for the condition included faradic electricity, wood, ivory, or glass pessaries worn internally to support the womb, sponges forced into the vagina to give support to the uterus, injections of alum in water or decoctions of red oak bark, tonic medicines, enemas, hip baths, and lying with the legs suspended in the air.[77] The practice of tight-

75. Cowl, "On Tight Lacing as Cause of Disease," 39–42; J. Nottingham, "Compression of the Female Waist by Stays," *Provincial Medical and Surgical Journal*, III (1841), 110–11; John Cleland, "Tight Lacing, Venous Congestion, and Atrophy of the Ovaries," *Glasgow Medical Journal*, XIII (1880), 89–92; Smith, "Corset-Wearing and Its Pathology," 324; Crutchfield, "Some Ill Effects of the Corset," 9.

76. A. M. Mauriceau, *The Married Woman's Private Medical Companion* (New York, 1847), 164; Dickinson, "The Corset: Questions of Pressure and Displacement," 513; Taliaferro, "The Corset in Its Relations to Uterine Diseases," 689–90.

77. Mauriceau, *The Married Woman's Private Medical Companion*, 164–66; Edward H. Dixon, *Woman and Her Diseases, from the Cradle to the Grave* (Philadelphia, 1860), 551–54; Henry S. Cunningham, *Lectures on the Physi-*

lacing, the wearing of heavy skirts suspended from the hips, and the relaxation of natural muscle supports had caused many women to suffer unbearably from prolapsus uteri. A glance at the advertisements for pessaries that appeared in both medical and popular journals, including, incidentally, the Sears Roebuck catalogs, confirms this. The typical American woman of the 1870s, wrote Marian Harland in *Eve's Daughters* (1882), was a stoic caricature—"Her hand on the lumbar region, eyes hollow and complexion chlorotic."[78] Dio Lewis, M.D., advised men to avoid marrying girls who had indulged in the practice of tight-lacing. While the girl may be a devoted wife, the husband would soon regret his marriage. "Physicians of experience know what is meant," he wrote, "while thousands of husbands will not only know, but deeply feel the meaning of this hint."[79]

"The history of the evolution of the corset," voiced one alarmed nineteenth-century practitioner, "is the record of diseases of the womb," which have undermined the health of the American woman. Lacing themselves as "tight as Dick's hatband," women cramped their waists to the point that it was all they could do "to keep the uterus inside the vagina."[80] One doctor recalled an incident in which a rather stout woman had dressed tightly in a new corset one Sunday, and on her way to church was seized with violent pains. Thinking the cause of her troubles required the services of a midwife, she called immediately for a local accoucheur and returned home to her bedroom to await the blessed event. After almost a day of fruitless labor pains, a physician was summoned, and on examination of the patient discovered that what was thought to be the movement of a child was really severe uterine conges-

---

ological Laws of Life, Hygiene and a General Outline of Diseases Peculiar to Females, Embracing a Revival of the Rights and Wrongs of Women, and a Treatise on Disease in General (Indianapolis, 1882), 264; Kingsford, *Health, Beauty and the Toilet*, 138–39; Robert R. Rentoul, *The Dignity of Woman's Health and the Nemesis of Its Neglect* (London, 1890), 65–70; Gustavus Cohen, *Helps and Hints to Mothers and Young Wives* (London, 1880), 84.

78. Harland, *Eve's Daughters; or Common Sense for Maid, Wife, and Mother*, 85.

79. Dio Lewis, "Health of the American Woman," *North American Review*, CXXXV (1882), 510; West, "The Corset, as a Factor in Pelvic Diseases," 210.

80. *Ibid.*, 220.

tion and a fallen womb. After prescribing a large dose of castor oil, to be followed by opium and hot poultices, the physician informed the embarrassed woman that if she wore that particular corset again, he just might "deliver" her womb.[81]

In a speech read before the Los Angeles County Medical Society in 1890, Theoda Wilkins, M.D., enveighed against the use of the corset, saying that it caused most of the pelvic congestion and invalidism in women of the day. Some women, she wrote, were such nervous creatures as a result of waist constriction that menstruation required the use of morphine and other strong narcotics to ease the pain. There were many women who were also victims of retroflexed and retroverted uteruses and were constantly obliged to depend upon tonics and opium for relief. "The sooner everyone concerned gets over the idea that healthy women's bodies need external support," she wrote, "the better for all humanity." But too many women, she added reluctantly, found the state of invalidism or semi-invalidism somehow fashionable in spite of the great mental and physical strains they endured in order to boast of "an elegant form."[82] Similarly, women's reformer, Frances Willard, warned that "a ligature at the smallest diameter of womanly figure means an impoverished blood supply in the brain, and may explain why women scream when they see a mouse." Unless women were willing to see that violations of physical laws were directly affecting the mental and spiritual element of the body, little could be done to insure complete emancipation or reform of the American woman. Indeed, unless one freedom kept pace with the other, there was little hope for the "new woman" other than in a purely rhetorical sense.[83]

The warnings and remonstrances of the nineteenth-century physician against the corset fell, for the most part, on deaf ears. Strangely allied with the newly emerging feminist movement in a stand against styles of dress, he found that his patients preferred to suffer the restrictions of fashionable apparel rather than heed advice offered by doctor and feminist alike.

81. Taliaferro, "The Corset in Its Relations to Uterine Diseases," 693.
82. Wilkins, "Pelvic Congestion from Moderate Compression of the Waist," 137–39.
83. Quoted in Greer, *Woman Know Thyself, Female Diseases, Their Prevention and Cure,* 43.

Perhaps the middle-class woman perversely asserted her independence from her male doctor and her aggressive female compatriot while at the same time unconsciously reaffirming her dependence upon fashion setters and society's mores. And perhaps she also reflected, quite unknowingly, Thorstein Veblen's theory that discomfort in woman's apparel, especially the corset and high heels, was evidence of her continuing economic dependence upon man. For certainly the corset prevented the woman from any practical activity and proclaimed her inability to do anything but look decorative. This symbol of newly acquired leisure and luxury satisfactorily and conspicuously proclaimed the urban woman's position in society, and not for mere reasons of health would she abandon a practice which so noticeably heralded the financial success which her husband, and vicariously, she herself, could claim.

Exercise and the Bicycle

In general, the medical profession seemed divided on the question of woman's exercise. Too many girls, wrote Lucy M. Hall, M.D., spent their hours indoors with little exercise. Drearily drumming out tunes upon a piano each day, working for hours in a bent position over intricate needlework, or laboring to add one more accessory to their toilet, they became more and more weighted with superfluous attire, poorly developed organs, and weakened nervous systems. She urged women to go outdoors and do exercises, such as rowing, walking, tennis, and regulated gymnastics.[84] But while there were any number of doctors who advised the woman to develop her muscles along with her brain, still others deplored physical exercise. Arabella Kenealy, M.D., wrote:

The spectacle of young women, with set jaws, eyes strained tensely on a ball, a fierce battle-look gripping their features, their hands clutching some or other implement, their arms engaged in striking and beating, their legs disposed in coarse ungainly attitudes, is an object-lesson in all that is ugly in action and unwomanly in mode. The so-called "tennis-

84. Lucy M. Hall, "The Physical Training of Women," *American Journal of Social Science*, XXI (1886), 103; S. P. White, "Modern Mannish Maidens," *Blackwood Magazine*, CXLVII (1890), 254; Nathan Allen, *The Education of Girls, as Connected with Their Growth and Physical Development* (Boston, 1879), 27.

grin," which on many women's faces does duty for smile, shows how the muscular tension of forceful effort permanently mars higher attributes. So too, the proverbial quarrelsomeness of tennis-playing women results from the combative habit of mind. Light and exhilarating, in place of strenuous competitive exercises, enable girls to develop their womanhood in healthy structure, efficient function, and beauty of body and mind.[85]

Indeed, there were those who could only portray the woman as a nerveless and asthenic nymph, fainting under a frown, and forever hanging on the arm of a male protector. Although lamenting the physical status of women, they seemed to cherish the frail woman who was spared the burdens of the energetic world. About the most active form of exercise prescribed was the massage ("passive exercise"), applied centripetally, in the direction of the heart. This was particularly helpful for the neurasthenic woman since it facilitated "the flow of the venous current, which in the arms and lower limbs has to struggle upwards against the force of gravitation."[86]

It was not without reason, then, that while the corset elicited the almost universal condemnation of the medical profession, there seemed to be far less unanimity with respect to exercises which precluded the harness altogether. Ironically, while doctors objected to the corset and tight stays, there were those who believed in limiting the woman's exercise nonetheless to only those sports in which some form of elastic support could still be worn.[87] Women were to avoid the bowling alley, for example, for fear of "broken corset bones under one-sided sudden strain." As for horseback riding, the problems of dress expense as well as modesty precluded its widespread use by women; it complicated pelvic troubles since the only acceptable form of riding (sidesaddle) was both awkward and destructive of body symmetry.[88]

Because there were so few other physical diversions, feminists as well as some physicians suggested that the bicycle offered the cheapest, safest, and most accessible exercise

85. Arabella Kenealy, *Feminism and Sex Extinction* (London, 1920), 139.
86. Finck, *Romantic Love and Personal Beauty*, 404.
87. Hall, "The Physical Training of Women," 103.
88. R. L. Dickinson, "Bicycling for Women from the Standpoint of the Gynecologist," *American Journal of Obstetrics*, XXI (1895), 25.

and transportation for the American woman. "After the first shyness from conspicuousness of position and garb has worn away," wrote physician R. L. Dickinson of New York, the bicycle would become an excellent form of exercise for the woman and "a means of comradeship in exercise with her husband"—perhaps the only outdoor sport which both husband and wife could participate in together.[89] Like Dickinson, other doctors in the 1890s saw in the cycle a veritable lifesaver for corseted women who for centuries had been virtual recluses in the home environment, forced to dress unhygienically and conform to harsh social conventionalities.[90] Weir Mitchell, a specialist in neurasthenia, along with Horatio C. Wood, M.D., William Pepper, and Lucy N. Tappan, were most enthusiastic about the bicycle's use as a therapeutic agent for neurasthenic women. It was the most reasonable solution to the sedentary life of many Victorian ladies suffering from nervous exhaustion.[91] Some doctors believed that it aided women with problems of prolapsus uteri, and still others thought it cured women with gout, diabetes, dyspepsia, constipation, functional and organic paralysis, and hysteria.[92] Those women who were "stout," "plethoric," or "lithemic," and whose habits tended to aggravate neurotic affections, would find comfort in moderate cycling. Still others with problems of digestion and "chronic constipation" could use the wheel as a medium for allaying their troubles. But physicians were cautious in advising its indiscriminate use and usually advised thorough examination of the pelvic and thoracic organs before permitting or prescribing bicycle riding.[93]

Most doctors recognized that the bicycle would entail a

89. *Ibid.*, 26, 30–31; James F. Prendergast, "The Bicycle for Women," *American Journal of Obstetrics*, XXXIV (1896), 247; (Anony.), "The Bicycle; Its Judicious and Injudicious Use," *Medical Review*, XXXII (1895), 210.

90. Prendergast, "The Bicycle for Women," 245; Crutchfield, "Some Ill Effects of the Corset," 3.

91. Prendergast, "The Bicycle for Women," 249.

92. Charles W. Townsend, "Bicycling for Women," *Boston Medical and Surgical Journal*, CXXXII (1895), 594; Graeme M. Hammond, "The Influence of the Bicycle in Health and in Disease," *Medical Record*, XLVII (1895), 132; Lewis Bauer, "The Bicycle Problem," *St. Louis Clinique of Physicians and Surgeons*, IX (1896), 161.

93. Thomas Lothrop and William Warren Potter, "Women and the Bicycle," *Buffalo Medical Journal*, XXXV (1896), 349.

certain amount of dress reform—the woman would ha[...]
adopt bloomers, wear knickerbockers, or dress in a skirt wh[...]
would reach to her boot tops and be "properly loaded to resis[...]
air currents and to protect her in case she is dismounted."
Naturally, the element of modesty had to predominate at all
times, but there were also hygienic factors involved. Physician
Mary Wood-Allen's remark that "many things in regard to a
girl's personal cleanliness could be learned by riding behind her
on a tandem" was not an idle one.[94] Doctors advised women to
wear a woolen union undergarment when riding in order to
absorb perspiration and to protect against catching cold. They
also cautioned against the use of stocking garters because they
caused the veins in the leg to swell while riding. Most important, however, the bicycle precluded the use of the corset.
The tight-laced woman would have to discard her harness
for either a "corded flexible waist," or a "well-adjusted abdominal band or supporter."[95] For those women whose breasts
were "large and flabby," doctors prescribed a breast support
hung from the shoulders; but in any case, the corset could be
avoided. The woman cyclist had the advantage of not having
to maintain the tailormade, hourglass figure which etiquette
still required of the woman on horseback.[96] "Through the general use of the wheel by women," wrote one practitioner, "we
look for a reform in dress, more exercise in the open air, better
muscular development, more stable nerves, easier labors, and
healthier children."[97] It would work wonders upon the mentally overworked and underexercised woman and eliminate
many of the causes of depression which at times verged on
melancholia.[98]

According to the editors of the *Buffalo Medical Journal* in
1896, the usefulness of the bicycle for the working girl was

94. Mary Wood-Allen, *What a Young Woman Ought to Know* (Philadelphia, 1898), 78.
95. Lothrop and Potter, "Women and the Bicycle," 350; J. Championniere, "Women and the Wheel," *Health Magazine for Every Family*, II (1894–95), 279.
96. Dickinson, "Bicycling for Women from the Standpoint of the Gynecol-ogist," 35.
97. Prendergast, "The Bicycle for Women," 253.
98. Francis Smith Nash, "A Plea for the New Woman and the Bicycle," *American Journal of Obstetrics*, XXXIII (1896), 557.

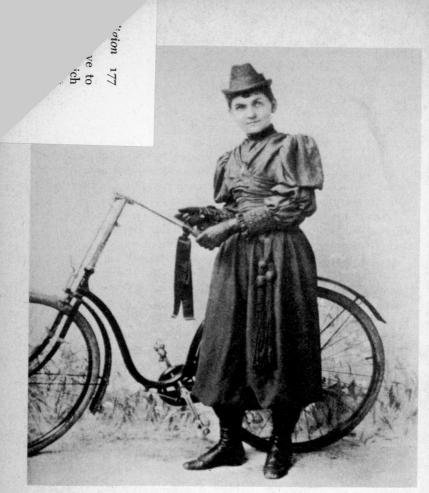

A woman cyclist, as shown in Mrs. Frances E. Russell, "The Rational Dress Movement in the Columbian Year," *Arena*, February, 1894. Indiana University.

beyond dispute. Young working-class women would find the wheel the best and healthiest method of transportation to and from their jobs, and certainly the most appealing for those who were employed far from their homes. It allowed them to avoid streetcars "when they [were] overcrowded, unhealthful, uncomfortable, [and] even dangerous." In addition, the bike refreshed them in the morning air, made them better able to cope with their work duties, and stimulated their appetites as well as improved their digestion. But as a form of transportation or recreation for the fashionable lady, the bicycle became a burning moral issue. While doctors accepted the bicycle as a necessary conveyance for the working girl, they thought it of dubious value for the woman or girl of "social position." For her, its use necessitated a stringent set of rules. Young ladies, the editors advised, "should be permitted to use the bike only under the strictest supervision of a competent parent or governess," and under no circumstances should they be allowed "to ride at evening with the opposite sex unaccompanied by a proper chaperone." "We have no doubt," the editors went on to say, "that a violation of this cardinal principle . . . has been fruitful of much social mischief and would easily lead to ruinous consequences."[99]

There were some skeptics and moralists both in and out of the medical profession who lamented the fact that woman had found yet another avenue through which she could escape the home circle. In Atlanta, for example, one Reverend Hawthorne spoke out vindictively against the wheel, charging the female cyclist with immodesty, indecency, and mannishness. Like many ministers of the late nineteenth century, Hawthorne's claim to medical etiology was confined to his recommendation for Royal Germetuer, a nostrum which claimed to cure everything from female irregularities to lockjaw. But Reverend Hawthorne notwithstanding, the editors of the *Atlanta Medical and Surgical Journal* went on record as saying that the quack minister had as much authority to discuss bicycles as "that of a sandfiddler on finance."[100] Unfortunately, Hawthorne was not alone in his

99. Lothrop and Potter, "Women and the Bicycle," 348–49.
100. Editorial, "Bicycling for Women," *Atlanta Medical and Surgical Journal*, XII (1895–96), 421.

Christian crusade against the woman cyclist. Allied with him were a good number of physicians and prudish women who saw the invention as "the advance agent of the devil." A very typical attitude was expressed by Miss Charlotte Smith, president of the Rescue League of Washington, D.C. According to her, the bicycle promoted libidinousness and immorality in the American woman. Specifically, her conclusions were as follows:

1. The most alarming increase of immorality among young women, in the United States, is most startling to those who have investigated the subject.

2. A great curse has been inflicted upon the people of this country because of the present bicycle craze; and, if a halt is not called soon, seventy-five per cent of the cyclists will be an army of invalids within the next ten years.

3. Immoderate bicycling by young women is to be deplored because of evil associations and opportunities offered by cycling sports.

4. Bicycling by young women has helped to swell the ranks of reckless girls, who finally drift into the standing army of outcast women of the United States, more than any other medium.

5. Bicycle runs for Christ, by the so-called Christians, should be termed bicycle runs for Satan; for the bicycle is the devil's advance agent, morally and physically, in thousands of instances.[101]

While the medical journals did not approve of the sanctimonious remarks of nostrum divines and alarmists like Miss Charlotte Smith, they were less than critical with members of their own profession who saw the wheel as a morally and physically destructive force, and who blamed it for everything from vibrated brains to the need for forceps to facilitate childbirth, to being employed as an abortifacient.[102] In the *St. Louis Journal of Homeopathy*, a physician lamented the sorrowful results of the wheel on the female population, particularly upon the destruction of their innate modesty. "We say most

101. Quoted in William C. Hatch, "Women and the Bicycle," *Massachusetts Medical Journal*, XVII (1897), 10.

102. (Anony.), "Cycling for Women," *British Medical Journal*, I (1896), 115–16; Thomas R. Evans, "Harmful Effects of the Bicycle upon the Girl's Pelvis," *American Journal of Obstetrics*, XXXIII (1896), 554; Prendergast, "The Bicycle for Women," 247; E. D. Page, "Women and the Bicycle," *Brooklyn Medical Journal*, XI (1897), 86–87; H. O. Carrington, "As to the Bicycle," *American Midwife*, II (1896), 16.

respectfully but plainly," he wrote, "that we think the attitude and costume necessary for women in the use of the bicycle saddle most unfortunate, trenching as they do upon good decorum and modesty of manner." He hoped that with a "sober second thought and wise conclusions which we are sure our matrons and older sisters will arrive at as soon as the furor and craze of novelty shall have subsided," women would return to the modest decency that so marked their nature and role in society. He blamed much of the wheel's popularity upon the poor level of education in the public schools. Too many girls lacked the moral character instilled by the older forms of education, and, tempted by the pleasures of the bicycle, willingly departed from their naturally modest instincts, clothing themselves in costumes which were both disagreeable to their figures and illustrative of a moral decadence. He suggested that part of the moral question involved in the riding of bicycles could be abated if women rode only on "private lawns" rather than through the public streets, but he suspected that such a solution was probably impossible to achieve. In time, he predicted, this fascination for the wheel would bear "fruit in the shape of impaired health both local and general." Women's recklessness with their physical hygiene and their morals would only subject them to serious illnesses on one hand and "rudeness by roughs and toughs" on the other. He blamed the indecencies of the bicycle on the revolution that had begun several years earlier by "progressive women" who had attempted to emancipate themselves from the home. While he admitted the validity of women's claim to the ballot, to greater independence, and to the right to earn money and hold property without male interference, he nonetheless felt that a prudent physician had to draw the line somewhere—and he chose to hold the line with the bicycle.[103]

One of the more elaborate criticisms of women cyclists came from E. D. Page, M.D., of Brooklyn. He declared as unfounded the claims that the wheel had been responsible for strengthening the weakened leg and abdominal muscles of women, for

103. W. A. Edmonds, "The Bicycle," *St. Louis Journal of Homeopathy*, II (1895–96), 406–7.

increasing respiration, and forcing a modification in the use of the corset. On the contrary, he argued, there was a distinct tendency for women to "run the flesh all off them" with the injudicious use of the horrible contraption. The bicycle was an insidious invention whose fascination had led many women to an immoderate use almost immediately. As for the argument that the bicycle encouraged increased respiration, Page pointed out that the limited muscle activity within the constricted saddle position of the rider tended to cramp chest and arm muscles as well as create a deformed, narrow chest. Page was similarly skeptical of the apparent revolution in dress and corset which the wheel seemed to propitiate. "We are bid to ask," he wrote, "if these changes are permanent, or only for the purpose of enabling her to ride the wheel more easily?" He believed that the modification of woman's dress to permit her to ride the cycle would in no way tend to modify her other forms of clothing. Women would only have to "work harder at night to bring [their] corsets together" after a day of riding in a looser fitting "cycle corset." Advanced civilization, he pointed out, demanded that the woman from the age of puberty should wear a dress reaching to the floor. Dress styles were determined in a large measure by the customs, conventions, and mores of society; and he speculated that in those countries where women wore shorter dresses, a large number of the inhabitants were probably illegitimate. Any degree of shortness in between, he inferred, caused a proportionate amount of immorality in the society. American women, becoming lax in their modesty by accepting the cycle dress, were encouraging the same promiscuity. According to Page, delicacy and modesty were necessary attributes of civilized woman—with the possible exceptions of actresses, eccentric Mary Walker, and the cyclist. (Miss Walker, a physician, spiritualist, and wearer of men's trousers, founded a colony for women in 1897 called "Adamless Eden.") If cycling would merely remove once and for all the horrors of the corset, that was to be applauded; but Page feared that the dress reform inaugurated by the cyclist would cause untold problems of decency for the "reformed woman." The variety of bloomers and open skirts which bicycle riders were adopting not only made them objects of ridicule, but the recipients of in-

decent remarks as well.[104] There were enough problems in the
way women mounted and dismounted from the bicycle
to cause any modest woman to blush. "The ability of a woman
to defend herself from insult is commendable," he wrote, "but
she forgets she invites the criticism by her dress, in the first
place, and her sensitiveness to criticism is acknowledgement of
its justness."

A married patient purchased her first pair of cycle boots. When the
shoeman had laced them to the height of her usual boots, she said:
"That will do." He stopped, looked her in the face, and said: "Young
woman, you'll show your legs a good deal higher than that before you
have rode a bicycle long." He then raised her dress to her knees and
laced the boot to the top, amid her confusion. Five years ago that would
have cost him his dismissal; to-day woman submits to it because it is a
fad. This is the first step in the loss of modesty and delicacy—elements of
character peculiarly woman's and which are her protection and her
charm.[105]

It seemed to Page that, all things considered, the moral and
intellectual side of woman's nature was irreparably damaged
by the use of the bicycle. It was the responsibility of the community to protect her from such harmful sources. He felt that
allowing woman this permissiveness in dress would only precipitate a further deterioration in her innate modesty. While
the health of the woman was the physician's responsibility,
Page pointed out that the medical profession had the added
burden of advising the community when deleterious changes
in woman's moral life threatened to destroy her physical well-
being. Visiting Coney Island, he observed hundreds of bicycle
riders, many of whom were girls, touring along the boulevard.
A good number of the women, he wrote, were under eighteen
and were "being followed by strange men until occasionally
their company was accepted." The bicycle as well as the bicycle skirt seemed to be undermining both proper modesty and
correct etiquette. In nearly all the summer resorts, women in
bicycle suits appeared in public about the hotels and parlors
"in an indifferent, careless sort of way, a bicycle-woman spirit,

104. Page, "Women and the Bicycle," 82–83; Robert Werlich, "Mary
Walker; from Union Army Surgeon to Sideshow Freak," *Civil War Times
Illustrated*, VI (1967), 46–49.
105. Page, "Women and the Bicycle," 84.

therefore permissible." The so-called "bicycle face" carried with it the connotation of permissiveness—the indifferent woman with hair undone and virtue ready for undoing. Her "fellow-feeling of bicyclists" had led her to accept the conversation of strange men, and Page's proof of this charge, while instructive of nineteenth-century morality, spoke little of his own Victorian chivalry.

One [young girl] about sixteen years of age we saw enticed by a beautifully dressed woman·(a prostitute in cycle suit) to take a glass of wine. One of the six young men who had joined in this scheme ordered the wine loaded. We heard him. The girl was soon in their power and was being marched off for immoral purposes, amid the delight of her captors, who agreed among themselves not to give it away. She looked like an innocent child, but was away from home influence. The girl, at that age, had not the power to resist all that influence, keen and friendly at first, but commanding as soon as she was intoxicated. Hundreds of girls slip down here by this means, unknown to their parents, and scores are ruined thereby. Those girls were not bad girls naturally, we believe, and would not have been so save for that visit there per wheel, and otherwise would have been at home, or at least elsewhere than being subjected to the vile influence of West End.[106]

The reason many physicians were reluctant to approve of the woman cyclist stemmed from their belief that those who used the wheel would find themselves outside the protective influence of the home circle and, in their weakness, tempted to become negligent in personal modesty. Apparently a good deal of the physicians' concern with personal modesty grew out of a discussion that had taken place in the Academy of Medicine of Paris. The debate, "whose echo was reproduced a thousand times in all parts of the civilized world," caused American doctors to begin spirited discussions on the morals of women cyclists.[107] Indeed, the single issue that seemed to dominate the whole question of women on bicycles was the fear that the wheel would "beget or foster the habit of masturbation" in the rider. "It certainly would not be desirable," wrote one physician, "for a young woman to get her first ideas of her sex from a bicycle ride."[108] Another physician observed a case of an

106. *Ibid.*, 85–86.
107. (Anony.), "The Bicycle; Its Judicious and Injudicious Use," 208.
108. Carrington, "As to the Bicycle," 16.

overwrought, emaciated girl of fifteen "whose saddle was arranged so that the front pommel rode upward at an angle of about 35 degrees, who stooped forward noticeably in riding, and whose actions . . . strongly suggested . . . the indulgence of masturbation." Even those who accepted the bicycle as a boon to the emancipated woman were fearful of the possibility that "under certain conditions the bicycle saddle could both engender and propagate this horrible habit."

The saddle can be tilted in every bicycle as desired, and the springs of the saddle can be so adjusted as to stiffen or relax the leather triangle. In this way a girl such as the one mentioned could, by carrying the front peak or pommel high, or by relaxing the stretched leather in order to let it form a deep, hammock-like concavity which would fit itself snugly over the entire vulva and reach up in front, bring about constant friction over the clitoris and labia. This pressure would be much increased by stooping forward, and the warmth generated from vigorous exercise might further increase the feeling.[109]

The real danger then was a moral one of greatest magnitude, and one which demanded immediate attention. The problem, according to many physicians, seemed to originate in the breakdown of the home circle and the loosening of those instincts of women which were best protected in the privacy of the home. The deplorable situation was made even worse because bicycle manufacturers had catered only to the needs of men rather than women. The ordinary saddle, "over which the rider is hung astride on the same principle as riding a rail," was wholly unsuited for the prudent woman. Such a saddle, warned one doctor, threw the woman's weight forward and gave rise at times "to friction and heating of the parts where it is very undesirable and may lead to dangerous practices."[110] A physician from Tennessee reported that one of his patients took up the bicycle for the purpose of masturbation and admitted to him that "it was no uncommon thing . . . to experience a sexual orgasm three or four times on a ride of one hour."[111]

109. Dickinson, "Bicycling for Women from the Standpoint of the Gynecologist," 33–34; Page, "Women and the Bicycle," 85.
110. Prendergast, "The Bicycle for Women," 250.
111. W. E. Fitch, "Bicycle Riding: Its Moral Effect upon Young Girls and Its Relation to Diseases of Women," *Georgia Journal of Medicine and Surgery*, IV (1899), 156.

Not all doctors worried over the possible practice of "self-pollution" by the female cyclist. "Possibly riding may produce amorous desire" in a woman, wrote H. O. Carrington, M.D., of New York, but he suspected that her "virtue . . . must be at a low ebb when such a cause can disintegrate it."[112] According to F. S. Nash, M.D., in a paper read before the Washington Obstetrical and Gynecological Society in 1895, a short ride after a day of hard work would relieve woman of "that tired feeling" which had led so many of them to the corner druggist for tonics and restoratives. There was, furthermore, no problem of "bicycle face" or eroticism as long as the woman used the cycle with judicious moderation. Obviously, this meant that she was to avoid "century runs" as well as the crooked, humped-over posture of a "scorcher" in an attempt to obtain high speeds. As long as she remained erect on the bike, with the support of the saddle touching only her tuber ischiorum and nowhere else, she would avoid the prurient desires that affected so many of her sister cyclists through saddle irritation. In the meantime, doctors advised manufacturers to remedy the saddle problem by taking a plaster or wax cast of the woman's seat and designing a proper saddle with that as its model.[113] But as long as the woman sat upright and had her saddle level with her weight resting upon the buttocks, there was little cause for alarm and little possibility for erotic pleasures.[114] One doctor from St. Louis was particularly caustic with the efforts of "preacher friends" and moralistic dilettantes in the medical profession who were railing against the wheel. "I am not yet persuaded," he wrote, "that [the bicycle] has any serpentine intentions upon the vulnerable parts of [our] daughters . . . with which perforce of circumstance its relations have been so close; no more do I believe that it is going to jolt their gray matter into a primitive jelly, nor fan it into a consuming fire."[115] According to Graeme M. Hammond, M.D., writing in the *Medi-*

112. Carrington, "As to the Bicycle," 16.
113. Nash, "A Plea for the New Woman and the Bicycle," 559; James R. Chadwick, "Bicycle Saddles for Women," *Boston Medical and Surgical Journal,* CXXXII (1895), 595; Championniere, "Women and the Wheel," 279.
114. Dickinson, "Bicycling for Women from the Standpoint of the Gynecologist," 34.
115. Frank R. Fry, "The Bicycle and the Nerves," *Medical Mirror,* VII (1896), 272.

cal Record for 1895, the suggestion that the bicycle threatened personal morality was merely another red herring thrown up to hinder the American woman and restrict her activities even more within the home circle. "She may ride for the purpose of obtaining genital irritation, or she may ride with perfectly proper motive," he maintained, "but she cannot do the both at the same time."[116]

116. Hammond, "The Influence of the Bicycle in Health and in Disease," 131.

Chapter V

THE FITTEST MAN

Of all the diseases or derangements which affect or which can affect the generative organs, there is none equal nor half so bad as Spermatorrhoea. All others together, or one after another, in a continuous round, are not capable of producing—and never have and never can produce—half so much mischief, derangement and ruined health, as this one evil of Spermatorrhoea or involuntary emission of Semen! It is a direct draft upon the vital energies of life itself, destroying both body and mind as it goes! And the longer it continues, the more difficult it becomes to overcome.

C. Bigelow, *Sexual Pathology*, 1875

In an industrial age whose sheer momentum seemed to guarantee material ascendancy if not uninterrupted progress, nineteenth-century physicians and purity writers gloried in the added responsibility of elevating each new generation above the last. They placed themselves at the center of national life, claiming to be the moral vortex of the century's power and progress, whose attitudes on religion, training of the will, exercise and diet, intellectual employment, amusement, and marriage helped to build national character. With lessons that seemed to have no end, manual writers responded to their own and society's visionary dreams by portraying the image of the century's male youth and establishing the sphere within which they could grow. In true Spencerian fashion, they promised continual victory for every challenge met. If sufficient effort were devoted to coaxing young men to acquire the speech and manners of gentlemen, if enough boys were encouraged to take to their studies (not so much for the sake of the lessons, but for moral and social goals), and if boys could be schooled with the precision of machinery, then order would eventually triumph over chaos, and progress and morality would become assured realities in the new age. Viewing their skills as decisive in the nation's future, manual writers became the archfriends of progress, painting with grandeur and drama the images of less-disciplined classes and peoples. The seriousness of the male's education was manifest, for within the belief that anything not exactly controllable was out of its proper order in the universe, such traits as laziness or indolence could only be despised— never ignored. Those minds either asleep, dreaming, or distracted to mischief were exposed to the ravages of evil upon evil. The privileges of the middle class were not to be taken for granted; privilege was to be modestly accepted, not for the edge it gave over the working class, but because it provided an opportunity for achieving greater progress and more material

A portion of this chapter has been previously published as "Bachelor's Disease: The Etiology, Pathology, and Treatment of Spermatorrhoea in the 19th Century," *New York State Journal of Medicine*, LXXIII (1973), 2076–82.

benefits for the nation. The white man's burden became the young man's burden, and on his slender shoulders the young male Caucasian had to carry the weight of the century's ideals, hopes, and goals.

Simone de Beauvoir's remark that "girls are weighted down with restrictions, boys with demands," could not have been more evident than in the nineteenth century, for the Victorian man-child felt himself watched, encouraged, cautioned, and threatened by every social force to achieve those values which were deemed necessary to his future manhood, and to eschew those which were either harmful or of no value in his struggle to become the fittest man.[1] Few dreamed of complaining or resisting. Promised that they would eventually assume the responsibilities of the age, they were expected, in the meantime, to live and think democratically, discovering and praising the nation's institutions without criticism. Responsive to the forces which both coaxed and led him, the man-child knew the boundaries which separated him from the gentler sex. While the young girl cultivated the protective camouflage of sentimentality, he was taught to avoid displays of emotion and instead, to spare no effort in developing those attributes, both real and artificial, which would ensure success in the competitive business world. "Many a boy has shot ahead of his fellows of equal merit," wrote Kate Upson Clark in *Bringing Up Boys* (1899), "by means of his ready manner, his bright face, or some other purely superficial quality."

The first object in the training of a child is, of course, to secure his moral integrity and a love for true religion. Second in importance comes the discipline of his mind; but next, the wise parent should surely consider the formation of those manners which will be most likely, when he shall be launched into the world outside his home, to gain for the boy a favorable consideration of his more solid qualities of heart and mind. Ungainly movements, a head habitually thrust forward, a heavy, lubberly step, and the painful self-consciousness which usually accompanies these defects when they are under inspection, are distinct and sometimes decisive handicaps upon an aspiring youth. Often they make a disagreeable first impression, which only the most brilliant inner gifts and the most heroic will-power suffice to overcome.[2]

1. Simone de Beauvoir, *The Mandarins; a Novel* (New York, 1956), 378.
2. Kate Upson Clark, *Bringing Up Boys; a Study* (New York, 1899), 62.

Each boy, she wrote, should understand the requirements of duty, the dangers of laziness, and the fact that the "evolution of a strong and forceful character" depended in the last analysis upon male energy, proper manliness, and self-reliance.[3]

The age was literally dotted with heroes to whom a young man could look for guidance—from Gladstone to Bismarck, from Lincoln to Livingstone, from Horatio Alger's little men to the giants of industry and statesmanship. Countless youth organizations catered to this hero-worship and demanded similar response in the coming generation. The Brotherhoods of St. Andrew seized upon romantic affections, the Captains of Ten, founded by Miss A. B. MacKintire, specialized in carving, weaving, and other skills, the Orders of the Knights of King Arthur encouraged hero-loving gallantry, and the Agassiz Association was devoted to science. Various temperance organizations such as the Band of Hope, Juvenile Good Templars, and the Loyal Temperance Legion aided the young boy in his struggle against the temptations of alcohol, while the popular Epworth League and the YMCA looked to the building of a "moral athlete." Believing that the growing boy reproduced successively the ideals of his race, educator H. M. Burr tailored his instructional courses at the YMCA in Springfield, Massachusetts, in an ascending order of seriousness:

1. Race stories, especially Teutonic myths, legends, and folklore.

2. Stories of nature; animal and plant stories.

3. Stories of individual prowess; hero tales—Samson, Hercules, etc. Stories of early inventions.

4. Stories of great leaders and patriots. Social heroes from Moses to Washington.

5. Stories of love; altruism; love of women; love of country and home; love of beauty, truth, and God.[4]

According to Joseph A. Conwell in his *Manhood's Morning* (1896), young men were the chief actors in the history of the world. "In their normal sphere they were the proteges of none, the protectors of all. To a remarkable degree it is true that

3. *Ibid.*, 83.
4. William B. Forbrush, *The Boy Problem; a Study in Social Pedagogy* (Philadelphia, 1902), 145.

young men have founded kingdoms, empires, and republics, and formulated laws and systems of government. They have championed the world's reforms, fought its battles and turned its contests into victories. . . . They have, through discoveries and inventions, kept the wheels of progress busy and turned the world into a thriving mart of commerce."[5] The responsibilities of the young man precluded any weakness, either physical, mental, or moral, for these would only hinder the struggle for an ever-ascending level of progress. His duty to push himself and his race to higher planes of achievement meant that his prime responsibility—to himself and posterity— was to keep mentally and physically fit at all times in order to deal with the ceaseless struggle of evolution. Anything which weakened his vital energy in youth detracted from his potential greatness in maturity. The evils of smoking, chewing, drinking, and swearing stood ominously in the doorway to progress. The plutocracy of wealth, whiskers, and stiff collars could be achieved only through the work ethic and moral strength of one of Horatio Alger's many heroes. Moral vices took their toll in physical suffering, and the sins of youth would be visited upon middle age. Taught from childhood that any sign of weakness or deviation from a restricted path of uprighteousness and conformity would doom him to a life of unproductive or counterproductive obscurity, the Victorian man-child bore the strictures and ever-watchful eyes of parents, teachers, and physicians as he strove toward manhood.

In their position as the moral preceptors of the age, physicians and purity writers undertook to guide the young boy in his search for a moral and physical ethic on which to base his future conduct in the bewildering morass of machinery, technocracy, and changing social values that comprised the Gilded Age. Medical men, steeped in the century's fear of moral weakness, stressed the horrors of sin more than the beauty of virtue. Images of hell seemed to be more impressive than those of heaven (or more easily created), and the vivid portrayals of the physical sufferings of the fallen assailed the

5. Joseph A. Conwell, *Manhood's Morning; or "Go It While You're Young."* *A Book to Young Men between 14 and 28 Years of Age* (New Jersey, 1896), 30; Tandy L. Dix, *The Healthy Infant, a Treatise on the Healthy Procreation of the Human Race* (Cincinnati, 1880), 26.

impressionable mind of the Victorian man-child. Faced at all sides by the horrors of vice and sin, he was made to bear stoically the potential for evil, inherited with Adam's guilt, that his elders assumed all men carried.

The Unmanly Habit

Medical concern with masturbation and other "unnatural" sexual disorders evolved from the century's obsession with the sanctity of the male semen. Nineteenth-century opinions regarding its source and content originated in ideas of the medical ancients, who believed that the seminal fluid (*cerebri stillicidium*) was a discharge of the brain and spinal marrow. Pythagoras called semen the "flower of the blood," while Epicurus looked upon it as a mixture of soul and body. Hippocrates, on the other hand, wrote that "the humours enter into a sort of fermentation, which separates what is most precious and balsamic, and this part, thus separated from the rest, is carried by the spinal marrow to the generative organs."[6] According to a medical treatise published in 1767, the *semen virile* was "the most elaborate and noble production of the whole body, except that of the nerves." Borrowing from Pythagoras, the author identified semen as "the flower and choicest part of the blood and nervous fluid," and for that reason, suggested that the male be judicious in its expenditure, since any great evacuation of the fluid would cause a corresponding decline in health.[7] While Aurelius Celsus spoke of the unnatural or involuntary losses of semen as a wasting of the spine (an opinion which became popular among the farming districts of England in the late nineteenth century), Hippocrates used the term *Tabes Dorsalis* (spinal consumption) to describe the evils attending the unnatural loss of semen from the body. The disease, he surmised, originated in the spinal marrow and attacked young men whose libidinous temperament led

6. Quoted in (A Court Physician), *Reproductive Disorders, Spermatorrhoea, Exhausted Brain, etc. Their Nature, Symptoms, Pathology, and Successful Treatment* (London, 1876), 57; C. Bigelow, *Sexual Pathology: A Practical and Popular Review of the Principal Diseases of the Reproductive Organs* (Chicago, 1875), 36.

7. (A Physician in the Country), *A Short Treatise on Onanism; or, the Detestable Vice of Self-Pollution* (London, 1767), 15, 17.

them to sexual excesses. Although no fever accompanied the disease, the individual lost weight and pined away.[8]

Rather than discount these early theories, medical writers in the first half of the nineteenth century merely added to the plethora of ideas by speaking of the semen as "the essential oil of animal liquors," the purest of the body humors, or the most "spirituous part of the animal frame."[9] As M. Venel wrote in his *Advice to the Nervous and Debilitated of Both Sexes* (1815), semen contained "the most ethereal or subtilized portion of the blood, a highly rectified and refined distillation from every part of the system, particularly the brain and spinal marrow."[10] And in his *Popular Treatise on Venereal Diseases* (1852), author Frederick Hollick drew from the writings of Celsus to support his thesis that the connection between the nervous and sexual systems in the male was not just sympathetic but, in fact, "the nervous substance and the seminal fluid are . . . essentially the same thing."[11] According to Hollick, while the brain and sexual apparatus were placed at opposite ends of the body, they were "like two poles of a Galvanic Pile," connected by the spinal marrow.[12] It was thus reasonable to assume that unnatural emissions would give the victim of self-abuse the sensation that "his mind is passing away," or that "his head was really empty." In fact, Hollick argued, persons who masturbated or suffered from nocturnal emissions did indeed experience mental imbecility or "softening of the brain."[13] The

8. John Davenport, *Curiosities Eroticae, Physiologiae; or Tabooed Subjects Freely Treated* (London, 1875), 68.

9. Sylvester Graham, *A Lecture to Young Men on Chastity. Intended also for the Serious Consideration of Parents and Guardians* (Boston, 1839), 51; Goss and Co., *The Aegis of Life, a Non-Medical Commentary on the Indiscretions Arising from Human Frailty, in which the Causes, Symptoms, and Baneful Effects of Lues, Venerea, Gonorrhoea, Stricture, Seminal Weakness, etc., Are Explained in a Familiar Way* (London, 1827), 72.

10. M. Venel, *Advice to the Nervous and Debilitated of Both Sexes; Containing a Series of Useful and Interesting Information on Subjects of Importance to Married People, or Those on the Eve of Marriage, but Whose Infirmities Are an Insurmountable Bar to Connubial Happiness* (London, 1815), 19.

11. Frederick Hollick, *A Popular Treatise on Venereal Diseases in All Their Forms. Embracing Their History, and Probable Origin; Their Consequences, Both to Individuals and to Society; and the Best Modes of Treating Them* (New York, 1852), 69.

12. *Ibid.*, 44.

13. *Ibid.*, 46.

man who misused his sexual organs in masturbation or became impotent for whatever reason was "in imminent danger of becoming Insane, or at least of weak Intellect," as a result of the drain of vital fluid from his system.[14]

The suggested causes of masturbation were almost legion—from eczema and worms to purgatives and gymnastics. There were even doctors who diagnosed self-abuse when children showed a particular disgust for foods they had previously enjoyed.[15] Eighteenth-century manual writers theorized that the eating of gravies, fish, jellies, and "other provocatives to lust" were contributing causes to the "carnal enjoyments" of youth.[16] By the early nineteenth century, doctors, food faddists, and purity authors had added to the list a number of forbidden foods and condiments. They condemned tea, coffee, chocolate, tobacco, and alcoholic beverages, along with flesh meats, oysters, and eggs as stimulants which irritated the nervous system and which, through their action on the brain, inflamed and excited sexual desires. Salt, pepper, mustard, carraway, cloves, ginger, mace, and fine-flour breads, on the other hand, encouraged constipation which irritated the nerves of the vas deferens and vesiculae seminales, producing morbid desires.[17] "The nicotine of tobacco, dissolved in the alcohol of beer and whiskey," wrote one concerned purity advocate, "finds its way to the deepest and innermost vitals. Thus comingled, they force each other into action, the whole body becomes poison-

14. *Ibid.*, 69; James Graham, *New and Curious Treatise of the Nature and Effects of Simple Earth, Water, and Air, when Applied to the Human Body . . . to Which Is Added, an Appendix Containing Pathetic Remonstrances and Advices to Young Persons, and to Old Men against the Abuse of Certain Debilitating and Degrading Pleasures* (London, 1793), 28–29.

15. Joseph W. Howe, "On the Etiology, Pathology and Treatment of Spermatorrhoea," *Medical Record*, XII (1877), 690; Bigelow, *Sexual Pathology*, 32–33; John Cowan, *The Science of a New Life* (New York, 1871), 359–60.

16. (Anony.), *Onanism Displayed: Being I. An Enquiry into the True Nature of Onan's Sin II. Of the Modern Onanists III. Of Self-Pollution, Its Causes, and Consequences; with Three Extraordinary Cases of Two Young Gentlemen and a Lady Who Were Very Much Addicted to This Crime IV. Of Nocturnal-Pollutions Natural and Forced V. The Great Sin of Self-Pollution with the Judgment of the Most Eminent Divines upon this Subject VI. A Dissertation concerning Generation with a Curious Description of the Parts and of Their Proper Functions, etc., according to the Latest, and Most Approved Anatomical Discoveries* (2nd ed.; London, 1719), 37.

17. Cowan, *The Science of a New Life*, 98–99; (A Physician), *Licentiousness and Its Effects upon Bodily and Mental Health* (New York, 1844), 34–35, 38.

HOWARD ASSOCIATION,

PHILADELPHIA.

IMPORTANT ANNOUNCEMENT

To all persons afflicted with Sexual Diseases, such as SPERMATORRHŒA, SEMINAL WEAKNESS, IMPOTENCE, GONORRHŒA, GLEET, SYPHILIS, the Vice of ONANISM or SELF-ABUSE, &c., &c.

The HOWARD ASSOCIATION of Philadelphia, in view of the awful destruction of human life and health, caused by sexual diseases, and the deceptions which are practised upon the unfortunate victims of such diseases by Quacks, have directed their Consulting Surgeon, as a CHARITABLE ACT worthy of their name, to give MEDICAL ADVICE GRATIS, to all persons thus afflicted (Male or Female,) who apply by letter, with a description of their condition (age, occupation, habits of life, &c.,) and in cases of extreme poverty and suffering, to FURNISH MEDICINES FREE OF CHARGE.

The Howard Association is a benevolent Institution, established by special endowment, for the relief of the sick and distressed, afflicted with "Virulent and Epidemic Diseases," and its funds can be used for no other purpose. It has now a surplus of means, which the Directors have voted to advertise the above notice. It is needless to add that the Association commands the highest Medical skill of the age, and will furnish the most approved modern treatment. Valuable advice also given to sick and nervous females, afflicted with Womb Complaint, Leucorrhœa, &c.

This Institution is appropriately named after HOWARD, the devoted APOSTLE OF HUMANITY, who spent his life and fortune in ministering to the sufferings of his fellow men (especially those "sick and in prison," or afflicted with virulent and pestilential diseases,) and who died at last of a malignant fever, contracted in the pursuit of his noble mission, a MARTYR to the cause he had espoused!

The name of the Association acquires a singular significance, when it is remembered that the only son of the celebrated Philanthropist, Howard, died, at an early age, a raving maniac in a Lunatic Asylum, the victim of gross sexual excesses and loathsome Venereal disease! While the noble father was travelling the world over, on errands of mercy, plunging into fever-haunted dungeons, and confronting the plague in its direst forms, with the hope of reducing the sum of human misery, this degenerate son was spending his days and nights in the brothels and hells of London, poisoning his blood with worse than pestilential taints—taints which destroy not only the body, but even the "immortal part" of man!

Address (post-paid,) Dr. GEO. R. CALHOUN, Consulting Surgeon, Howard Association, No. 2 South NINTH Street, Philadelphia, Pa.

By order of the Directors,

EZRA D. HEARTWELL, PRESIDENT.

GEO. FAIRCHILD, SECRETARY.

The back page of George R. Calhoun, *Report of the Consulting Surgeon on Spermatorrhoea, Seminal Weakness, Impotence, the Vice of Onanism, Masturbation, or Self-Abuse, and Other Diseases of the Sexual Organs,* 1858. National Library of Medicine, Bethesda.

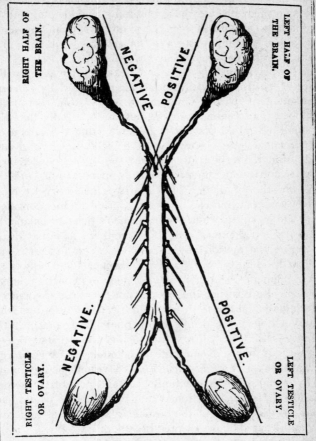

CONNECTION BETWEEN THE
BRAIN AND THE SEXUAL ORGANS.

RIGHT HALF OF THE BRAIN.

LEFT HALF OF THE BRAIN.

NEGATIVE

POSITIVE

NEGATIVE.

POSITIVE.

RIGHT TESTICLE OR OVARY.

LEFT TESTICLE OR OVARY.

The two halves of the Brain are separated, to show they are distinct from each other, and to show their connec-nection with the Sexual Centres.

A medical diagram used to demonstrate the dangers of mas-turbation and spermatorrhea, from F. Hollick, *A Popular Treatise on Venereal Diseases, in All Their Forms, Embracing Their History, and Probable Origin; Their Consequences both to Individuals and to Society; and the Best Modes of Treating Them,* 1852. National Library of Medicine, Bethesda.

soaked and pickled, and only the shadow of the original man is retained. Within the vitals of the young men of America, these two elements are daily poisoning and devitalizing untold millions of human beings yet unborn, inflicting an inevitable curse upon posterity, the result of which will be children with debilitated nerves, impaired intellects, abnormal appetites and passions, and weakened powers of will."[18] Delicate youths were constantly being tortured by concupiscence, wrote Sylvester Graham, by stimulating diets which developed their "animal propensities" more rapidly than their "rational and moral powers."[19] Believing that the semen of a continent male was absorbed by the blood stream and circulated through the body to produce the deeper voice, beard, muscles, and temperament of a truly manly adult, and that, moreover, the circulation of semen was necessary by reason of the "continual increase of seed," purity authors considered the diet a most important factor in man's delicate balance between virtue and animal lust. "It is true that a man may disturb and injure the motion of the seed by excess in diet," wrote William Brodum in 1801, "and various meats and liquors that either augment the quantity of semen too much, render it sharp, or else obstruct the vessels, and so cause a corruption and stagnation of the seed," resulted in various disorders which incited problems of priapism, spermatorrhea, masturbation, and satyriasis.[20] "Very few young men can use cheese, or eggs, or asparagus for the evening meal," commented W. F. Morgan, M.D., in the *New York Medical Times*, "without being annoyed the following night by erections . . . and possibly by seminal emissions." He even cautioned that watermelons would cause unnatural excitement of the sexual organs, "a fact said to be fully appreciated by our colored breathern."[21]

One early manual writer, Bernhard Christian Faust, M.D., in his work *How to Regulate the Sexual Impulse* (1791), blamed masturbation on the custom of wearing breeches at an early

18. Conwell, *Manhood's Morning*, 78–79.
19. Graham, *A Lecture to Young Men on Chastity*, 60–61.
20. William Brodum, *A Guide to Old Age: Or, a Cure for the Indiscretions of Youth* (London, 1801), 135–36.
21. Walter F. Morgan, "Talks with Young Men on the Sexual Function," *New York Medical Times*, XXIV (1896), 334.

age, which produced "a great and damp warmth, which is especially marked in the region of the sexual organs, where the shirt falls into folds." Because the young boy usually encountered difficulties in taking the penis out of his breeches for urinating, he depended upon older children, maids, and manservants to manage for him. "By this handling, pulling, and playing . . . which others do for him, with his sexual organs, the boy is led . . . into constant acquaintanceship with parts which he would otherwise have regarded as sacred, unclean and shameful."[22] Still other medical men blamed "foreign nurses" (usually French or Irish) for inciting the habit among young children by tickling their sexual organs to pacify them.[23] In some cases, fathers were accused of initiating their sons to the practice by testing them for "robustness."[24]

Purity writers in the nineteenth century taught that the healthy male could live until marriage without the loss of a single drop of seminal fluid. "A perfectly healthy, continent man, living a right life socially, morally and physically," remarked John Cowan in his *Science of a New Life* (1871), "does not and cannot have seminal emissions. Health does not absolutely require that there should ever be an emission of semen from puberty to death, though the individual live a hundred years."[25] As Orson Fowler wrote, "only lust creates semen; pure love, never any."[26] On the other hand, each time that the male lost his seed in an "unnatural manner," either by masturbation or by nocturnal emission, he threatened the health of his mind

22. Quoted in Iwan Bloch, *The Sexual Life of Our Time in Its Relations to Modern Civilization* (London, 1909), 427.

23. William Acton, *The Functions and Disorders of the Reproductive Organs in Childhood, Youth, Adult Age, and Advanced Life Considered in Their Physiological, Social, and Moral Relations* (3rd Am. ed., Philadelphia, 1871), 25.

24. Henry N. Guernsey, *Plain Talks on Avoided Subjects* (Philadelphia, 1882), 25.

25. Cowan, *The Science of a New Life*, 120–21.

26. Orson S. Fowler, *Creative and Sexual Science: Or Manhood, Womanhood, and Their Mutual Interrelations: Love, Its Laws, Power, etc., Selection, or Mutual Adaption; Courtship, Married Life, and Perfect Children; Their Generation, Endowment, Paternity, Maternity, Bearing, Nursing, and Rearing; Together with Puberty, Boyhood, Girlhood, etc.; Sexual Impairments Restored, Male Vigor and Female Health and Beauty Perpetuated and Augmented, etc., as Taught by Phrenology and Physiology* (Cincinnati, 1870), 891; Daniel W. Cathell, *Physician Himself, and What He Should Add to His Scientific Acquirements* (Boston, 1882), 111.

and soul because the act sprang "from a willful prostitution of these higher powers."[27] Purity authors regarded unnatural emissions as a more serious loss of vital energy than coition, since the polluter, without an object of love, was forced to invent his pleasure and sensation through the enjoyment of an "imaginary mistress."[28]

> But what more base, more noxious to the body,
> Than by the power of fancy to excite
> Such lewd ideas of an absent object,
> As rouse the organs form'd for nobler ends,
> To rush into th' embraces of a phantom,
> And do the deed of personal enjoyment![29]

"It is not the beautiful Goddess of Love," remarked an author in 1876, "but Circe, the wanton one, and the floating forms are Sirens who allure him—the luckless, the headless, within their deadly embrace." Unless self-control mastered the enticing charms of the sirens, the youth would be left chasing a "fleeing mirage of happiness" and in the dawn of his manhood, sink into a morass of disease and self-hatred. "As the worm silently bores the dyke, and the hidden termite honeycombs the giant timbers, so his strength is sapped and his constitution undermined, and a thousand secret channels afford an inlet to the flood of disease, which could never otherwise have forced nature's barrier."[30]

Besides the pleasurable inventions of the imagination, medical writers blamed the novel for inciting much of what they considered the almost epidemic predilection for self-pollution among young men. The romantic novel tended to excite the emotions, allowing young men to stimulate their feelings without sufficient physical activity to compensate for their excited nervous state. Romantic books sapped the vital energies of the body and besieged the imagination during its idle hours,

27. Guernsey, *Plain Talks on Avoided Subjects*, 61; (A Physician), *Licentiousness and Its Effects upon Bodily and Mental Health*, 17–18.

28. Leopold Deslandes, *Manhood; the Causes of Its Premature Decline, with Directions for Its Perfect Restoration; Addressed to Those Suffering from the Destructive Effects of Excessive Indulgence, Solitary Habits, etc.* (Boston, 1843), 31.

29. (A Physician in the Country), *A Short Treatise on Onanism*, i.

30. (A Court Physician), *Reproductive Disorders*, 66–67; G. M. Phillips, "Sexual Infelicity," *General Practitioner*, II (1896), 155–59.

tempting the mind from its proper responsibilities. "The fancies, once turned in this direction, wear a channel, down which dash the thoughts, gathering force like a river as they move away from the fountain-head."[31] Not without reason, purity writers ruled that no man be permitted to read a novel before his twenty-fifth birthday.[32]

Discussion of the evils of masturbation gained impetus from the publication of a sensational report on idiocy presented to the Massachusetts state legislature in 1848 by the superintendent of the lunatic asylum at Worcester, who claimed that 32 percent of admissions to the hospital were insane because of self-pollution.[33] Within a few years, medical writers had incorporated the report in almost every purity pamphlet and book for young men, and superintendents of asylums across the country were besieged with requests to substantiate the claims of the Massachusetts report. Few were willing to challenge the superintendent's claim, and soon the whole issue became exaggerated out of proportion by purity crusaders and medical quacks who took the opportunity to expound upon their own private analysis of the national disease. The clarion call by the superintendent of the Massachusetts asylum, however, was no idle statement; rather it represented what seemed to be the majority opinion in the medical profession at that time, or at least the majority opinion of doctors writing on the subject. Those few who remained skeptical of the relationship between self-abuse and insanity all too often became the pariahs of the profession.

W. S. Chipley's *A Warning to Fathers, Teachers and Young Men, in Relation to a Fruitful Cause of Insanity and Other Serious Disorders of Youth* (1861) was one of the many books published in the aftermath of the Massachusetts report which related masturbation to insanity and other equally frightful diseases. As medical superintendent of the Eastern Lunatic Asylum in Lexington, Kentucky, Chipley pointed to the high number of insane who practiced self-pollution, and then argued

---

31. Anthony Comstock, *Traps for the Young* (New York, 1883), 11.
32. Sylvanus Stall, *What a Young Man Ought to Know* (Philadelphia, 1897), 33.
33. Bigelow, *Sexual Pathology*, 50.

that masturbation had been the main cause of their insanity. In addition to insanity, however, the superintendent warned that epilepsy and allied paroxysms preyed upon the mental powers of self-polluters. "The subjects rapidly sink into the most hopeless state of drivelling idiocy," he wrote, "some find a lower level than that occupied by the most senseless brutes; or, their stupidity is interrupted only by outbursts of uncontrollable and destructive violence, during which they seem to lose all consciousness of surrounding objects; they appear to neither hear, see nor feel, but strike indifferently at every thing within their reach."[34] The paroxysms of insanity and epilepsy resulted from the willful transgression of nature's laws. "It seemed impious to attribute to the Creator," commented William M. Cornell, M.D., "any such glaring imperfection" in God's handiwork as insanity. The existence of large numbers of idiots in every generation was the consequence of violations of the natural law and, believing that every violation brought retribution, physicians felt that the sin of self-abuse had been met with the most serious physical consequences.

It is the immutable decree of the Almighty that fire shall burn, and the person who puts his hand into it will be burned. So it is just as immutable in the divine economy of this world that "abusers of themselves" shall suffer. They may murmur, and repine against Providence; they may say God gave them passions to be indulged, and they will indulge them; they may sit in sullen despair when the consequences of transgression begin to overtake them; but it will all be to no purpose. No natural law of God will be changed for their convenience or accommodation. The whips and scourges, the idiotic and insane minds, epilepsies, spasms, consumptions, loss of vision, hearing, feeling, paralysis, asthma, catarrh, and the thousands of other weaknesses and deformities of body and mind that follow a violated law of our being, will continue to follow it—by day and by night, in youth and in age. As long as men sin, so long they shall suffer, and they may be sure their sin will find them out.[35]

Unlike any other vice, warned Joseph Conwell, the ravages of masturbation were "written in the countenance"; the symp-

34. W. S. Chipley, *A Warning to Fathers, Teachers and Young Men, in Relation to a Frightful Cause of Insanity and Other Serious Disorders of Youth* (Louisville, Ky., 1861), 117.

35. William M. Cornell, *The Beacon: Or, a Warning to Young and Old* (Philadelphia, 1865), 41; Chipley, *A Warning to Fathers, Teachers, and Young Men*, 64–69.

toms were self-evident and designed to arouse suspicion in parents and friends as well as frighten the polluter with the torments of endless suffering.[36] By his shy and retiring mannerisms, his display of "unusual sadness," and his suspicions of those around him, the polluter publicly admitted his guilt. Confused by defective memory and hearing, he soon became negligent in his personal habits and acted dull and stupid before other people. In conversation, the masturbator could never look a person in the face, but averted his eyes. He avoided the glances of women, yet stole every opportunity to look at them. He was known for his pallid, bloodless, countenance, hollow and "half-ghastly eyes." When the habit continued for any length of time, however, his eyes acquired black and blue semicircles popularly known as "plague-spots." Eventually his memory failed, he lost his power to concentrate, ceased to be self-reliant, and succumbed slowly to the poisonous venom of pollution. This changed the color of his skin and made his muscles flabby, he avoided work as distasteful, and complained of backaches, dizziness, and indigestion. Soon, the stooping hollow-chested skeleton of the former man wasted away, succumbing after long illness to consumption, diabetes, jaundice, or general blood diseases. Physicians believed that self-pollution was often an indirect cause of death, and indeed, in some cases, was a direct cause.[37]

> In vain we scan the springs of human woe,
> To find a deadlier or more cruel foe
> To erring man, than this sad self-pollution,
> This damning wrecker of his constitution.
>
> In its foul march it tramples vigor down,
> Darkens the soul, usurps the mental throne,
> Preys upon the vitals of its filthy slave,
> And drags him early to a hopeless grave.
> Could this truth to all be known and foreseen,

36. Conwell, *Manhood's Morning*, 79.

37. Roberts Bartholow, *On Spermatorrhoea: Its Causes, Symptomatology, Pathology, Prognosis, Diagnosis, and Treatment* (New York, 1866), 19–20; Orson S. Fowler, *Amativeness: Or Evils and Remedies of Excessive and Perverted Sexuality: Including Warning and Advice to the Married and Single* (New York, 1846), 51–52; Bigelow, *Sexual Pathology*, 48; C. S. Eldridge, *Self-Enervation: Its Consequences and Treatment* (Chicago, 1869), 16–19.

A sea of misery would be spared the world,
And hell's own engine from the land be hurled.

The fire of heaven on Onan quickly fell,
Cursed was the culprit ere he sank to hell,
Brief was the period 'twixt the noxious deed
And the dread chastisement, pollution's meed.
Just as certain now as then, is the indulger undone,
Not by ethereal stroke as there we see,
But equal in effect and certainty,
For death results although by slow degree.[38]

In order to guard against the possibility of self-pollution,
purity writers continually advised parents to keep boys occupied in useful work. If this was accomplished, William Acton
observed, the properly educated child would grow to adult-
hood without any sexual notions or feelings entering his head,
"even in the way of speculation."[39] To ensure this, boys were
not to be pampered, and any sedentary habits should be
quickly ended—they were not to lie in bed after awaking, nor
were they to sleep on their stomachs for fear of heating the
genital parts. Precocious development, long hours working at
school without proper exercise, tight clothes, desire for flagel-
lation by teachers, love of dancing, or sliding on poles or trees
were considered dangerous signs of self-pollution. Pure-minded
parents were encouraged to be ever watchful of their children
when they undressed, bathed, went to the privy, or slept.
"Watch his motions as the child lies with covered head," wrote
another author, "listen to his breathing. Is it quick, hurried,
gasping, sighing? There is danger lurking there." In boarding
schools, there should be no private rooms, and the common
sleeping chambers were to be always lighted to assist watch-
fulness. "In some schools the doors to the privies are open at
the top, so that an adult can look into them. Need we add that
persons who are suspected should be watched in the bath."[40]

Occasionally, medical writers prescribed marriage as the
only proper cure for masturbation. Total suppression of the
habit without a "natural" evacuation of semen, they warned,

---

38. R. N. Barr, "Spermatorrhoea," *Ohio Medical and Surgical Journal,* VII
(1855), 174–75.
39. Acton, *The Functions and Disorders of the Reproductive Organs,* 17–18.
40. Chipley, *A Warning to Fathers, Teachers and Young Men,* 176–77.

would cause satyriasis, and swelling and inflammation of the testicles. Total abstinence without recourse to marriage could only be accomplished with the continuous use of cathartics and other evacuants. "There is no fact more certain," wrote one physician in the 1870s, "than that an organ which has been unduly excited, and is partially exhausted, will atrophy if relegated to inaction." Youths who were given to unnatural excesses and then "suddenly reigned up" and forced to live in a state of continence were liable to become impotent. For these persons, an "occasional connexion," local electrization, or aphrodisiacs were considered helpful until more regular intercourse in marriage could be obtained.[41]

Treatment for masturbation reflected a potpourri of medical folklore, mechanical gadgetry, and medieval torture, all designed to simultaneously control the vice and punish the sinner. Although some practitioners merely recommended pure thoughts, early rising, a brisk walk before breakfast, and marriage, most looked to more ingenious cures such as ice or cold cataplasms to the sexual parts at bedtime, electromagnetism, and hydrotherapeutic techniques. One water cure, the so-called "sweating process," consisted of encouraging perspiration and then alternating it with cold air or baths; in another method, a wet sheet was wrapped around the person and as soon as he became warm, the sheet was replaced with another.[42] More mechanically inclined doctors constructed special beds to prevent the sleeper from turning over, sold "handbags" which were tied to the side of the bed at night, and designed a chemise which reached below the feet and was drawn together at the bottom to prevent the careless exploring of hands.[43] In Sylvanus Stall's *What a Young Boy Ought to Know*, the author suggested straitjackets for masturbators to sleep in; he also recommended tying the hands to the posts of

41. (A Court Physician), *Reproductive Disorders*, 205–6.

42. (A Physician), *Licentiousness and Its Effects upon Bodily and Mental Health*, 94–102.

43. Deslandes, *Manhood*, 233; Homer Bostwick, *A Treatise on the Nature and Treatment of Seminal Diseases, Impotency, and Other Kindred Affections; with Practical Directions for the Management and Removal of the Cause Producing Them; Together with Hints to Young Men* (New York, 1848), 62–63; L. D. Fleming, *Self-Pollution, the Cause of Youthful Decay: Showing the Dangers and Remedy of Venereal Excess* (New York, 1846), 15–20.

the bed, or to rings in the wall.[44] These procedures were originally suggested in the 1840s by Deslandes, who not only prescribed the "straight waistcoat fastened behind, which may force the arms to rest on the chest," but also, in the event that the measure was not quite sufficient, ordered parents to tie the feet so that the thighs would remain separated. In some instances, he contrived "cork cushions" which he placed on the inside of the thighs to keep them apart. In addition, he fashioned a metal truss of silver (or tin) in which the penis and scrotum were placed and held by springs, and to add to the security of the truss, he prescribed clothes which opened only from behind.[45] These so-called "genital cages" were a nineteenth-century derivative of the chastity belts of the Middle Ages, and could be purchased from a variety of suppliers who advertised in popular journals and newspapers.[46] R. J. Culverwell advertised in his *Professional Records* (1846) a special chair designed to serve as a douche bidet for the masturbator. The contraption consisted of an arm chair with an open seat, beneath which was a zinc pan filled with cold water or a "medicated refrigerant fluid." By means of a pump, the masturbator could direct the fluid to his genitals, thereby "cooling" his sexual ardor during those moments when he was most susceptible to acts of unnatural venery.[47] Other doctors treated the habit by blood-letting, or applying leeches and cups around the sexual parts to remove "congestion." Still others perforated the foreskin of the penis and inserted a ring, or cut the foreskin

44. Sylvanus Stall, *What a Young Boy Ought to Know* (Philadelphia, 1909), 117.

45. Deslandes, *Manhood,* 234.

46. John Moodie, *Medical Treatise; with Principles and Observations, to Preserve Chastity and Morality* (Edinburgh, 1848), 69–72; Eric J. Dingwall, *The Girdle of Chastity; a Medico-Historical Study* (London, 1931), 124–28. The U.S. Patent Office lists several "genital cage" inventions for men.
    (1) Michael McCormick of San Francisco (1897) no. 587,994.
    (2) Joseph Lees of Pennsylvania (1900) no. 641,979. This particular device sounded an electrical alarm in the event of an erection.
    (3) Raphael Sonn of Georgia (1906) no. 827,377.
    (4) Ellen E. Perkins of Minnesota (1906) no. 875,845.
For a brief description of these inventions see James L. Harte, "When Men Wore Chastity Belts," *Real Life Guide,* I (1957), 3–5.

47. Robert J. Culverwell, *Professional Records. The Institutes of Marriage, Its Intent, Obligations, and Physical and Constitutional Disqualifications* (New York, 1846), 75.

with jagged scissors.[48] Drugs included applications of red iron, tartar emetic ointment, or a Spanish fly-blister to make the genitals tender to the touch.[49] "It is better to go to any amount of trouble and to endure any physical discomfort," wrote Henry Guernsey, M.D., in his *Plain Talks on Avoided Subjects,* "than to sacrifice one's chastity, the loss of which can never be replaced."[50]

In 1875, Orson Fowler, whose popular books on love and marriage touched on everything from animal magnetism to phrenology, birthmarks, and health foods, presented what he called the "Life-Boat Resolution" for persons addicted to self-abuse. The prayer had all the fervor of a biblical psalm.

I wash away the stain of the past in the reformation of the future. Born with capabilities thus exalted, I will yet be the man, no longer the grovelling sensualist. Forgetting the past, I once more put on the garments of hope, and press forward in pursuit of those noble life-ends to which I once aspired, but from which this Delilah allured me. On the bended knees of contrition and supplications I bow before Jehovah's mercy-seat: On the altar of this hour I lay my vow of abstinence and purity. No more will I sacrilegiously prostitute those glorious gifts with which Thou hast graciously crowned me. I abjure forever this loathsome sin, and take again the oath of allegiance to duty and to Thee. O, "deliver me from temptation!" Of myself I am weak, but in Thy strength I am strong. Do Thou work in me to "will and to do" only what is pure and holy. I have served "the lusts of the flesh;" but O, forgive and restore a repentant prodigal, and accept this entire consecration of my every power and faculty to Thee. O gracious God, forgive, and save, and accept; and Thine shall be the glory forever, Amen.

I rise a renewed man. My vow is recorded before God. I will keep it inviolate. I will banish all unclean thoughts and feelings, and indulge only in holy wedlock. I will "press forward" on the road of intellectual attainment and moral progression; and the more eagerly because of this hindrance. I drop but this one tear over the past, and then bury both my sin and shame in future efforts of self-improvement and labors of love. I yet will rise. As mourning over my fall does not restore, but unnerves resolution and cripples effort, I cast the mantle of forgetfulness over the past, have now to do only with the future, but must not remain

48. Deslandes, *Manhood,* 186; Bloch, *The Sexual Life of Our Time,* 427–28.
49. Bostwick, *A Treatise on the Nature and Treatment of Seminal Diseases,* 62–63; Henry M. Lyman, *et al., The Practical Home Physician* (Chicago, 1883), 541–42.
50. Guernsey, *Plain Talks on Avoided Subjects,* 62–63.

a moment passive or idle. I have a great work before me, to repair my shattered constitution, which is the work not of a day, and also to recover my mental stamina and moral standing, and, if possible, to soar higher still.[51]

There were a few physicians in the nineteenth century willing to challenge popular beliefs concerning masturbation. Samuel W. Gross, in his *Practical Treatise on Sterility, and Allied Disorders of the Male Sexual Organs* (1881), remarked that he had never known an instance of insanity, dementia, or phthisis to follow masturbation. Similarly, Sir James Paget, in his *Clinical Lectures and Essays* (1875), stated that "masturbation does neither more nor less harm than sexual intercourse practiced with the same frequency in the same conditions of general health, and age, and circumstances." Whatever ills ensued, he suggested, resulted from the "quantity, not the method."[52] T. F. Lockwood, M.D., writing in 1904, found it strange that "this long-practiced art . . . has waited these many years for someone to take a stand in defense of its rights." Far too many practitioners, he reminded the medical profession, had been reluctant to speak of the practice for fear of being classed as advocates of immorality. The generative organs required the same exercise demanded by other bodily parts. "Surely," he wrote, "a testicle that has descended from its congenital moorings and lies dormant in its secluded sac, and is never called into question or duty upon any occasion, will become useless." Unable to eject his secretion in a normal sexual function, a man would find the fluid passed involuntarily during "phantom copulation" in sleep. But although nocturnal emission was the usual manner of ejecting stored-up fluid, masturbation was by no means unnatural. "I do believe it is wrong to condemn the whole function as a blast to the rising young because some poor weak-willed Willie has abused the privilege," he wrote. "It is not the physical exertion in the process of masturbation that causes the evil effect, if there be any, for it matters not what means are utilized to bring about an orgasm; it is the too frequent orgasm that may sap the life from the body; and if

51. Orson S. Fowler, *Sexual Science* (Philadelphia, 1875), 382–83.
52. Samuel W. Gross, *A Practical Treatise on Impotence, Sterility, and Allied Disorders of the Male Sexual Organs* (Philadelphia, 1881), 28; Sir James Paget, *Clinical Lectures and Essays* (London, 1875), 284.

the masturbator does not indulge any oftener than he would in natural intercourse, there is no more danger in it than in the former." Lockwood was particularly disgusted with the purity-minded jeremiads who predicted physical and mental retribution on those who transgressed the sacred laws of sex. "So, dear hearer," he concluded, "if you find yourself [either sterile or impotent] blame no one for it but self-modesty and rare opportunities to cultivate the little pitiful appendage that now adorns the middle anterior portion of your anatomy."[53]

The views of men like Lockwood and Paget, however, were drowned out in the lamentations of Deslandes, Acton, Lallemand, and a host of others, who did not believe the male organ would shrink if not properly exercised. "When any such decrease in size does occur," one wrote, "it will be found to be caused by exactly the reverse—namely, excessive exercise by self-abuse."[54] In his chapter outline on self-abuse, purity author Sylvanus Stall reflected the prevailing opinion on the matter: "God Intended Man to Work—Many Seem to Be Born Lazy—All Must Learn to Work—Some Forms of Labor Call into Service Only a Few Muscles—Every Muscle Should Do Service—Importance of Exercise—The Boy's Bible and Dum-Bells—The Muscles Developed by Exercise—This Not True of the Sexual Member."[55]

Bachelor's Disease

With the possible exception of masturbation, spermatorrhea, first described by French surgeon Claude-Francois Lallemand in his *Des pertes seminales involontaires* (1836), was the single most discussed problem in instructional books for boys and young men. Although many eighteenth- and early nineteenth-century physicians diagnosed the urethral discharge as a form of contagious clap ("gonorrhea dormientium") and immediately doused their patients with salivatory doses of mercury, Lalle-

53. T. F. Lockwood, "Sexual Orgasm a Physiological Function Requisite to Maintain Healthy Sexual Capacity," *Medical Record,* XXI (1904), 146–47.

54. Cowan, *The Science of a New Life,* 118; E. L. Keys, "The Sexual Necessity," *Medical News,* LXXXVII (1905), 72–74; R. C. Bankston, "Man's Predominant Passion—Sexual Instinct and Its Control," *Alabama Medical Journal,* XII (1901), 473–85.

55. Stall, *What a Young Boy Ought to Know,* 142.

mand believed that many sufferers had never experienced sexual relations and suspected that their peculiar "seminal leakage" resulted from the initial practice of masturbation. A large number of young men inflamed their minds by reading lascivious books and dreaming of sexual pleasures, and having begun self-pollution to gratify their morbid thoughts, they found themselves not only demanding sexual relief during the day but at night also. "Under both circumstances," wrote a physician in 1845, "the gratification derived by contemplating the image, on the one hand, and by the physical excitement, on the other, keeps up a constant irritation" to the point that seminal secretions became chronic. Before the vigilant parent or physician could discover the nature of the youth's problem, his body became debilitated, his sexual organs impotent, and both the generative fluids and the vital forces of the body drained to such an alarming degree that the victim all too often succumbed to consumption, epilepsy, insanity, or an early grave.[56] One popular nineteenth-century sex manual for men even explained that the real reason for Samson's weakness in the Old Testament story was the involuntary loss of seminal fluid resulting from his prurient thoughts of Delilah.[57]

Writers on spermatorrhea warned against delay in seeking medical attention. "Whoever finds that he is, even but in the smallest degree, subject to emissions . . . or is even troubled with nightly erections of the penis," wrote C. Bigelow in his *Sexual Pathology* (1875), "should seek advice and assistance from some good physician, and that without delay."[58] Taking his cue from a multitude of earlier jeremiads on the masturbation problem, Bigelow warned that untreated spermatorrhea caused a weakness of the mind, and its victims tended to become dull and listless, substituting "shadowy dreams" and "erratic phantasms" for intellectual labor. Taking less and less interest in their business affairs, they found themselves becoming increasingly tired, with poor respiration and irregular

56. Claude-Francois Lallemand, *A Practical Treatise on the Causes, Symptoms, and Treatment of Spermatorrhoea* (Philadelphia, 1853), xiv; Bostwick, *A Treatise on the Nature and Treatment of Seminal Diseases*, 46–47; Goss and Co., *The Aegis of Life*, 14.

57. Stall, *What a Young Man Ought to Know*, 77.

58. Bigelow, *Sexual Pathology*, 72.

heat beat.[59] Indeed, the medical prognosis for unattended spermatorrhea was tantalizingly macabre, with the victim sliding nightmarishly from one disaster into another. In the early stages, the male would complain of weakness and listlessness; nervous and shy, he tended to avoid company and conversation. Soon, his complexion became pale and he showed signs of emaciation. These latter signs were followed by dull pains in the loins and lower extremities, fatigue at the slightest exertion, constipation, watery eyes, and memory losses. As the seminal emissions continued, they were accompanied not only by libidinous dreams but by diminished erections and decreased pleasure as well. Ultimately, emissions occurred without erection or sensation at all, and any attempt at natural connection resulted in impotency.

The disrelish for society increases; dyspeptic symptoms become more evident; inexplicable pains in all parts of the body; the mind more enfeebled and incapable of attention; the memory more fallacious; the disposition more morose; a general sadness, even to tears, upon trivial occasions. The aspect becomes dejected; the patient rarely raises his eyes from the ground, even when addressed; conscious of his wretched condition, and fearful of discovery, he prefers solitude, and in many cases will not acknowledge his affliction, even on the repeated inquiries of the physician. The tendency to constipation generally increases with the disease; the urine is passed more frequently; the genital organs decrease in size, and denote feebleness; the testicles hang pendulous in the scrotum, which is void of rugae; erections after a time cease altogether, the most exciting positions failing to produce them, or, if produced, are so transient a nature that the act cannot be consummated; debility and loss of flesh increase; severe headache, giddiness, cough, and palpitation are added to the catalogue of symptoms; and the patient frequently wishing for death, without the courage to destroy himself, exposes himself to dangers avoided by other men, trusting that chance will accomplish that which he has not the daring although the desire to effect. At length, epilepsy, catalepsy, mania, or some other disease of the nervous system, makes its appearance, and the patient is relieved from his horrid state of existence by a premature death, the cause of which had frequently been entirely overlooked by his unsuspecting physician.[60]

Lallemand's theory of spermatorrhea was not confined to the medical profession alone. Almost immediately, sections of his

59. *Ibid.*, 58–59.
60. George N. Dangerfield, "The Symptoms, Pathology, Causes and Treatment of Spermatorrhoea," *Lancet*, I (1843), 211.

works were quoted and misquoted in journals, pamphlets, newspapers, and magazines throughout Europe and America. Spermatorrhea became a familiar if not a household word, with almost every sexual hypochondriac diagnosing his real or imagined generative problems in terms of the alarming new disease. From the professional medical journal to the popular magazine, he could read of the near-epidemic character of the disease and find some cure proportional to his pocketbook and as accessible as the corner drugstore, mailbox, or local nostrum vendor. Distraught males, believing themselves victims of the dreaded disease after having a single wet dream, wrote impassioned letters to medical men, itinerant quacks, and proprietors of anatomical galleries or museums who dispensed their miracle drugs and devices from basements or backyard laboratories. Feeding upon the fears of an adolescent population, and using every means short of extortion to fleece their victims, these self-styled specialists in the treatment of generative disorders plied their trade by offering cures at a "modest" or "self-sacrificing" price. Claiming a humanitarian desire to prevent further misfortune, nostrum sellers encouraged thousands of young men who were guilt-ridden with the horrors of their private disease to seek their special services.

In many instances, the spermatorrhea victim found it easier to confess his private habits to an itinerant quack than to face his family physician with the evidence. In correspondence with these specialists, the victim usually admitted to self-abuse and the subsequent fear engendered by the first nocturnal emission. In addition, he sent a urine specimen so that an examination could be made for the presence of semen. The patient was usually informed that he not only suffered from nocturnal leakage (by his own admission) but that his semen was escaping diurnally through the urine, and unless the condition was treated immediately, his spinal marrow would waste away, his brain would soften, and he would end his days in an insane asylum. Struck by such warnings, patients willingly gave their fortunes in medical fees to correct the problem and contracted with the specialist to supply the proper amount of cure. One skeptical prankster sent a vial of cider instead of urine to a quack and was informed in the most serious language that it contained "a very large proportion of seminal fluid!"[61] According to the Chicago Vice Commission report, quacks sometimes offered to return a patient's money in the event that he was not cured, but the patient first had to secure the signatures of his minister, "a principal business man in his community," a member of his family, and have the signatures notarized, certifying that the habit existed before treatment and that the treatment had not affected a cure.[62]

Treatment for spermatorrhea ranged from an electric alarm which sounded under the sleeper's pillow when the penis expanded by erection and completed an electrical circuit; to Lallemand's cauterization of the urethra. A most popular device was the four-pointed urethral ring consisting of a leather or silk sheath with steel points turned inwards. The points of the steel ring remained flat against the penis until erection, when they arose and pressed against the skin to awaken the sleeper. Some of these sheaths were secured by small locks so that the sleeper could not remove them at night. Armand Trousseau (1801–67) recommended the insertion into the rectum of a wooden ovoid cylinder the size of a pigeon's egg, large enough to compress the prostate gland. The egg, worn both day and night, was not designed to prevent erection or ejaculation, but was thought to redirect emission by forcing the semen backwards into the bladder.[63] Although the device was more popular in Europe than America, there were metal, rubber, and porcelain "eggs" sold in the St. Louis area during the 1860s and 1870s.[64] There were other more barbaric mechanisms which applied pressure to the penis in order to forcibly prevent emission. Frank Harris, in his autobiography *My Life and Loves,* mentioned tying a piece of leather whipcord around his penis at night. "As soon as the organ began to swell and stiffen in excitement," he wrote, "the cord would grow tight and awake me with pain."[65] This device, remarked

61. (A Court Physician), *Reproductive Disorders,* 199.
62. Vice Commission of Chicago, *The Social Evil of Chicago* (Chicago, 1911), 221–22.
63. Bartholow, *On Spermatorrhoea,* 85–86.
64. A. P. Lankford, "Some Practical Suggestions about Spermatorrhoea," *Medical Herald,* V (1871), 295.
65. Frank Harris, *My Life and Loves* (New York, 1963), 52.

one medical skeptic, had as much success as stopping a man from vomiting by compressing his throat.[66] William Acton, whose study of sexual disorders received wide currency in both Europe and America, prescribed a very simple and inexpensive procedure of tying a towel around the waist with a large knot to prevent the sleeper from lying on his back. Other physicians contrived preventatives such as tying the patient's hands to a bedpost, or the use of a thin sheet of lead spread over the mattress, on which was fastened a piece of wood, which, in turn, connected to a girdle about the sleeper's loins to prevent him from moving in bed.[67]

Internal remedial agents included ergot (used by physicians in the last stages of labor and by some women to induce abortion in the early months of pregnancy) to induce the contraction of the inter-rachidian vessels, quinine, bromide of potassium, chalybeate waters, squills, digitalis, strychnia with iron, belladonna, cimicifuga, cannabis indica, and opium.[68] In addition, doctors prescribed nightly purging, injections of tepid water into the rectum, drafts of unsweetened gin in hot water, hemlock poultices to the perineum, strenuous exercise, galvanism, electromagnetism, "electric baths" of static electricity along the spinal column and genitals, and even suction cups to the perineum to draw blood, after which the region was blistered with cantharides.[69]

The book, *Reproductive Disorders, Spermatorrhoea, Exhausted Brain, etc.; Their Nature, Symptoms, Pathology and Successful Treatment*, written in 1876 by "a court physician," was a typical example of nineteenth-century medical terrorism.

66. (A Court Physician), *Reproductive Disorders*, 175.
67. Bartholow, *On Spermatorrhoea*, 103–4; Acton, *The Functions and Disorders of the Reproductive Organs*, 233.
68. John L. Milton, "On the Nature and Treatment of Spermatorrhoea," *Lancet*, I (1854), 244–45.
69. Cowan, *The Science of a New Life*, 346; Culverwell, *Professional Records*, 198–99; Dangerfield, "The Symptoms, Pathology, Causes and Treatment of Spermatorrhoea," 215; Bartholow, *On Spermatorrhoea*, 106; George G. Gascoyen, "On Spermatorrhoea and Its Treatment," *British Medical Journal*, I (1872), 96; Barr, "Spermatorrhoea," 180; Wesley Grindle, *New Medical Revelations, Being a Popular Work on the Reproductive System, Its Debility and Disease* (Philadelphia, 1857), 120–21; John S. Haller, Jr., "The Glass Leech: Wet and Dry Cupping Practices in the Nineteenth Century," *New York State Journal of Medicine*, LXXIII (1973), 583–92.

Although published in London, it sold widely in America and the anonymous author made frequent references to American medical men and the problems of their patients. He began by stressing the increasing evidence of nervous and sexual exhaustion among the urban business class. Borrowing many of his ideas from New York physician George M. Beard, who introduced the term "neurasthenia" to the Western world, the author claimed that brain-workers in the advanced countries of the world were reaping the bitter harvest of sexual excesses in youth and overzealous passions in married life. With their systems already taxed by the responsibilities of state and the pressures of the money market, they now succumbed to depression, impotency, and the involuntary loss of spermatic fluid. Supporting the thesis that semen was a superior quality of nerve substance and that its essence was equivalent to forty times its weight in blood, the author warned of the disastrous effects involuntary leakage would have on the brain and spinal cord.[70] In order to cure spermatorrhea, he encouraged cold bathing, outdoor exercise, wearing an urethral ring, sleeping on a hair mattress with little covering over the genitals, and avoiding erotic novels or dallying with questionable women. In addition, brain-workers were to shun intimate dinners, spiced foods, oysters, and alcoholic beverages. He also suggested occasional intercourse, which he felt would cause less depression than that which followed an "unnatural" emission. As for drugs, he prescribed both depressants and aphrodisiacs.[71] Ultimately, however, success could only be obtained so long as the rays of the moon were not permitted to fall upon the sleeper![72]

A number of institutes and museums of anatomy existed on the fringe of medical respectability, publishing booklets on disorders of the nervous system and reproductive organs and offering "private treatment." The Peabody Medical Institute of Boston, staffed by physicians Albert Hayes and Willard Parker, and the New York Museum of Anatomy, run by L. Henry

70. (A Court Physician), *Reproductive Disorders*, 57.
71. *Ibid.*, 205.
72. *Ibid.*, 184.

Jordan, guaranteed the utmost secrecy for patients suffering from masturbation or seminal losses. In the event the patient wished to have a personal consultation, the booklets informed him that the office was "free from observation (no idlers hanging around the doorway, so common to other localities), and patients . . . will see no one but the Doctor himself, as his numerous parlors are specially adapted to this purpose." Those who preferred to be "corresponding patients" were likewise promised secrecy; all letters would be either returned to the sender or burned upon completion of treatment—provided the consultation fee of five dollars was included in each letter or "specimen box."[73] In numerous instances, however, the patient's letters were simply published in future pamphlets designed to alarm the public of the seriousness of the disease, or were sold to patent drug companies as potential buyers of bogus cures.[74]

The creation of philanthropic organizations such as the Howard Association of Philadelphia, dedicated to the work of English prison, hospital, and asylum reformer, John Howard (1726–90), was an example of early efforts to reform the near monopoly which medical quacks and nostrum sellers held on sexual disorders. But even the reform agencies placed a premium on secrecy. Believing that private rather than public agencies had the greater opportunity for correcting the misfortunes of the sexually diseased, the association encouraged persons to write to its medical board describing their condition and history of treatment. With this information the directors of the association promised to consider each individual case and write out their pharmaceutical prescriptions "in plain English . . . in order that [the patients] may obtain and use the drugs themselves, without being subject to the deceptions of drug-

---

73. Albert H. Hayes, *The Science of Life: Or Self-Preservation* (Boston, 1868), appendix; Jordan and Beck, *The Philosophy of Marriage, Being Four Important Lectures on the Functions and Disorders of the Nervous System and Reproductive Organs* (New York, 1863); L. H. Jordan, *Man's Mission on Earth! A Treatise on Nervous Debility and Physical Exhaustion* (New York, 1871), 178–81; J. Hamilton, *Nervous-Exhaustion, Hints of Vital Importance to Youth and Manhood* (London, n.d.), 29–31; Anthony Comstock, *Frauds Exposed; or How the People Are Deceived and Robbed, and Youth Corrupted* (New York, 1880), chaps. 28 and 29.

74. M. L. Stevens, "Chastity and Health," *Southern Medicine and Surgery*, XXX (1907), 138.

gists, who often wilfully mislead them in respect to recipes which they cannot understand."[75]

Medical journals in the nineteenth century carried numerous charges that doctors were advising illicit sex for unmarried men in order to prevent spermatorrhea. A majority of those who spoke out felt that such irregular prescriptions infringed on the laws of religion and morality and demanded strict continence as the only cure for seminal losses. "The frequency of involuntary nocturnal emissions," wrote a medical adviser in 1874, "is an indubitable proof that the parts . . . are suffering under a debility and morbid irritability utterly incompatible with the general welfare of the system, and the mental faculties are always debilitated and impaired by such indulgence."[76] Many physicians who took seriously the early theories on the nature and source of spermatic fluid believed that healthy and virtuous men reabsorbed the spermatic fluid so that it not only enriched the blood but brought added vitality to the brain as well. "The young man who would secure the highest and best development of his physical and intellectual powers," wrote the author of one sex manual, "will carefully seek to avoid, as far as possible, all loss of sexual fluid, either in the form of emissions or even in the form of lawful sexual intercourse."[77] Indeed, many manuals referred to John Locke and William Pitt as men of enormous intelligence who never married and yet "never in any way gratified the sexual desire," and the statement by Sir Isaac Newton that he never lost a single drop of seminal fluid. Frank Harris repeated a conversation concerning Balzac, as told by the French poet and novelist Theophile Gautier:

"What's the matter?" asked Gautier.
"Matter enough," replied Balzac; "another masterpiece lost to French Literature!"
"What do you mean?" cried Gautier.
"I had a wet dream last night," Balzac replied, "and consequently shall

75. George R. Calhoun, *Report of the Consulting Surgeon on Spermatorrhoea, or Seminal Weakness, Impotence, the Vice of Onanism, Masturbation, or Self-Abuse, and Other Diseases of the Sexual Organs* (Philadelphia, 1858), 22.
  76. Cowan, *The Science of a New Life,* 120–21.
  77. Stall, *What a Young Man Ought to Know,* 76–77.

not be able to conceive any good story for at least a fortnight; yet I could certainly write a masterpiece in that time."[78]

Not all physicians, however, were inclined to accept strict continence. "If we consider the subject without reference to religion," wrote W. H. Ranking, M.D., in *Lancet*, "the opinion of Lallemand appears to be rational in that the occasional employment of the organs would conduce to their vigor, upon the principle that a muscular organ is invigorated by moderate exercise."[79] English physician John Chatto was similarly inclined to discredit the moralists on this issue. "An organ unexercised," he wrote, "remains insufficiently developed, or falls into a greater or less state of decay. . . . Promiscuous sexual intercourse is only the lesser of two evils which the unfortunate arrangements of society force upon us, and if it is to be sternly prohibited, rely upon it, nature will find a substitute too often, even though all happiness and all moral considerations must become eventually undermined by the use of such substitute."[80]

The controversy over continence versus sexual intercourse as a cure for spermatorrhea continued well into the late nineteenth century. For many medical skeptics, continence was productive only of further evil consequences.[81] Like John Chatto, physician Robert E. Dudgeon was inclined to look upon continence as the actual cause of most cases of seminal emissions. "I venture to say," he wrote, "that all surgeons who have had any considerable number of patients under their care affected with seminal discharges, must have met with some who could ascribe their complaints to nothing but the most absolute continence." Furthermore, according to Dudgeon, spermatorrhea victims who accepted continence as the first

78. Harris, *My Life and Loves*, 247; Cowan, *The Science of a New Life*, 118; William A. Hammond, *Sexual Impotence in the Male and Female* (Detroit, 1887), 16.
79. W. H. Ranking, "Observations of Spermatorrhoea, or the Involuntary Discharge of the Seminal Fluid," *Lancet*, I (1843), 51; Amicus Veritatis, "On the Prevention of Spermatorrhoea and the Salutory Effects of Early Marriage," *Lancet*, I (1843), 384; Lallemand, *A Practical Treatise on the Causes, Symptoms, and Treatment of Spermatorrhoea*, 327.
80. John Chatto, "Continence Not a Preventive of Spermatorrhoea," *Lancet*, I (1843), 400; G. N. Dangerfield, "Spermatorrhoea; Reply by Dr. Dangerfield to Dr. Bull," *Lancet*, I (1843), 398–99.
81. Henry Graves Bull, "Continence, Never the Cause of Spermatorrhoea," *Lancet*, I (1843), 330.

priority of cure often were wretched in their rigorous efforts
to prevent recurring emissions. By purchasing devices to prevent contact between their genitals and their garments while
walking, tying their hands at night, and inserting wooden
cylinders in their rectums, they became obsessively morbid
in their sexual fears. Some of these victims, he wrote, were so
consumed with guilt that they dreaded marriage or even conversation with a member of the opposite sex for fear of further
endangering their health.[82] The following letter to one of the
popular writers on spermatorrhea is a good example of this
state of mind.

Boston, Jan. 10, 1845

Dr. Bostwick,

Dear Sir:—Oh! with what interest, and at the same time hopeless
despondency, I have read for months past your monthly reports. I say
with interest, because I have need of your services. Oh! Sir, I am in a
terrible condition. I am on the point of giving up all hope of recovery,
and dying the most miserable of all deaths by my own hands. I cannot
live long. What shall I do? I have been troubled with emissions for over
four years. I am sad, lonely, and hopeless. I have so far continued to
attend to my business, 'tis true, but oh! that I could adequately describe to you my feelings. You would pity me. My emissions take place
as often as three times a week, and for the sake of humanity, if nothing
else, will you do something for me? In addition to the emissions, I am
troubled, in urinating, with a burning sensation in the urethra; and on
going to stool, I observe a dribbling of semen. My appetite is tolerably
good except when it is destroyed by sadness. I am troubled with pain
over the eyes, in the back part of my head, in my joints, and a weakness
in my limbs. You cannot conceive the misery and deplorable state of my
mind and body. Perhaps I should say that the emissions sometimes occur
with an erection, and sometimes without; sometimes during lascivious
dreams, and sometimes I have no recollection of any dream.

I have seen many days and weeks that I did not wish to live. The
emissions affect me more and more. I feel prostrated and greatly debilitated, and have almost a constant and deep-seated pain in the space between the anus and scrotum, and shooting through the loins.

I have been paying attention to a lady that I love, and what am I to
do? Would it not be insulting for me to propose marriage in my present
condition? Would she not feel imposed upon? Oh! Sir, if I could but

82. Robert E. Dudgeon, "Continence Not a Cure for Spermatorrhoea,"
Lancet, I (1843), 401; Benjamin Phillips, "Observations on Seminal and Other
Discharges from the Urethra," *London Medical Gazette*, XXI (1843–44), 456;
Lankford, "Some Practical Suggestions about Spermatorrhoea," 292.

banish these feelings, and once more be restored to health, what is there that I would not give? I ought to have consulted some respectable medical man long before, instead of spending so much money in purchasing quack nostrums; but the fact is, I was so ashamed of myself, that I never could make up my mind to do it. This habit produces most singular results, in spite of one's self. It makes a man a great coward—afraid even of his own shadow. It makes him feel that he is the meanest of all God's creatures, and as though he never again wanted to look his fellow-man in the face. It makes him shun society, and lose all confidence in mankind. What can be more horrible? Would to God I had never been born![83]

Ironically, both physicians and quacks unanimously agreed on the last stage of treatment of spermatorrhea. While they disputed the efficacy of endless contraptions designed to prevent seminal emission and while they prescribed a variety of physiologically antagonistic drugs to bring the system back to normal, they nevertheless recommended marriage at the completion of treatment. "After the age of puberty," wrote Lallemand, "the semen cannot be suspended or sensibly diminished without more or less injury to the health; the accumulation of this fluid in the seminal vesicles must naturally produce importunate erections, inevitable relapses, or nocturnal or diurnal pollutions, all of which cannot be prevented but by sexual intercourse." Only coitus, he advised, could keep the patient in a healthy state of generative normalcy and deter the "morbid sensibility of the organs." Marriage was the sole effectual means of reforming the unnatural habits of the male and enabling him "to perceive the immense distance which separates his melancholy and disgusting pleasures from those naturally and physiologically procured."[84] For most medical practitioners, the only difficulty lay in determining the point at which the patient was ready for this last element of the cure. Most felt that patients first had to be brought along through an almost interminable number of treatments with drugs, sexual continence, special foods, hair mattresses, and assorted devices before they could graduate to normal intercourse.

83. Bostwick, *A Treatise on the Nature and Treatment of Seminal Diseases,* 124–26.
84. Quoted in Dangerfield, "The Symptoms, Pathology, Causes and Treatment of Spermatorrhoea," 216.

Although marriage marked the end of treatment for the bachelor victims of spermatorrhea, the "irregular" practitioner continued to treat numerous obstructions in the patient's path.

Hartford, January, 1847

Dr. Bostwick,

Dear sir:—About a year ago last November, I consulted you concerning my case of nocturnal emissions, debility, etc., and obtained some medicines which I took with me, and after I had taken it I wrote you from New Orleans; you answered me, and gave me a prescription, and further directions, all of which I strictly obeyed. I have improved in every particular; my emissions are not so frequent, and when they do occur, they do not debilitate me so much as they formerly did.

I came back from the south last spring, and called on you again, obtained some more medicine, and returned home. I have just finished taking the last box of pills, and am slowly, but decidedly on the mend, with the single exception of these dark or blue spots under my eyes. What is this? is it in the blood, skin, or where? Can it be removed? I still have emissions, but very seldom. I do not think they hurt me now at all; perhaps they do not occur oftener than they would in one who had never been addicted to the habit that brought them on.

You recommended me the last time I saw you to get married; your advice is good; I have not yet taken it, but have determined to do so in the spring. I feel quite relieved from all my former apprehensions on that interesting subject. I do not discover but what my erections are as strong and healthy as they ever were. I shall be passing through your city in April after a wife. The only remains of my former troubles are spots under my eyes. If I can get rid of them I shall be perfectly happy; but they seem to cling to me like a guilty conscience.

Sex manuals for the male identified these so-called "plague-spots" as the telltale evidence of masturbation. They were the outward sign of a morally bankrupt individual and were said to disappear only after Nature was convinced that the masturbator had completely forsaken his evil habit. Bostwick treated the patient's plague spots by prescribing the splashing of cold water on the genitals every morning, sitz baths, douches, a diet of fresh vegetables and fruit, sleeping on a hair mattress, early rising, prohibition of lascivious books, Bible reading, and the wearing of a suspensory bandage and bag (containing camphor and wheat bran) over the genitals.[85]

To be sure, there were physicians who looked upon seminal

85. Bostwick, *A Treatise on the Nature and Treatment of Seminal Diseases*, 78–82.

emission as the "greatest bugbear of young men."[86] As early as the 1840s, Benjamin Phillips, surgeon to Westminster Hospital, concluded that spermatorrhea was not nearly as serious as the picture drawn by Lallemand and others; and even William Acton considered nocturnal emissions as natural and in most instances a sign of manly vigor. Phillips believed that seminal discharges after puberty operated in the same manner that the menstrual period and the glands of Bartholin functioned for the female uterus. All brought periodic relief to "embarrassed" sexual organs. Unless the seminal vesicles were relieved through normal sexual activity or unnaturally through self-pollution, he wrote, the body would find a way to eliminate the fluid through involuntary emissions.[87] Noted physician Elizabeth Blackwell was inclined to view spermatorrhea in similar fashion. In *The Human Element in Sex* (1884), she stated that both menstruation and sperm emission were "natural healthy actions of self-balance, and established by the economy for preserving the mastership of each individual over her or his own nature."[88] She suggested that ignorance on the part of parents (especially mothers), adolescents, and physicians tended to exaggerate the consequences of this natural function. Similarly, Henry M. Lyman in his *Practical Home Physician* (1883) stated that it was "perfectly natural and healthy for the fluid to escape without the usual provocation"; and while some men could have an emission of this type once in two weeks, others might well have several in a week and yet remain perfectly healthy.[89] But despite these remarks, self-appointed guardians of youth concluded that unless halted quickly, spermatorrhea would act as a drain on the male's vital system, with life and virility departing the body along with the involuntary escape of semen. Few doctors were inclined to question the

86. Lyman, *The Practical Home Physician*, 535.

87. Benjamin Phillips, "Further Observations on Spermatic Discharges," *London Medical Gazette*, XLI (1848), 489; Joseph W. Howe, "On the Etiology, Pathology, and Treatment of Spermatorrhoea and Impotence," *Medical Record*, XII (1877), 689; Ranking, "Observations of Spermatorrhoea, or the Involuntary Discharge of the Seminal Fluid," 46; Acton, *The Functions and Disorders of the Reproductive Organs*, 54–55.

88. Elizabeth Blackwell, *The Human Element in Sex* (London, 1884), 26.

89. Lyman, *The Practical Home Physician*, 535.

nature of Lallemand's claim, and those who did were for the most part unsuccessful in placating the sexual fears of worried parents and young men. That a healthy man could have vigorous sexual activity in married life without brain damage seemed to matter little to those whose minds were filled with the awesome spectacle of destruction following a single wet dream.

Choosing a Wife

Manual writers were usually cautious in advising marriage as the only alternative for "sexual distress" in youth. "It has always struck me as very degrading," commented physician Charles L. Dana, "for a man to purposely select a wife to relieve him of the results of a weak will and vicious sensual indulgence. If marriage comes in the natural course of events, as it often does, so much the better; but to select a wife as a remedial agent for masturbation [or spermatorrhea] is unjust to the woman and a confession of a moral and mental feebleness."[90] According to William Acton, perfect continence and not marriage was the only solution to a young man's problems, and for anyone under the age of twenty-five, he prescribed the chaste life.[91] The man who married earlier might well arrest the growth of his body, weaken his system, and fall prey to disease and premature aging. Early marriage, like self-abuse, weakened the nervous system and the brain became "oppressed and clogged." Children born of early unions were more susceptible to disease and evidenced a higher mortality rate. Although they gave an appearance of health, wrote John Cowan, "they seldom reached the age of manhood, and old age was out of the question."[92] Manual authors also suggested that there should be a seven to ten year difference in ages between the man and his wife. "Women age much more rapidly than men," Acton observed, "and as the reproductive functions should cease in both

90. B. G. Carleton, "The Causes and Treatment of the So-Called Sexual Neuroses of the Male," *Medical Times*, XXV (1897), 69.

91. Acton, *The Functions and Disorders of the Reproductive Organs*, 91; Stall, *What a Young Man Ought to Know*, 33.

92. Cowan, *The Science of a New Life*, 32.

partners about the same time, some such interval as this is evidently desirable."[93]

Manual writers cautioned the young man to choose only a healthy woman; a scrofulous or consumptive family history, despite the appearance of health in the woman, meant early death for the wife and sickly and short-lived children. In addition, the man was to avoid women with hysterical temperaments. Although a few tears were expected of a woman, particularly during the honeymoon phase of the marriage, there was no greater misery than to be married to a woman of delicate temperament who "upon all and no occasions throws herself into that incurable and misery-causing malady—a fit of hysterics." Another indication of an abnormal and unhealthy woman was a small waist, caused by the wearing of corsets. "Avoid them as you would the plagues of Egypt," wrote one author, "for they encompass sickness, premature decay and death." Wasp-waisted women were capable of neither love nor right judgment, and since their souls were "malformed in harmony with their bodies," children of the union would be unhealthy and often mentally deranged. Agreeing with Orson Fowler, he cautioned men to make as their marriage rule: "Natural waists, or no wives."[94] Manuals assured men that in the long run a pleasant manner and cheerful disposition were far superior to any intellectual accomplishments a woman might have, particularly since "great accomplishments so seldom survive the first year of married life."[95] The strong-minded woman must be passed by for the woman accomplished in everyday duties of household management; couples "unequally yoked" because of a "wrongly-educated" wife would suffer unhappiness and grief.[96] Writers recommended that the couple be as nearly as possible from the same rank of society. If a difference existed, however, it was better for the husband to select a wife from a class above him. "Men can and often do rise from a humble origin to a social status far above that of

93. Acton, *The Functions and Disorders of the Reproductive Organs,* 126; John C. Bayley, *Marriage as It Is and as It Should Be* (New York, 1857), 70–71.

94. Cowan, *The Science of a New Life,* 51–52.

95. Acton, *The Functions and Disorders of the Reproductive Organs,* 127.

96. Cowan, *The Science of a New Life,* 51–52.

their wives, however great the disparity was originally," Acton wrote, "but this is very seldom the case as regards women." Money and a husband's rank would help a prospective bride, but her vulgar or low-born position would seldom enable her to climb a single step in the social ladder.[97]

Most of the popular manuals in the 1870s and 1880s stressed the importance of phrenology in choosing marriage partners, which would enable men and women to seek those of similar thought and feeling through a searching analysis of the brain's "soul-chambers."[98] Orson Fowler devoted hundreds of pages in his marriage manual to head analysis and depicted exemplary head shapes from among the distinguished personages of the day. Most marriage difficulties, he contended, could be avoided if the parties entering the contract would take time to discover their peculiar traits and check them against those of their companion. The wise bachelor in search of a wife would have an analysis made of his character and a chart constructed of his head which he could use for comparison. Then, he could look among only those women who appeared to approximate his own character analysis. Some manuals advised the male to advertise his character analysis in the newspaper "inviting replies from only those who imagine they approach your standard of character." The man was to request a phrenological analysis from each woman who answered his advertisement, and then determine the one most similar in analysis to himself. The woman, of course, was not to advertise; rather, she was to "wait patiently and hopefully" for the right man.[99]

William Alcott, in his manual *The Young Husband* (1839), stressed the need for both husband and wife to keep a journal, where each person's most private thoughts and feelings could be expressed. Like so many other aspects of nineteenth-century behavior, the journal became a substitute for direct discussion of personal problems which were considered beyond the pale of polite conversation, even between married couples. Just as

97. Acton, *The Functions and Disorders of the Reproductive Organs*, 128.
98. Cowan, *The Science of a New Life*, 43.
99. *Ibid.*, 59, 61, 71; Culverwell, *Professional Records*, 139–41; Orson S. Fowler, *Matrimony: Or Phrenology and Physiology Applied to the Selection of Congenial Companions for Life: Including Directions to the Married for Living Together Affectionately and Happily* (New York, 1851).

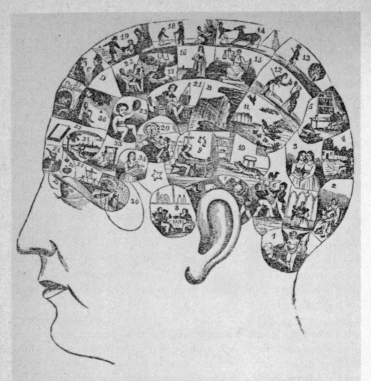

NUMBERING AND DEFINITION OF THE ORGANS

1. AMATIVENESS, Sexual and connubial love.
2. PHILOPROGENITIVENESS, Parental love.
3. ADHESIVENESS, Friendship—sociability.
4. UNION FOR LIFE, Love of one only.
5. INHABITIVENESS, Love of home.
6. CONTINUITY, One thing at a time.
7. COMBATIVENESS, Resistance—defence.
8. DESTRUCTIVENESS, Executiveness—force.
9. ALIMENTIVENESS, Appetite, hunger.
10. ACQUISITIVENESS, Accumulation.
11. SECRETIVENESS, Policy—management.
12. CAUTIOUSNESS, Prudence, provision.
13. APPROBATIVENESS, Ambition—display.
14. SELF-ESTEEM, Self-respect—dignity.
15. FIRMNESS, Decision—perseverance.
16. CONSCIENTIOUSNESS, Justice—equity.
17. HOPE, Expectation—enterprise.
18. SPIRITUALITY, Intuition—spiritual revery.
19. VENERATION, Devotion—respect.
20. BENEVOLENCE, Kindness—goodness.
21. CONSTRUCTIVNESS, Mechanics, ingenuity

21. IDEALITY, Refinement—taste purity
B. SUBLIMITY, Love of grandeur.
22. IMITATION, Copying—patterning.
23. MIRTHFULNESS, Jocoseness—wit—fun.
24. INDIVIDUALITY, Observation.
25. FORM, Recollection of shape.
26. SIZE, Measuring by the eye.
27. WEIGHT, Balancing—climbing.
28. COLOR, Judgment of colors.
29. ORDER, Method—system—arrangement
30. CALCULATION, Mental arithmetic.
31. LOCALITY, Recollection of places.
32. EVENTUALITY, Memory of facts.
33. TIME, Cognizance of duration.
34. TUNE, Music—melody by ear.
35. LANGUAGE, Expression of ideas.
36. CAUSALITY, Applying causes to effects
37. COMPARISON, inductive reasoning.
C. HUMAN NATURE, perception of motives
D. AGREEABLENESS, Pleasantness—suavity

A phrenological chart depicting human traits and character, from O. S. Fowler, *Love and Parentage Applied to the Improvement of Offspring, including Important Directions and Suggestions to Lovers and the Married,* 1868. National Library of Medicine, Bethesda.

the young man and his parents had an unspoken understanding concerning the vices of self-pollution and spermatorrhea, so the married couple were to observe the signs of courteous formality in dealing with personal expectations or misgivings of the other's character. On the other hand, each was expected to make observations on the marriage, with frank discussion of its virtues and vices. "There is a certain backwardness—better known than accounted for—on the part of the husband and wife, intimate as the relation is," wrote Alcott, "to express the inmost feelings, and desires, and purposes, and regrets, in conversation; and this, too, when the fullest confidence is felt that it will not come before the world." It was thus that the private journal acted as the medium for the married couple. Each was to have access to the other's private thoughts, and their unspoken review of these most private relations could thus be expressed with openness yet with proper reserve.[100]

Lost Manhood

Whether real or imaginary, permanent or temporary, sexual impotency was a source of great anxiety for the nineteenth-century male, and his apprehensions furnished a lucrative market for unscrupulous quacks, clairvoyants, mesmerizers, natural healers, faith-curers, anatomical museums, and layers-on-hand in his search for recovery of his sexual powers. Although victims of this blight have been noted in all eras—from Egyptian king Amasis and Roman emperors Nero and Honorius to Frankish monarch Charlemagne—the disorder was particularly disturbing for the highly wrought neurasthenics and hypochondriacs of the nineteenth century who, having accepted the prevailing medical opinions on excessive masturbation and spermatorrhea, withdrew from matrimonial attempts or marriage rights from fear of impotence. The male whose sexual emotions were interrupted by fears of incapacity, timidity, disappointment, and general anxiety because of the damage done to his system by self-abuse and nocturnal emission now sought medical advice to recover his lost manhood.[101]

100. William A. Alcott, *The Young Husband, or Duties of Man in the Marriage Relation* (Boston, 1839), 18.

101. James R. Smyth, "Impotence and Sterility," *Lancet*, II (1841), 783–84;

Physicians employed stomachics, aromatics, odoriferous gums, balsams, resins, essential and volatile oils, perfumes (particularly musk), phosphorous, opium, and cantharides to raise the sexual ardor of the impotent male. Cantharides remained the "sheet-anchor" of the nostrum trade, especially in France and Italy, where it formed the main ingredient of the Venetian *pastilles de serail* and the *diavolini;* in addition, it formed the basis of the pastes and the opiates of the Orient which were in so much demand by Western travelers. A favorite of the East was a combination of opium, musk, and ambergris which when taken daily promised to excite venereal desire.[102] Ants were popular as a remedy for impotence in France and Germany and were also employed for sterility in certain parts of Africa. Then, too, Victorians used electricity and ozone as aphrodisiacs to cure feeble erections. Physicians sometimes advised the "sexually bankrupt" to drink warm fresh blood each morning before breakfast. Koumiss, a fermented liquor made from mare's or camel's milk, was an expensive aphrodisiac of Russia; imitators found English cow koumiss a lucrative commodity. There were any number of recommended fish diets to restore the phosphoric elements in the body and tonics containing a mixture of alcohol and strychnine to restore sexual power. Charles Knowlton in his *Fruits of Philosophy* suggested a variety of aphrodisiacs including two teaspoonsful of cayenne every day, Dewees's Volatile Tincture of Guaiac (gum Guaiacum), carbonate of potash, saleratus and allspice in an alcoholic fluid, and tincture of Spanish flies.[103]

Physicians sometimes gave special dietary instructions for the sexually impotent in the hope of improving virile strength. Although denying them to the young male because they contributed to masturbation and spermatorrhea, physicians recom-

---

W. A. Hammond, "Some Remarks on Sexual Excesses in Adult Life as a Cause of Impotence," *Virginia Medical Monthly,* X (1883–84), 147; John Harvey, *The Restoration of Nervous Exhaustion* (London, 1865), 52–60.

102. Thomas E. Beatty, "Impotence," *Cyclopaedia of Practical Medicine,* IV (1847), 602.

103. Charles Knowlton, *The Fruits of Philosophy. A Treatise on the Population Question* (Chicago, n.d.), 36–37; Edward H. Dixon, *Some Abnormal Conditions of the Sexual and Pelvic Organs, Which Impair Virility* (New York, n.d.), 5–8; (A Court Physician), *Reproductive Disorders,* 163–67.

mended saffron, mustard, cinnamon, sage, carrots, turnips, marjoram, nutmeg, cardamom, arrowroot, laurel, leek, ginger, onions, cloves, peppers, parsnips, celery, fennel, vanilla, oysters, fish, game, and pork as aphrodisiac foods.[104] They hoped, of course, that their suggestive diets would not so much encourage the worn-out libertine to continue in debauchery, but rather introduce "tropical heat into matrimonial refrigerators."[105] Whether intended or not, however, aphrodisiacal suggestions formed the basis of hundreds of pamphlets entitled "Lost Manhood," "Premature Decay," or "The Errors of Youth" which promised salvation to the impotent and happiness to the latent roué. Their diets, nostrums, and appliances literally staggered the imagination. Drugs included gold chloride, arsenic, platinum chloride, phosphorus, hypodermic injections of ergot, strychnine, damiana, saw-palmetto, agnus castus, caladium, capsicum, china, conium, digitalis, gelsemium, picric acid, platina, stramonium, sulfur, and zincum. In addition, doctors prescribed circumcision, local faradization, galvanism, and franklinization.[106]

Physicians as well as quacks were quick to discern that psychological problems commonly attended the impotent male. "Every physician who has had much experience in this department of medicine," wrote Henry M. Lyman in 1883, "knows how many cases there are in which the patient fails to perform the act merely from lack of confidence; and how many instances occur in which the use of some mysterious remedy, or the application of instruments in parts of the body which are to the patient mysterious, results in perfect cures of impotency, even though these medicines and these instruments have

104. V. G. Vecki, "How to Feed the Sexually Impotent," *Pacific Medical Journal*, XLIV (1901), 92.

105. C. N. Cowden, "The Sexual Bankrupt; What Shall We Do with Him?," *Nashville Journal of Medicine and Surgery*, XCVI (1904), 674.

106. (Editorial), "Sexual Hygiene," *Alkaloidal Clinic*, VI (1899), 647; G. M. Beard, "Impotence of the First Stage, of One Year's Standing," *New York Medical Journal*, XIX (1874), 398; L. W. Reading, "The Electrical Treatment of a Few Sexual Disturbances," *Physical Therapeutics*, XIX (1901), 47–53; E. D. Chipman, "Some Observations on the More Common Forms of Sexual Impotence," *Yale Medical Journal*, VI (1899–1900), 128; John J. Caldwell, "Impotence and Sterility—Their Causes and Treatment by Electricity and Damiana," *Virginia Medical Monthly*, VI (1879–80), 436–46; J. Henry Simes, "Three Lectures on Impotence," *Philadelphia Polyclinic*, IV (1886–87), 196–99, 228–30, 260–62.

really not affected the individual in the least." Most such victims suffered from a distraught imagination and not from a diseased sexual organ. Having failed in their first attempt at intercourse or perhaps frightened by the popular beliefs concerning the results of self-abuse and spermatorrhea, they became disheartened and demoralized and imagined themselves in such a predicament that they were afraid to repeat the act.[107] One eighteenth-century quack, a Dr. James Graham of Edinburgh who was an enthusiast of Benjamin Franklin's electrical experiments, understood the influence of the imagination, and in his promise of fruitful connection, opened an establishment in London in 1780 called the "Temple of Health," which advertised a number of "electrical beds" designed to "awaken the dormant generative powers" of the couple. His "celestial beds" were provided with costly draperies and perfumes, and stood on glass legs to insulate the magnetic currents generated by two sexual batteries. Sterility, impotence, and other assorted difficulties could be overcome and the couple blessed with beautiful progeny, and although Graham reportedly charged a hundred pounds per night for the use of his "celestial beds," there were a sufficient number of interested clients to make his temple a profitable success.[108]

Of course, there were a surprising number of variations of this celestial bed adopted by eighteenth- and nineteenth-century physicians to overcome psychological impotence. It was reported, for example, that John Hunter prescribed that impotent males spend six nights in bed with a young woman without attempting sexual intercourse; usually, before the allotted time, the patient found himself surprisingly virile.[109] One California physician writing in 1899 recalled a patient who worked himself into a complete state of anaphrodisia or impotence following the use of camphor and bromides to treat a severe case of gonorrhea. He attempted to employ nervous

107. Lyman, *The Practical Home Physician*, 531; M. G. Thompson, "Impotence in the Male," *Memphis Medical Monthly*, XVII (1897), 71; John Lindsay, "Sexual Hypochondriasis in the Male," *Philadelphia Polyclinic*, XLII (1896), 413.

108. Bartholow, *On Spermatorrhoea*, 60; Beatty, "Impotence," 606.

109. Beatty, "Impotence," 602; Michael Ryan, *The Philosophy of Marriage, in Its Social, Moral, and Physical Relations* (London, 1839), 343.

tonics and later aphrodisiacs to cure the man's difficulty, but to no avail. He turned then to hygienic recreation, cold douches, massage, horseback riding, and other fresh air exercise, but all proved to be fruitless. Having reached the end of his therapeutic rope, he made one last suggestion to save his patient, who was rapidly becoming a wild-eyed paranoic, contemplating suicide.

Upon the next visit I inquired of my patient whether he knew of a voluptuously developed girl, young and good-looking, and of sufficient elastic morality to play a passive role in a physiological experiment. I promised that he should secure the services of such a person—who would of necessity be highly magnetic—for three successive nights. They were to sleep in an insulated broad bed, glass disks being used to insulate each bedstead leg from the floor. The bed itself was to be two feet removed from the walls, the head to the east, and my impotent invalid to occupy the southerly edge of the bed and the experimental maid the northerly side, the parties not to approach each other nearer than two feet. The maid, it was further stipulated, should disrobe on the right side of the bed—the patient might look on this disrobing if so inclined—but that under no condition or for any purpose whatever should my impotent patient transgress or trespass even a finger beyond his boundary of the neutral zone of two feet that was to remain between the two persons. The treatment was to be platonically moral as well as magnetic, the impotent receiving the full current of magnetism as it left the maid's body in its southwardly journey, while the insulation of the bedstead enabled him to store up the much-needed magnetism in his body. Three nights were to be devoted to this treatment, at the expiration of which time I assured my patient that he would be as puissant as Daniel Webster or an Augustus the Strong.

Rather than wait the three days before reporting the results, the patient turned up early at the office the next morning "with his former lacklusterless eyes beaming like two shiny jet beads," admitting that the treatment had repaired his system in just ten minutes, and that had he been compelled to wait the three nights "he would certainly have exploded from the storing magnetism as it traveled from north to south."[110]

That the man often failed as a "moral athlete" only mirrored the brittleness of Victorian ideals. The real and imagined sexual problems of the Victorian male were a natural eruption

110. P. C. Remondino, "Some Observations on the History, Psychology and Therapeutics of Impotence," *Urologic and Cutaneous Review*, III (1899), 255–56.

of the tremendous pressures of the age. If public decorum required woman to remain motionless upon her pedestal for fear that any slight movement might send her toppling, it likewise circumscribed the male with a welter of responsibilities to support that edifice. Already instructed to support the weight of the century's achievements on his shoulders, he had also to absorb the woman's deficiencies, for in her weakness lay a need for his strength, and the Victorian male acted in full knowledge that he bore the burden for both sexes as he struggled to ever higher planes of evolution. Beset on all sides by evidences of civilization's past achievements, he knew that any slight failing on his part would reflect upon his family, nation, and race in the struggle for survival of the fittest; he could admit of no weakness, for to do so would deny his very role and stigmatize him as less than a "fittest man." Anointed with the hopes and dreams of a century of materialistic progress, and promised by evolutionary ideas that every challenge could be met successfully, yet marked with the taint of Adam's sin, the young Victorian struggled against impossible ideals, and when he stumbled, he carried both the onus of personal failure and the knowledge that he had failed to carry forward the torch of his civilization.

Chapter VI

A NIGHT WITH VENUS,
A MOON WITH MERCURY

Deplorable as are the effects of adultery upon man, both philosophy and experience clearly demonstrate that its consequences are still worse upon woman whenever she becomes a willing participant to the act. For in this act she combines within herself the depraved conditions of all with whom she holds criminal commerce; and what is still worse, each paramour conveys to her every sphere with which he has previously been connected, so that she becomes the cess-pool of the combined forces of their evils. . . . This is true in both a literal and a spiritual sense; for moral diseases are no less infectious than physical. These mingling, as sin inevitably must, in antagonistic confusion upon the sensitive plane of life, but with feeble moral vitality to counteract their influence, have proved too demoralizing to be overcome by human efforts. Here is the origin of syphilitic diseases, springing from the rottenness of the soul in crime, and reacting upon man with terrific conseqences.

B. F. Hatch, M.D., *The Constitution of Man, Physically, Morally and Spiritually Considered,* 1866

Although purity writers made every effort to prevent a single unchaste thought from sullying the mind of the "fittest man," there was nonetheless a certain ambivalence in society's definition of the term which discreetly permitted a certain amount of undisciplined vitality to emerge now and again, if only to add another dimension to the already disparaging inequality in the role of the sexes. While woman reigned safe and sovereign in the home circle, imbibing only those maxims which kept her virtue and respect intact, society assuaged the male ego by allowing occasional lapses in virtue as he struggled amid the untamed forces of the city, tempted by real as well as imaginary dangers. "Unless men have a greater degree of admiration for the good and beautiful, than is inculcated in the common course of education," wrote the author of a manual for men in 1818, "the passions will, during the period of youth, occasionally usurp and sway."[1] There was a note of sensuality in the nineteenth-century male's notion of happiness and it became a form of manly self-assertion amid an otherwise docile acceptance of his regimented upbringing. Outwardly a purist in politics and morals, who spoke contemptuously of the weak and imprudent, he nonetheless courted a certain defiance of social requirements, and in his more private understanding of the complex passions of life, he sometimes attempted to sustain a balance between propriety and the necessity of the moment. His pretension to moralism gave to the age an assurance of stability which only weakly concealed a more hedonistic solipsism; his instincts merged more nakedly as he drew a distinction between love and sex in his cultivation of the joys of Venus.

Sporting Life

It was commonly understood in nineteenth-century society that man, because of his physical diversity, could not commit

1. (Anony.), *A Popular Dissertation on the Venereal Diseases, and Their Sequels; with the Mode of Prevention and Cure* (London, 1818), 4.

marital infidelity in the same sense that woman could. His unfaithfulness, wrote an American physician in the 1860s, introduced no new blood into the home and therefore caused no hereditary defects as did the same act by the woman. The liability of the adulterous woman, on the other hand, lay in the possibility of her introducing illegitimate blood into the family circle "which must either be maintained by a man not its father, or cruelly driven from the household for a sin not its own." If the wife chose to conceal her guilt, she was forced to live a falsehood which would be "fearfully disastrous to her physical and spiritual well being." This was not the case for the male, however, who could "live in adulterous relations, to a greater or less extent, all his life, and still maintain his marital attachment." Although the husband's infidelity would naturally lessen the "oneness of soul essential to true conjugal enjoyment," the husband would find "renewed fondness" and respect for his wife since, in truth, he could have only loathing and disgust for the woman who administered to his lust. Furthermore, "though the husband may allow a courtesan sphere to intercept between him and his wife, he does not incorporate into his constitution, as does the wife, the prolific forces by which an entire change is effected towards her." Society, for its part, seemed willing to accept this logic, and was thus more willing to hold woman in stricter account than man. In fact, the logic of the argument seemed to suggest that husbands who were unfaithful had all the more reason to respect the sanctity of the home circle and the purity of their wives. When all was said and done, men were better (indeed "fitter") for their actions.[2]

Besides the "casual friendships" or waiting mistresses which brought a happy interlude to the male's private hours, brothels and assignation houses enabled him to revel in a more pedestrian liberty amid a trained and hardened staff of professionals. From the elegant bordellos of New Orleans's Storyville district to the parlor houses and dance halls of Chicago and New York, and from the covered wagons on the outskirts of

2. Benjamin F. Hatch, *The Constitution of Man, Physically, Morally, and Spiritually Considered* (New York, 1866), 405–6; Edward D. Cope, "On the Material Relations of Sex in Human Society," *Monist*, I (1890–91), 41.

Eldorado, Kansas, to the lumber camps of Michigan and Wisconsin, commercialized sex posed an agreeable alternative to the exacting demands for virginity in prudish nineteenth-century culture.[3] The same society which boasted of "Comstockery," strict continence, and Horatio Alger's little heroes, looked with less than public pride on statistics which estimated more than 40,000 prostitutes in New York City in 1893, from 10,000 to 20,000 in Chicago and Philadelphia, and similar figures for cities both large and small across America. Yet, despite the crusades of Charles H. Parkhurst and the Lexow Commission in New York, of W. T. Stead, the Chicago Vice Commission, Anthony Comstock, and the avenging angels of the WCTU's Purity Department, prostitution flourished, not as a counterculture, but rather as an intimate part of the Gilded Age—a sort of psychic drainage system for an otherwise proper and respectable era.[4] "An inevitable attendant upon civilized, and especially closely-packed, population," observed William Acton, "it is, and I believe ever will be, ineradicable."[5]

Acton somewhat shocked Victorian society by maintaining that prostitution was a transitory state through which thousands of women passed. Since many of them became wives in respectable households, he urged that rather than condemn them as society had done traditionally, it was in the interest of every nation to help these women "through that state, so as to

3. Joseph H. Greer, *The Social Evil; Its Cause, Effect and Cure* (Chicago, 1909), 49–50; Stephen Longstreet, *Sportin' House; a History of the New Orleans Sinners and the Birth of Jazz* (Los Angeles, 1965); Charles Winick and Paul M. Kinsie, *The Lively Commerce: Prostitution in the United States* (Chicago, 1971). William Allen White remarked in his autobiography: "And one summer day we discovered a camping place deep in the woods above the town where there was often a covered wagon and some strange girls. We used to peek through the brush at what was going on there until Merz Young, who was the protector of the innocent, came and chased us off with yells and curses, throwing rocks. And the knowledge of good and evil came to us, even as to the Pair in the Garden." See his *Autobiography of William Allen White* (New York, 1846), 40.

4. James T. Jelks, "The Prevention of Venereal Diseases," *Journal,* Arkansas Medical Society, III (1893), 353; Charles H. Parkhurst, *My Forty Years in New York* (New York, 1923); Lincoln Steffens, *Autobiography* (New York, 1931), 215–20; W. T. Stead, *If Christ Came to Chicago!* (Chicago, 1894); Herbert Asbury, *The Gangs of New York* (New York, 1927); Egal Feldman, "Prostitution, the Alien Woman and the Progressive Imagination, 1910–1915," *American Quarterly,* XIX (1967), 192–206.

5. William Acton, *Prostitution in Relation to Public Health* (London, 1851), 32.

save as much as may be of the bodies and souls of them."[6]
Although Acton was every bit a Victorian, especially when it
came to his views concerning the role of women and marriage,
his attitude toward prostitution was out of step with a public
morality which relied upon a variety of suppressive and regulatory devices derived from ancient times. Society in the nineteenth century was divided between abolitionist dreams and
regulatory measures, the former promising to cleanse the
troubled conscience and the latter offering a token compromise
with reality. Elaborate regulatory steps were undertaken in
France, Germany, Russia, Austria, Belgium, Hungary, Spain,
and Portugal to register prostitutes and examine them periodically. Between 1860 and 1888, similar experiments in regulation were imposed in England, Norway, Switzerland, and Italy;
but the results were less than encouraging, since regulation simply led to clandestine prostitution. The number of brothels in
Marseilles during its period of regulation, for example, dropped
from 120 households and 600 women in 1875 to 12 houses
and 60 women in 1895. The reluctance of prostitutes to be
registered and examined resulted in an underworld of un-
registered houses with an even greater incidence of venereal
disease.[7] On the other hand, the abolitionist efforts of Prussia,
Rome, Bavaria, Stockholm, and most countries where prohibition had been tried, remarked one syphilologist, demonstrated
"not only the futility of the repressive measures, but their positively bad effect in the increase of venereal disease and the
demoralization of society."[8]

In 1859, William Sanger, resident physician in the venereal
wards in Blackwell's Island in New York, published one of the
early documentaries on prostitution in America. In his study of
New York City, he found that of the 2,000 prostitutes in his

6. *Ibid.*, 75.
7. Marshall H. Bailey, "Some Problems concerning Venereal Diseases," *New England Journal of Medicine*, CXLVI (1902), 594.
8. W. F. Monroe, "On the Prevention of Venereal Diseases," *New England Journal of Medicine*, V (1870), 373; Frederic Bierhoff, "Police Methods for the Sanitary Control of Prostitution in Some of the Cities of Germany," *New York Medical Journal*, LXXXVI (1907), 298–305; Sheldon Amos, *A Comparative Survey of Laws in Force for the Prohibition, Regulation, and Licensing of Vice in England and Other Countries* (London, 1877); (Anony.), "Review of European Legislation for the Control of Prostitution," *Journal*, Louisiana State Medical Society, XI (1854–55), 667–705.

survey, nearly 63 percent were foreign born, most from the British Isles. A nativist at heart, he placed much of the blame for prostitution on what he felt were unwholesome foreign influences on American morality—fashionable novel reading, lascivious waltzes, low-necked dresses, and the aura of romanticism which encouraged a search for adventure and intrigue. Many of these denigrating influences had been brought to America by her own native sons and daughters who, in traveling to Europe to improve their minds, had returned "to our shores with ideas calculated to be anything but beneficial to their native country in a social or moral point of view." In ignorance of their own indigenous culture, they attempted to ape European manners and morals—"and to this cause must be assigned the gradual approximation of our fashionable society to the vices of the European capitals, their ladylike and gentlemanlike frailties, their genteel peccadilloes and affections." According to the New York syphilologist, American society could protect itself from these distasteful foreign influences by creating "a phrenological and psychological bureau, armed with full powers to examine all persons desiring to travel, so as to ascertain whether they may safely make the grand tour, and have sufficient strength of intellect and firmness of principle to resist the vitiating influences and examples which will surround them there." As another important line of defense, Sanger urged Americans to guard themselves from European immigrants who were teeming into the cities and bringing in their baggage the degraded state of morals existing in their native towns and cities.

That we are rapidly introducing many of the most absurd follies and worst vices of Europe is a patent fact. Almost every one can specify acts now tolerated in respectable families which, so far as being permitted fifteen years ago, would have been thought by our plain common-sense parents amply sufficient to warrant the exclusion of the offender from the domestic circle; and it is an equally conspicuous fact that our social morality is deteriorating in a direct ratio to the introduction of these habits. Every day makes the system of New York more like that of the most depraved capitals of continental Europe, and it remains for the good innate sense of the bulk of the American people to say how much farther we shall proceed in this frivolous, intriguing, and despicable manner of living; or whether they will not strive to perpetuate the stern morality of the Puritan fathers, our great moral safeguard so far, and thus put an effectual barrier against the inroads of a torrent which must undermine our whole social fabric, and finally crush us beneath the ruins.[9]

Sanger felt that traditional abolitionist restraints and punishments were useless in dealing with prostitution. Throughout the ages, women had been scourged, banished, executed, deprived of their civil rights, proclaimed immoral in public, and made to suffer innumerable indecencies, all without any noticeable effect. In place of these inhuman practices, he urged American sanitarians to consider regulatory measures similar to those in force in various European cities. Ironically, despite his nativist sentiments, Sanger commended the high-class sporting houses of New York City kept by European madames who, being accustomed to medical inspection laws in the old world, preferred to continue the practice in the United States by paying physicians to visit their women every few days and check for disease. Borrowing from European regulatory measures, he recommended the construction of hospitals for the treatment of venereal disease, the legal authorization for medical men to visit all known houses and to remove any woman found to be infected, and last, the power to detain persons having venereal disease until cured. He hoped that the Paris hospitals and their medical visitation plan would become the eventual model for American reform.[10]

The spasmodic attempts to control prostitution in the United States were all too frequently in the hands of religious fanatics or social zealots whose limited experience in the real world left them defenseless as the institution changed to accommodate to their moral crusades. The country's first attempt at regulation, tried in St. Louis between 1872 and 1874, failed miserably. Borrowing from Paris regulations, the Missouri legislature required that all prostitutes be registered in one of three classes: inmates of houses, the occupants of rooms outside of such

9. William Sanger, *The History of Prostitution* (New York, 1858), 570–72.
10. *Ibid.*, 644–46; Arthur C. Bauer, "The Regulation of Prostitution as a Hygienic Measure," *Lancet-Clinic,* n.s., XXXIII (1894), 411–16; J. F. Herrick, "Some Ways of Lessening the Social Evil," *Iowa Medical Journal,* XI (1905), 233–37; Alfred W. Herzog, "A Plan to Regulate Prostitution," *Medical Brief,* XXXIII (1905), 381–83.

houses, and those known as "kept women" or mistresses. The law made no distinction between a mistress and her unfortunate sister in a disorderly house. Women were forbidden to change their place of business without proper notification to authorities; solicitation on the street or from a window or door was prohibited, nor could a red light be allowed outside a house to attract customers. Registered women were required to have weekly medical examinations from "social-evil examiners" and the fee collected helped to maintain a hospital open to all registered women.[11] Supporters of the regulation looked with pride on the evidence that there were 238 fewer prostitutes in the city a year after its passage. They based this on statistics showing that only 480 women registered out of 718 known prostitutes. But what the bare statistics failed to indicate, however, was that the law had merely led to clandestine prostitution. More important, however, the regulatory measures threatened to endanger the incomes of public officials who had learned to depend upon protection money over the years. Ultimately, the politicians and policemen joined forces with concerned clergy and purity leaders who were prophesying a worse fate for St. Louis than had been meted out to Sodom and Gomorrah. Refusing to compromise with sin, they staged a "moral uprising" that demanded the repeal of the law licensing the vice. Petitions were presented to the state legislature in wheelbarrows decorated in ribbons and accompanied by young girls attired in white gowns and followed by an ever-present contingent of mothers and clergy. Americans preferred abolition to regulation, but it was the type of abolition that could soothe the stricken conscience while simultaneously filling the pockets of graft.[12] Further attempts at regulation were made in Buffalo and Philadelphia in 1902, and in Detroit and Cincinnati. Pittsburgh's abolitionist zeal, which culminated in the closing of sporting houses and turning the inmates into the streets without food or lodging, ironically resulted in a counter-

11. L. Lustgarten, "The Question of Legal Control of Prostitution in America," *Medical Record*, LVII (1900), 57; James E. Washington, "A Social Evil Act Needed," *Nashville Journal of Medicine and Surgery*, XX (1877), 175–83.
12. Lustgarten, "The Question of Legal Control of Prostitution in America," 58; W. E. Whitehead, "The Social Evil," *Pacific Medical Journal*, V (1871–72), 56.

wave of moral outrage which brought the institution back as strong as ever. Similarly, the Reverend Parkhurst's efforts to reform New York in 1891 and 1892 resulted in cleaning out a localized institution by spreading it over an area several times as large as it had been originally, and filling the thoroughfares with streetwalkers for the first time.[13]

By the 1870s and 1880s, urban prostitution had begun to change in character. The independent bordello, under the aegis of a madame, continued to exist and prosper, but prostitution became more and more a highly organized business with male managers of a string of girls. According to muckraker George Kibbe Turner, prostitution had become a function of slum politics, establishing a position which proved impossible to dislodge; progressive efforts to rid New York of the vice, for example, inevitably came up against the stone front of Tammany Hall. The association between prostitution and political machines grew first in New York, then spread to other large cities as young men, recruited by the machine from sweatshops and apprenticeships, were hired to lure young immigrant girls into the profession. By the last two decades of the century, according to Turner, prostitution had replaced saloon halls and gambling parlors as the major source of the machine's revenue. The young pimps, or "cadets," strengthened their power within the machine by doubling as "repeater voters," and by 1900 had acquired high status in local wards by acting as musclemen in elections, controlling large sectors of voters, and often holding the balance of power in key areas of New York, Newark, Philadelphia, and Chicago. The efforts by reformers to eliminate prostitution thus became tied to ousting corrupt political machines, and the diffusion of objectives that characterized such reform efforts assured that the profitable trade in female flesh would continue to prosper.

13. Isadore Dyer, "The Municipal Control of Prostitution in the United States. Some Opinions as to Methods Adapted to Municipal Care and Control of Prostitution and for the Prophylaxis of Venereal Diseases," *New Orleans Medical and Surgical Journal*, LII (1899), 316; Richard H. Thomas, "A Few Observations on State Regulation of Prostitution," *Maryland Medical Journal*, VIII (1881–82), 469–72; M. L. Heidingsfeld, "The Control of Prostitution and the Prevention of the Spread of Venereal Disease," *Journal*, American Medical Association, XLII (1904), 305–9; George Gould, comp., *Digest of State and Federal Laws Dealing with Prostitution and Other Sex Offences* (New York, 1942).

As was historically true, the procurers preyed on the weak—the poor, the newly arrived immigrant, the exploited shop girl, or domestic servant. Nationalities of girls lured into prostitution followed immigration patterns—Irish and German in the 1850s, Jewish, Polish, and Slovak in the 1880s, and Italian after the turn of the century. Most of the procurers of the late nineteenth century were Jewish, and as immigrant population increased, they recruited girls from the lower East Side Jewish tenements. These "Jewish businessmen" formed associations, the best known of which was the New York Independent Benevolent Association, to fight opposition from religious groups and to protect their fast-prospering interests from criminal prosecution. The associations set up ethnic dance halls for the newly arrived immigrants; here, the young girl could for five cents buy an evening's enjoyment, one of the very few cheap amusements available to her. And here, unfamiliar with new customs, unable even to speak the language, she was approached by the cadet, only slightly older than herself and projecting the aura of a hero, and she was easily secured by the promise of marriage to engage in prostitution. Once caught up in the horrors of the trade, the girls had no way to escape, for families literally cast them off as dead, and most grew desperate and hardened in the profession. After the turn of the century, as demand for Italian prostitutes grew, procurers introduced a new method to lure girls to the profession. Unable to attract the Italian-American daughters of very protective families, they turned to young Italian laborers, who, returning to their native land for the winter, would persuade young girls to accompany them to the United States the next year, on promise of marriage. Once ashore, the girls, unprotected by family structures, were turned over to dealers by their erstwhile lovers for the sum of their passage. Since the average "life" of a girl in the trade was five years, new "supplies" had constantly to be found, but the slum tenements provided an endless number of ignorant, innocent victims. The trade soon spread from the highly profitable New York center to other cities as the cadets took their girls and their organizing abilities to as yet untapped sources of supply and demand. It was estimated that at the turn of the century one-half of the prostitutes in the United States began their profession in New York and were carried by their managers to other cities.[14]

Aside from comprehensive investigations carried out by Parent-Duchâtelet on Parisian prostitutes in 1836, by Sanger in 1858, and by Michael Ryan, William Acton, and Henry Mayhew on the English "horizontal trade" in 1839, 1851, and 1862, there was also an important investigation made in New York City between 1900 and 1902 by the Committee of Fifteen.[15] A member of the committee, Alvin S. Johnson, classified the prostitutes queried in the study into three groups. The first consisted of women or girls who "having been brought up in the very atmosphere of ignorance, squalor, and immorality, in our slums, may be said to have been trained for prostitution from earliest childhood." According to Johnson this first group grew up without proper moral training, were "little better than animals and fell easy victims to their vicious male associates while they were only half matured." The second group consisted of large numbers of women who, being employed as shop girls, domestics, and factory-hands in the cities, found themselves unable to earn a living. These were the salesgirls in New York and Chicago department stores who earned from two to five dollars a week; yet management required that they attire themselves in clothes attractive to customers. These women were "expected by their employers to eke out their starvation wages through the generosity of a 'gentleman friend.'" On any given evening when the shops were closing, "gentlemen friends" could be seen outside the stores "waiting to entrap

14. George K. Turner, "The Daughters of the Poor; a Plain Story of the Development of New York City as a Leading Center of the White Slave Trade of the World, under Tammany Hall," *McClure's Magazine*, XXXIV (1909), 45–61; J. D. Ball and H. G. Thomas, "A Sociological, Neurological, Serological, and Psychiatrical Study of a Group of Prostitutes," *American Journal of Psychiatry*, LXXIV (1918), 647–66; Ludwig Weiss, "The Prostitution and Its Relation to Law and Medicine," *Journal*, American Medical Association, XLVII (1906), 2073; Denslow Lewis, "The Social Evil," *Buffalo Medical Journal*, LXII (1906), 249–57; George B. H. Swayze, "Hardships of Social Vice," *Medical Times*, XXXIII (1905), 356–60.

15. Henry Mayhew, *London Labour and London Poor* (4 vols; London, 1861–62), IV; Acton, *Prostitution in Relation to Public Health;* William Acton, *Prostitution, Considered in Its Moral, Social, and Sanitary Aspects, in London and Other Large Cities and Garrison Towns* (London, 1870); Michael Ryan, *Prostitution in London, with a Comparative View of that of Paris and New York* (London, 1839).

some girl for a dinner and debauchery." Few of the thousands of customers "who flock to these emporiums after bargains," commented syphilologist Prince A. Morrow of New York, "know or suspect that they are moral hells, places where poor girls are forced and tempted to sell their bodies and souls in order that the owners may keep the trade by selling cheap and yet make a good profit on a large capital." A third class of prostitutes were not forced into the profession to avoid starvation, wrote Johnson, "but they cannot otherwise get more than a bare existence, which is not worth living for."

They find they can never have pretty clothes, can rarely go to the theatre and then must take the worst seats, can never buy pretty books or pictures, candy or any of the other innocent pleasures which are dear to every girl's heart, and hardest of all cannot have a comfortable and private place to receive their friends. These young women have a strong human instinct for "life, liberty, and the pursuit of happiness," which our Declaration of Independence declared to be the inalienable right of every one; they have little hope of marriage for a long time to come, for they know that few or none of their men friends could support a family decently; they see their working companions enjoying good clothes, good dinners, good seats at the theatre, and they know how easily these good things of life may be obtained; they know nothing of the horrors of venereal diseases and believe it is easy to avoid pregnancy; and finally, they have no strong religious or moral principles to keep chaste, nor do they fear the loss of social standing in their set. Is it then to be wondered at that the tens of thousands of working-girls who belong to this class allow themselves to be seduced by the "gentleman friend," the smooth-spoken flattering "cadet," who is a human hyena in the clothing of a "gentleman?"[16]

An example of this was depicted by Theodore Dreiser in *Sister Carrie* (1900), in which a young girl of eighteen set out for Chicago with four dollars and her sister's address on Van Buren Street in her pocket. Within a few weeks, she turned from the drabness of her sister's virtuous but impoverished life to that offered by her "gentleman friend" Drouet. When forced to choose between bare subsistence as a stitcher in a shoe fac-

16. Quoted in William L. Holt, "Etiology of the Venereal Plagues and Some New Methods of Prevention," *Southern California Practitioner,* XXIV (1909), 618–19; Prince A. Morrow, *Social Diseases and Marriage* (New York, 1904); Ernest A. Bell, *War on the White Slave Trade, a Book Designed to Awaken the Sleeping and to Protect the Innocent* (Chicago, 1909); George T. Kneeland, *Commercialized Prostitution in New York City* (New York, 1913).

tory, or living with material possessions and a sense of security, the selling of her body was of little or no concern. In fact, a large part of the criticism Dreiser received for his novel grew directly from the fact that Carrie's virtue was never an issue. Given the alternatives of poverty and security, virginity was extraneous. Carrie was one of countless clandestine women who were much preferred over prostitutes since men considered coition with them safer, more select, and less likely to result in exposure or infection.

The crusading efforts of vigilance committees, the Purity Department of the WCTU, the American Purity Alliance, and a host of supportive societies resulted in local and state efforts to control prostitution in the United States. The American Society of Sanitary and Moral Prophylaxis organized in New York in 1905, and similar societies in Chicago, Philadelphia, and elsewhere, strove to educate the public on the growing social evil. The efforts of these reform agencies, which were composed of medical men, social workers, and the idle elite, seldom advanced beyond the written word. At best, they dragged an assortment of venereal catalysts before the public eye: dance halls (nearly 300 in Chicago alone), department-store wage policies, theaters, manicure and massage parlors, Turkish baths, employment agencies (which frequently sent unemployed girls to assignation houses), tenement living, drug addiction, immigrant adjustment problems, lack of proper sex hygiene, and saloons. The Chicago Vice Commission reported in 1911 that "the whole tendency of modern industrialism is to place too heavy a strain on the nervous system of all classes, men and women alike. How much more serious is this, when the strain is placed on the growing girl at the period of adolescence when the child has to assume the burden of self-support and self-direction, and often aid in the support of her family." Since legitimate wages for women averaged less than five dollars a week, the young worker naturally became discouraged and either lost ambition or undertook "some adventure more or less hazardous, to supplement her meager wages."[17]

Those elements of the medical profession most involved with

17. Vice Commission of Chicago, *The Social Evil in Chicago* (Chicago, 1911), 269–70.

venereal prophylaxis were sometimes outspoken in their analysis and criticism of society. Compelled to examine the
causes, both direct and indirect, that lay behind the disease,
medical researchers found themselves face to face with many
of the more brutalizing inequalities of Victorian society. In a
speech before the Southern California Health Association
meeting in Los Angeles in 1909, W. L. Holt, M.D., reminded
the profession that modern prostitution bore the double stamp
of social and industrial injustices. It was one of the greatest
cruelties of modern society that women found themselves in a
one-sided world where all the repressive measures, sanitary
regulations, and persecution-oriented laws dealing with the
institution concerned them alone. He believed that this one-
sided sanitary legislation was as illogical as if a quarantine
officer had isolated all the women and female rats on a plague-
infested ship, allowing the men and male rats to move about
unencumbered. From a social standpoint, men were more
directly responsible for prostitution by their rapacious demand
for sexual gratification outside marriage. Through seduction
and desertion, discharge and starvation, kidnapping and "forc-
ible detention in a brothel," but most important, "by employment at impossible wages combined with the offer of comfort
and luxuries in exchange for her soul and body," man had
driven woman into becoming a slave to a morally bankrupt
civilization.[18]

Part of the problem, according to Holt, lay in the narrow attitude of society toward divorce and contraception. Many
marriages between incompatible couples were unnecessarily
maintained without happy sexual relations only because of the
negative public attitude toward divorce. This situation had led
many men to seek sexual compatibility outside marriage. Holt
likewise condemned the "bigoted moral censor" Anthony Comstock for placing punitive legislation in the way of pertinent
contraception information. Incompatible marriages, unwanted
children, and the resulting wholesale "slaughter of the innocent" through abortion were as much the products of Comstock's blind prudery as that of ignorance and thoughtless laws.

18. Holt, "Etiology of the Venereal Plagues and Some New Methods of
Prevention," 620.

Holt was equally disheartened by the "elective system" begun at Harvard and spreading among the colleges and universities of the country, fearing that it would permit "lazy men to choose studies which will require very little work besides attending the lectures," leading them to the cultivation of other, more sensuous interests. But he placed the major onus for prostitution squarely on the rich and influential citizens of the state and their social and industrial ignorance of society's problems. "If these rulers of society really wish to abolish prostitution," he wrote, "they can do so by giving back to the workers the wealth they have taken from them, and so making it possible for every young man and woman who is able and willing to work, to marry young and establish a comfortable and happy home."[19]

Holt recommended first that laws be passed granting divorce for sexual incompatibility, venereal disease, and further, that states follow the example of North Dakota by requiring every candidate for marriage to secure an affadavit certifying his or her freedom from venereal disease. He also advocated laws which would make it a crime to transmit venereal disease to another person. He hoped society would emancipate the working girls and women from their poverty and degradation and also raise the income of male workers "so that they can marry reasonably early and support a wife and a few children in comfort." But this could only be achieved, he believed, when people acquired ownership of the public industries. Borrowing from the reform ideas of Henry George, he recommended that all the manufacturing and distributing trusts, the railroads, mines, telegraph and telephone systems come under public control. Then, no man could "take the wealth produced by others, or own the very means of living of others, but all men will have to work to produce wealth . . . and each will get his due share of the wealth he has helped to produce, in proportion to his needs and his usefulness." Last, Holt included under moral measures the need to properly educate people

19. *Ibid.*, 622–25; Robert N. Wilson, "The Social Evil in University Life: A Talk with Students of the University of Pennsylvania," *Medical News*, LXXXIV (1904), 97–105.

concerning the evils of prostitution and venereal disease; this included full information on sexual hygiene and marriage reform. Most of all, society had to teach that man and not woman was responsible for the existence of the brothel and therefore, "in plain justice, the same moral standard should be demanded for him as for woman."[20] Holt was not alone in reflecting the influence of Henry George and other social reformers of the age. Physician Joseph Greer, in his book on prostitution published in 1909, wrote that nothing could eliminate the evil except a "complete change in the social and economic institutions and systems of our civilization." By that he meant that men must "get together in one great, cooperative, fraternal whole. . . . The earth and all its resources must not be owned and monopolized by a few—it must belong to all alike, and every man and woman must have an equal opportunity to labor and create upon it."[21]

By the turn of the century, reformers such as Jane Addams, Lillian Wald of New York, and physician Abraham Flexner of the New York Bureau of Social Hygiene, along with muckraker George Kibbe Turner, had sparked serious discussion of prostitution at all levels of government, resulting in state and national legislation, most prominently the Mann Act of 1910. In expressing their deepening concern for the problem, medical men sought a greater public role by advocating that physicians report venereal diseases, fulfilling the role as family and community advisers in promoting a single standard of morals for the sexes, seeking the creation of state boards of health with adequate facilities for venereal detection, advocating educational hygiene lectures for the working classes, requesting greater participation in parent-teacher associations, providing courses on sex hygiene in the universities and public schools, and promoting better instruction for medical and theological students to combat future problems. But the age which brought venereal disease and prostitution before the public eye also disturbed the dirty linen of countless other problems,

20. Holt, "Etiology of the Venereal Plagues and Some New Methods of Prevention," 626–27; Bailey, "Some Problems concerning Venereal Disease," 596.
21. Greer, *The Social Evil; Its Cause, Effect and Cure,* 63.

all of which demanded similar attention. Concern for prostitution and its attendant venereal diseases quickly degenerated into a diffused offensive along a wide front, each group picking and choosing its enemy from among an assortment of contributing evils—taverns, Tammany Hall, coeducation, capitalism, romantic literature, or dancing of the "terpsichorean whirl." In time, the forces coalesced, but under the "monistic therapeutics" of prohibition crusaders who diagnosed all of the nation's ills as stemming entirely from the "alcohol virus." Only when this disease was properly destroyed, they promised, would prostitution, venereal disease, and concomitant problems be eliminated and health and vigor return to the body politic.[22]

The Private Disease

The early ignorance concerning syphilis, soft chancre, and gonorrhea has made it difficult to trace the true history of venereal diseases, especially that of syphilis. Lepra, herpes, scabies, pemphigus, impetigo, eczema, lichen ruber, psoriasis, along with leukorrhea and catarrhal discharges were all confused at one time or another with venereal disease, and those who claimed that syphilis existed in Europe prior to the discovery of America found themselves having to face that confusion. Disorders resembling syphilis and identified as "pudendagra" prevailed in many areas of western Europe and the Mediterranean, and were detailed by the tenth-century Arabian physician Rhazes, the Arabic translator Johannes Mesüe, by Michael Scott in 1214, and by the early English

22. Noah E. Aronstam, "The Prevention of Venereal Diseases," *Medical Age*, XXIII (1905), 483–84; L. D. Bulkley, "For Young Men of the Working Classes," *Charities*, XV (1905–1906), 718–21; Margaret Cleaves, "Education in Sexual Hygiene for Young Working Women," *Charities*, XV (1905–1906), 721–73; B. L. W. Floyd, "Our Social and Moral Scourge," *Lancet-Clinic*, CVII (1912), 270–76; Frederic H. Gerrish, "The Duties of the Medical Profession concerning Prostitution and Its Allied Vices," *Transactions*, Maine Medical Association (1878), 331–50; Edgar G. Ballenger, "The Social Evil," *Southern Medicine and Surgery*, XXX (1907), 21–24; H. A. Kelly, "What Is the Right Attitude of the Medical Profession toward the Social Evil," *Journal*, American Medical Association, XLIV (1905), 677–81; Jane Addams, *A New Conscience and an Ancient Evil* (New York, 1912); Alex W. Stirling, "Education and the Social Evil," *Journal-Record of Medicine*, IX (1908), 637–45.

surgeon John of Arderne in 1371.[23] Valentine Mott, in his *Travels in Europe and Asia* (1842), associated the disease with leprosy which he claimed was the true progenitor of modern syphilis. Mott, along with other early medical writers, probably confused leprosy with syphilis since both were considered highly contagious and were thought to respond to mercury treatment.[24] Authors in the fifteenth and sixteenth centuries, including Gasparo Torella (1497), Peter Maynard (1518), and Girolamo Fracastoro (1530), suspected that syphilis originated in the conjunctions of Venus and Mars or of Jupiter and Venus; Fracastoro (1484–1553), a physician, poet, and astronomer, wrote a celebrated poem "Syphilidis Sive de Morbo Gallico Libre Tres" which gave the disease its name. Others acknowledged it to be a contagious malady carried in the air, which could give rise to epidemics. Jean Baptiste Van Helmont (1577–1644) claimed that it originated from an unnatural connection between a man and a horse sick with "farcy" or "glanders"; but there were those who blamed it on sodomy between men and monkeys, or satyrs.[25] Of course, theologians had long indicated that syphilis was a punishment ("flagellum Dei") inflicted upon man for adulterous sexual intercourse. In fact, it was claimed to be among the illnesses alluded to by Moses in *Leviticus* (15:2) when he prescribed rules for those afflicted with "a running issue out of the flesh." Samuel Solly, president of the Royal Medical and Chirurgical Society of London in 1867, voiced the views of many physicians and laymen in the nineteenth century when he referred to syphilis as

23. Freeman Josiah Bumstead, *The Pathology and Treatment of Venereal Diseases; Including the Results of Recent Investigations upon the Subject* (Philadelphia, 1870), 17–18.

24. Frederick Hollick, *A Popular Treatise on Venereal Diseases, in All Their Forms. Embracing Their History, and Probable Origin; Their Consequences, Both to Individuals and to Society; and the Best Modes of Treating Them* (New York, 1852), 21; C. B. Godfrey, *An Historical and Practical Treatise on the Venereal Disease* (London, 1797), 52.

25. William Acton, *A Complete Practical Treatise on Venereal Diseases, and Their Immediate and Remote Consequences* (London, 1841), 13–14; Hollick, *A Popular Treatise on Venereal Diseases*, 23; Homer Bostwick, *A Complete Practical Work on the Nature and Treatment of Venereal Diseases, and Other Affections of the Genito-Urinary Organs of the Male and Female* (New York, 1848), 68; William Van Wyck, *The Sinister Shepherd: A Translation of Girolamo Fracastoro's Syphilidis Sive de Morbo Gallico Libre Tres* (Los Angeles, 1934); Girolamo Fracastoro, *Fracastor Syphilis; or the French Disease* (London, 1935).

a "blessing . . . inflicted by the Almighty to act as a restraint upon indulgence of evil passions."[26]

The theory given widest credence attributed the disease to the return voyage of Columbus to Barcelona in 1493, the year before its epidemic appearance in Italy. This idea, first suggested by Leonhard Schmaus in 1518 and reinforced in the writings of Ulrich von Hutten in 1519 and Fracastoro in 1530, prevailed through most of the nineteenth century.[27] Jean Astruc (1684–1766) reported that syphilis had been endemic in the Antilles, particularly on the island of Santo Domingo where the disease, generally mild among the Indian population, severely afflicted the Spaniards who contracted it. How the virus came to originate in the West Indies was not entirely clear to these early theorists. Although some attributed it to the climate, skeptics noted that in that case it surely would have remained in the tropics and not spread to Europe. Some imagined it to have resulted from cannibalism among the Carib tribes, and one theory even suggested that it originated in consequence of a turtle feast.[28] Astruc pinpointed the "seed-plots" of venereal disease in Peru, New Spain, Florida, Africa below the equator (here medical men related the disease to the yaws), Java, the Molucca Islands, and China. Furthermore, he blamed the source of the disease on the particular diet, the immoderate venery of the people, and the "virulent acrimony of the menstrual flux." The disease then, had been communicated to the Spaniards in sexual intercourse and imported to Europe, where it spread rapidly.[29]

One of the vessels in the return fleet of Columbus reportedly carried more than 200 men infected with syphilis. From them, it allegedly spread through Spain and then Italy, where it infected the mercenary armies of Charles VIII in their un-

26. Quoted in Acton, *Prostitution in Relation to Public Health*, 7; Sylvanus Stall, *What a Young Man Ought to Know* (Philadelphia, 1897), 136.

27. Bumstead, *The Pathology and Treatment of Venereal Diseases*, 23–24.

28. H. Deacon, *A Compendious Treatise on the Venereal Disease, Gleets, etc., Divested of the Technical Terms; with the Best Methods of Cure, so Explained as to Render Medical Advice, in the Cure of Most Venereal Cases, Unnecessary. In Which Is Given a Lotion for the Prevention of that Disagreeable Complaint* (London, 1789), 3; Bostwick, *A Complete Practical Work on the Nature and Treatment of Venereal Diseases*, 68.

29. Acton, *A Complete Practical Treatise on Venereal Diseases*, 14–15; Deacon, *A Compendious Treatise on the Venereal Disease*, 1.

successful siege of Naples. The French claimed that the army acquired the disease from women sent from within the walls of the besieged city to entertain the troops—women who supposedly first contracted the disease from the sailors of Columbus's fleet. The French called the disease "mal de Naples" inasmuch as it had been unknown to them before the Neapolitan expedition, while the Italians ascribed it to the French and called it the "French Pox," or "Morbus Gallicus." Whether it was a modification of a pre-existing syphilitic virus or entirely new, by the end of the century it had spread throughout Italy, and then into Switzerland, France, and northern Europe, encouraged by the widespread social and political upheaval of the time. The English and Scottish mercenaries who fought with Charles VIII in Italy returned to England by way of Bordeaux in 1498 and the disease was thus named "Morbus Burligalensis." In Scotland, those who contracted "gore" or "glengore" were ordered by the Privy Council to be quarantined on the island of Inchkeith near Leith. Similarly, the infected persons of Paris were ordered to leave the city in 1497.[30]

According to William Acton, the "non-virulent" diseases existed throughout history and the more virulent affections, particularly syphilis, probably existed in Europe before the return of Columbus's ships, but proper information and an informed etiology of the disease was lacking. "I believe that the disease has had various phases," he wrote, "at one period it has assumed a very mild character, in consequence of attention to cleanliness and peace. On the other hand, in time of war and famine, it has assumed aggravated forms depending upon evanescent causes."[31] Karl Sudhoff, in a masterful study published in 1912, cast similar doubt on the Columbian origin of syphilis, claiming that the Neapolitan epidemic was probably an outbreak of typhoid or paratyphoid infection. "The end-result of Sudhoff's investigations," wrote medical historian Fielding Garrison, "is to the effect that from the twelfth century on, medieval physicians were richly supplied with mer-

30. David Newman, "The History and Prevention of Venereal Disease," *Glasgow Medical Journal*, LXXXI (1914), 92.
31. Acton, *A Complete Practical Treatise on Venereal Diseases*, 17.

curial recipes against an anomalous group of chronic skin affections, which, from their very names—scabies grossa, variola grossa, grosse vérole, scabies mala, böse Blattern, mal franzoso—were most likely syphilitic."[32] Sudhoff considered "scabies grossa," known in Italy in the thirteenth century, and treated with mercury, as sound evidence that syphilis predated the Columbian voyage.[33] Furthermore, as was pointed out by William Sanger, diseases very similar to what was later described as syphilis had been subject to public regulations in the 1430s in London. Police were required "to keep constant watch over such as should show symptoms of this *infirmitas nefanda*," and prevent them from entering houses of prostitution.[34] Sudhoff blamed part of the confusion surrounding the origin of syphilis on the polemical nature of pamphlet literature spreading through Italy and Germany, a result of the recent invention of the printing press. The literature on syphilis, enhanced by the art of printing, gave the disease a recognition none had experienced before. "It was printing," he argued, "that established and diffused the knowledge of the existence and nature of syphilis."[35]

Investigators in the first decades of the twentieth century testing the claim that syphilis had been brought to Spain by the sailors of Columbus looked for syphilitic bones in the grave mounds of America. "During recent investigations amongst the graves of the mound builders in the southern part of the United States," wrote physician David Newman in 1914, in a speech before the faculty of the University of Glasgow, "bones with lesions resembling those of tertiary syphilis have been found in abundance among the skeletons discovered in these mounds." Furthermore, the age of the mounds was established as pre-Columbian. On the other hand, studies made of bones in the lake and cave dwellings and barrows of western Europe showed no signs of syphilitic lesions. It seemed therefore certain to many in the early twentieth century

32. Fielding H. Garrison, *An Introduction to the History of Medicine* (4th ed.; Philadelphia, 1929), 191.

33. Karl Sudhoff, *The Earliest Printed Literature on Syphilis* (Florence, 1925), xxxiv.

34. Sanger, *The History of Prostitution*, 132.

35. Sudhoff, *The Earliest Printed Literature on Syphilis*, x–xi.

that syphilis had spread to western Europe from eastern America; however, this did not rule out the possibility that America had received the disease from Asia at a still earlier date, since there existed very graphic accounts among the Chinese ancients of apparent syphilitic disorders.[36] The Chinese medical writer Hoang-ty (2637 B.C.) gave the following description:

A corroding ulcer produced by a poison of a particular kind, and communicable by direct contact, is met with in the genital organs of the male and female: it generally appears from the third to the ninth day, either singly or accompanied by a number of other lesions of the same kind. It begins as a small red spot raised at its centre, and causing either pain or itching. In a short time a white spot appears at the centre, and forms a cavity, and increases insensibly in size and depth. At the base is seen and felt a kind of hard thick skin of whitish colour, the edges become equally hard with irregular notches. The consequent ulcers of the mouth, throat and nose, the mucous patches of the anal region.[37]

Until the early decades of the nineteenth century, many practitioners were treating the secondary and tertiary stages of syphilis without being fully aware of the actual cause. Because the primary sore was probably "small and insignificant," observed one syphilologist, "sexual intercourse was not suspected as the source of contagion."[38] John Hunter (1728–93), one of the founders of experimental pathology, added to the confusion by contending that gonorrhea and syphilis were produced by a single virus. To prove his thesis, and in an attempt to refute the views of Giovanni Morgagni (1682–1771), who had identified syphilis as the result of lesions of the cerebral vessels, Hunter inoculated himself with the discharge of a gonorrhea victim. The patient, however, was also suffering from syphilis; when Hunter contracted both diseases and proved to his satisfaction that they derived from a single origin, his claims retarded medical studies of syphilis for many decades. Hunter's thesis was not successfully challenged until

36. Although there was evidence of treponematosis found in the skeletal remains of pre-Columbian Indians the medical scientist Ellis Herndon Hudson, in his book *Treponematosis* (New York, 1946), argued against the American origin theory.

37. Newman, "The History and Prevention of Venereal Disease," 89.

38. *Ibid.*, 93.

Philippe Ricord's investigations in the 1830s at the Hospital du Midi in Paris. In his famous *Traité pratique des maladies vénériennes* (1838), Ricord not only established the autonomy of syphilis and gonorrhea, but he also characterized the primary, secondary, and tertiary stages of syphilis. He likewise described the distinction between the soft, nonsyphilitic chancre (chancroid) and the hard, syphilitic chancre. Subsequent investigations by Barensprung and Rudolph Virchow on hard and soft chancres and the contagion of secondary syphilis greatly aided medical knowledge. Advances in morbid histology brought greater understanding of the peculiar nature of venereal diseases and led to Albert Neisser's discovery of diplococcus of gonorrhea in 1879, soon followed in 1889 by Ducrey's and Paul Unna's discovery of the bacillus of soft chancre. The experiments of Eli Metchnikoff and Lassar on animals laid the foundation for the researches of Schaudinn and Hoffman on the spirochaeta pallida of syphilis in 1905. With that major hurdle completed, German bacteriologist August von Wassermann, Neisser, and C. Bruck were able to diagnose through blood tests the different stages of syphilis.[39]

The statistics on venereal disease in the nineteenth century were alarming. The city of Cincinnati, which instituted a system of medical licensing and regular physical examinations in 1893, reported that of the 625 licensed prostitutes, half were infected at least once during the year. Frederick R. Sturgis, in a paper read before the American Public Health Association in 1874, estimated that one out of every 18.5 persons in New York City was suffering from syphilis; in another paper read before the American Medical Association meeting in Detroit, a doctor claimed that one out of every 22 persons in the United States was syphilitic.[40] Statistics drawn up by the Army and Navy were no less encouraging.[41]

39. *Ibid.*, 96–97; William A. Pusey, *The History and Epidemiology of Syphilis* (Baltimore, 1933); Iwan Bloch, *The Sexual Life of Our Time in Its Relations to Modern Civilization* (London, 1909), 354–56; Gerald Dalton, *A Practical Manual of Venereal and Generative Diseases* (London, 1913), 1.

40. William L. Holt, "A Popular Treatise on Venereal Diseases," *Medico-Pharmaceutical Critic and Guide*, XI (1908), 149.

41. Albert L. Gihon, "Report of the Committee on the Prevention of Venereal Diseases," *Papers and Reports*, American Public Health Association, VI (1881), 405–6.

Venereal Disease in the United States Navy

YEAR	TOTAL FORCE AFLOAT	TOTAL SICK FROM ALL CAUSES ON BOARD MEN-OF-WAR	NO. OF CASES OF VENEREAL DISEASE	NO. OF CASES OF SYPHILIS	PER 1,000 OF FORCE Venereal	PER 1,000 OF FORCE Syphilis	PER 1,000 OF SICK Venereal	PER 1,000 OF SICK Syphilis	PERCENT OF SYPHILIS TO VENEREAL
1873	12,723	8,837	1,029	595	81	46	116	67	57.82
1874	13,870	9,995	963	562	69	40	96	56	58.36
1875	10,141	7,832	956	500	94	49	122	64	52.30
1876	11,138	7,797	889	437	79	39	114	56	49.15
1877	7,461	6,748	703	342	94	45	104	51	48.65
1878	7,806	6,873	751	341	96	54	109	50	45.40
1879	8,869	10,488	1,101	490	124	45	105	47	44.50
Average	10,287	8,367	913	467	88	45	109	56	51.15

Venereal Disease in United States Army

YEARS	TOTAL FORCE		TOTAL SICK FROM ALL CAUSES	NO. OF CASES OF VENEREAL DISEASE	NO. OF CASES OF SYPHILIS	PER 1,000 OF FORCE Venereal	PER 1,000 OF FORCE Syphilis	PER 1,000 OF SICK Venereal	PER 1,000 OF SICK Syphilis	PERCENT OF SYPHILIS TO VENEREAL
1875–76	White	21,718	32,523	2,262	1,147	104	53	69	35	50.70
	Colored	2,014	2,971	364	198	181	98	126	67	54.40
	Total	23,732	35,494	2,626	1,345	110	57	74	38	51.22
1876–77	White	23,383	34,683	2,463	1,283	105	55	71	37	52.09
	Colored	2,083	3,779	351	170	169	82	93	45	48.43
	Total	25,466	38,462	2,814	1,453	110	57	73	38	51.64
1877–78	White	20,812	26,398	1,840	954	88	46	69	36	51.84
	Colored	1,895	3,048	321	146	169	77	105	48	45.84
	Total	22,707	29,446	2,161	1,100	95	48	73	37	50.90
1878–79	White	21,847	32,814	1,902	885	87	41	58	27	46.53
	Colored	1,964	3,455	281	155	143	79	81	45	55.15
	Total	23,811	36,269	2,183	1,040	92	44	60	29	47.64
1879–80	White	22,087	33,645	1,957	960	89	43	58	29	49.05
	Colored	2,387	3,669	309	152	129	64	84	41	49.09
	Total	24,474	37,314	2,266	1,112	92	45	60	29	49.08
Mean	White	21,969	32,013	2,085	1,046	95	48	65	33	50.17
	Colored	2,069	3,384	325	164	157	79	96	48	50.
	Total	24,038	35,397	2,410	1,210	103	50	68	34	50.

The statistics of the United States Army and Navy, however, fell far behind those of the British Army in India. In a report of H. S. Cunningham for the year 1895, it was noted that of a standing force of 68,331 soldiers, there were no less than 36,881 hospital cases of venereal disease.[42]

Medical writers from the ancients into the nineteenth century attributed less virulent forms of venereal disease to such things as gout, rheumatism, bladder stones, exposure to dampness, the overuse of spices, snuff, Spanish flies, uncleanliness, and even the cutting of a tooth.[43] Many of the early theories were first introduced by Astruc, whose six-volume treatise on the diseases of women in the 1760s blamed the drinking of strong beer, riding, and "immoderate venery, though pure," as contributing causes.[44] Alexander Weill contended that if a man had intercourse with two different women in brief succession, he could acquire venereal disease, since "any kind of libertinism in sexual intercourse suffices by itself to give rise to this disease."[45] Physicians throughout most of the nineteenth century held that gonorrhea could be contracted from perfectly pure sexual relations, even between faithful married couples. It was thought by some, for example, that intercourse during menstruation could incite the severest form of gonorrhea. Then too, it could arise from simple excess in sexual intercourse, principally from the repetition of the act within a short space of time. "The physician is sometimes called in by the husband of a few weeks' standing," wrote Henry Lyman, M.D., "to determine whether or not the bride has communicated the gonorrhea which has attacked him in the second week of wedded life. . . . In the great majority of such cases it will be found upon close examination that the disease is merely the result of the youthful husband's impetuosity."[46]

Nineteenth-century manual writers continually reminded the male that intemperate venereal indulgences would destroy

42. Bailey, "Some Problems concerning Venereal Diseases," 592.
43. Deacon, *A Compendious Treatise on the Venereal Disease*, 3.
44. Quoted in (Anony.), *A Familiar Essay, Explanatory of the Theory and Practice of Prevention of Venereal Contagion, Interspersed with Observations on the Nature and Treatment of Gonorrhoea* (London, 1810), 45.
45. Bloch, *The Sexual Life of Our Time*, 351.
46. Henry M. Lyman, *et al.*, *The Practical Home Physician. A Popular Guide for the Household Management of Disease* (Chicago, 1883), 516.

the vigor of his manhood, impairing his faculties with weakness and disease. Only in the legitimate connubial embrace permitted by matrimony would the evil propensities of sex and its attendant physical disorders be safely avoided. Yet, while setting forth the only true state of sexual relationships, writers found themselves faced with the realities of prostitution and venereal disease, and rather than serve as literary midwives to happily married couples, many chose to teach preventive medicine for those occasionally remiss in virtue. Books which sold under the titles "Self-Preservation," "Life-Renovater," "Secret Sorrow—Certain Help," and "Manhood" gave careful instructions to the young man on how best to guard against disease. Davy's Lac-Elephantis, a medicated milk supposedly extracted from elephants, promised to cure venereal disease if taken within twenty-four hours of an "illicit connexion."[47] One famous preventive lotion sold by Messrs. Perry of London claimed to combine chemically with the venereal virus and destroy its power over the system. "How can a young man indulge his natural feelings and desires, without danger?", they advertised. "The *Preventive Lotion* will enable him to have connexion with the fair but frail Cyprians who perambulate our streets, without any fear or reason to dread the consequences in the shape of the venereal disease, in any of its forms, such as gonorrhea, clap, or syphilis. It will effectually prevent all danger from *indiscriminate sexual intercourse.*"[48]

Dedicated "votaries of Venus" not only applied washes and glutinous adhesives to the penis before and after coition, but washed the parts with caustics, and injected solutions such as mercury, water, and spirit of niter into the urethra to discharge whatever foul contagion might have entered during intercourse. An early preventive consisted of mucilages of gum arabic, isinglass, gum tragacanth, quince seeds, starch, and other glutinous substances which were mixed with calomel and applied to the penis before coition. A variation of

47. (Anony.), *Davy's Lac-Elephantis; or, Medicated Milk of Elephants. An Effectual Cure for . . . Venereal Disease, in Both Sexes, with a Plain Prescription* (London, 1815), 24.

48. Quoted in (Anony.), "The Anatomy of Quackery," *Medical Circular*, II (1853), 284.

this consisted of melted plasters applied to the penis before intercourse. The Venetian physician Nikolaus Massa in his *De Morbo Gallico* (1532) prescribed postcoitus washes of vinegar or white wine. Fracastoro recommended a lemon juice solution, while Petronius (1564) introduced a wine of camphor mixed with urine. Hermann Boerhaave (1668–1738), on the other hand, cautioned men to wash their genitals with lemon juice and salt before engaging with a suspicious woman. The application of the acids would constrict the opening of the urethra so that, despite ejaculation, the male would not absorb infected particles. In the seventeenth and eighteenth centuries, popular antivenereals included alum washes, mixtures of white wine and turpentine, or guaiac and wine, but the poor man's preventive was usually an alcoholic beverage splashed on the genitals before or after intercourse.[49] Although the condom, made of linen, fish bladder, lamb skin, and eventually rubber, was sold as a preventative of venereal disease, it was probably used more frequently in middle-class households or by kept mistresses than in the sporting houses, because of its reputation for detracting from the pleasure of the moment. Buret reported in *Syphilis in the Middle Ages and in Modern Times* (1895) that sporting houses preferred a salve of vaseline and boric acid to the condom. Parent-Duchâtelet noted in his study of Parisian prostitutes the use of a bottle of oil to facilitate intercourse and prevent abrasion of the vaginal walls, and a solution of caustic soda to guard against disease and prevent conception.[50]

Once a person showed signs of venereal infection, he could choose from literally a storehouse of reputed cures—from decoctions of marshmallow roots to salves of lard and tar. The Spanish introduced soaps, pills, and tinctures of guaiac (1508), a stimulant and alterative, as a cure for the venereal plague; China root (Galangal) was imported from China and Japan around 1535; this, in turn, was followed by American sarsapa-

49. Robert A. Bachman, "Venereal Prophylaxis—Past and Present," *Medical Record*, LXXXIV (1913), 602; Deacon, *A Compendious Treatise on the Venereal Disease*, 128–29; (Anony.), *A Familiar Essay, Explanatory of the Theory and Practice of Prevention of Venereal Contagion*, 117–18.

50. Frederic Buret, *Syphilis in the Middle Ages and in Modern Times* (Philadelphia, 1895), 130.

rilla and sassafras in the 1550s. Sarsaparilla fell into disrepute until 1757 when it was again revived by John Fordyce. Other remedies included Syrup de St. Ambroise, introduced by French physician Julian Palmier and consisting mainly of branches of a fig tree, but there were also remedies of camphor and antimony, linseed tea, purges of Epsom salts, linens soaked in acetate of lead, calomel, and limewater, pills of opium and henbane, as well as leeches and venesection. Some physicians even prescribed pouring scalding water over the genitals, drinking large drafts of salt water, or consuming "heroic" doses of prunes and figs.[51]

From the fifteenth century into the nineteenth, much of the odium connected with venereal disease extended even to the medical men who treated it. "As a consequence," wrote one doctor in 1895, "this department of medicine was largely relegated to the charlatan, who, under the control of ignorance and avarice, contributed to the exaggeration and confusion which still cloud the minds of many when they consider the subject."[52] For the same reason, statistics on venereal disease in the nineteenth century were sometimes grossly inaccurate, since they did not take into account the fact that most public institutions, except those which made a specialty of dealing with the "private disease," held it a disgrace to treat venereal patients. The same public morality which drove venereal victims out of the cities of London and Paris in the fifteenth and sixteenth centuries, and later heard from papal pronouncements that syphilis was God's punishment for incontinence, survived in institutions supported by public donations in the nineteenth century. Many hospitals in New York and elsewhere had rules prohibiting the treatment of gonorrhea or syphilis. With such public feeling, venereal victims usually resorted to "private specialists" and empirics who advertised in the daily papers. Of course, persons of respectable social standing preferred private treatment to public hospitals, but they paid a high price for secrecy, since a large number of the medical

51. (Anony.), *A Familiar Essay, Explanatory of the Theory and Practice of Prevention of Venereal Contagion*, 60–65, 68–70.

52. James N. Hyde and Frank H. Montgomery, *A Manual of Syphilis and the Venereal Diseases* (Philadelphia, 1895), 18.

parlors or institutions which catered to this clientele merely sold useless or harmful cures. Some gullible victims, having purchased pamphlets promising a cheap, drugless cure, were instructed to avoid exercise, walk slow, "keep the penis defended from the cold, never making water in a place exposed to the rigor of the cold north or easterly wind," consume water-gruel, bathe frequently, and rest.[53]

In any major city in Europe or America, one could find bathing rooms where people suffering from venereal problems could take warm fresh baths, salt-water showers, shampoos, sulfur fumigating, ferrous salts, medicated vapors, douches, and other "cures." Numerous medical pamphlets gave a brief history of sexual disorders from masturbation and spermatorrhea to clap and syphilis, and then offered information on consultation hours, forms of treatment, case histories of successfully treated patients, and price lists for special drugs or devices. Advertisements for curing the male's private diseases appeared in magazines and newspapers of the day, on signs pasted on the walls of toilets, and even on matchbox covers, praising the effects of a nostrum or providing addresses of local specialists.[54] Numerous proprietors of patent medicines wrote books to advertise their own particular cure for venereal diseases. Medicines packaged under the name of Curtis's Manhood, Sir Samuel Hannay's Specific, Dr. Brodum's Botanical Syrup, or Dr. Morse's Invigorating Cordial, or sold as "anti-venereal lotion," "life-drops," "preventive wash," "purific pills," "blood purifiers," or "compound renal pills" promised protection and cure for the infected victim. There were specifics such as Naples soap (named after the city where syphilis had reportedly become epidemic), The Boss, Armenian Pills, Big G, Bumstead's Gleet Cure, Lafayette Mixture, and Hot Springs Prescription. Two favorite drugstore remedies were sold under the name of Red Drops (corrosive sublimate, alcohol, and spirits of lavender) and Unfortunate's Friend (a decoction of sarsaparilla, guaiacum, burdock, parsley, and licorice roots, and a half-dozen other ingredients in alcohol). Another popular cure, known as Pine Knot Bitters, could be

53. Deacon, *A Compendious Treatise on the Venereal Disease,* 36–37.
54. Vice Commission of Chicago, *The Social Evil of Chicago,* 131.

purchased in both drugstores and liquor stores in the nineteenth century.

The monistic systematists in medicine who reduced all human complaints to single sources—humors, gastro-enteritis, fevers, or nervous force—gave rise to their counterparts in the world of pharmacy, and the hundreds of cures pledged to treat all the ills of man. A glance at the patent medicine shelves of the day would have demonstrated the universality of the vendor's claims. Since there was but one disease, so there was but one remedy. The monistic reasoning used to sell Morison's Vegetable Medicine could be applied to hundreds of others on the druggist's shelves.

All animals consist of fluids and solids!
All embryo animals consist entirely of fluids.
The chief fluid is the blood, from which all others are derived.
Blood forms the body—air gives it life.
All constitutions are radically the same.
All diseases arise from impurity of the blood.
All diseases arise from one source, and therefore require but one medicine.
Proper purgation by vegetables is the only effectual way of curing all diseases.
This vegetable purgative must be capable of being digested, and mixing with the blood, so as to rid the body of all superfluous humors (disease).

The only question that remained for the purchaser was how to choose from among the countless nostrums claiming to be the sole dispenser of health. From Vaughn's Vegetable Lithontriptic to Morison's Vegetable Medicine to Dr. Ward's Unfortunate's Friend, the claims covered everything from split toenails to syphilis, bilious fever, and insanity.[55]

Within fifty years of the Italian epidemic, mercury had become the most prevalent antisyphilitic remedy. Administered in the form of blue mass, gray powder (mercury and chalk),

55. (Anony.), "The Anatomy of Quackery," 25; (Anony.), *General Treatise on the Nature and Cause of Disease in the Human Body; Together with Proofs of the Efficacy of Vaughn's Vegetable Lithontriptic Mixture, as a General Restorer of the System, and Purifier of the Blood* (Buffalo, 1845), 12; William Buchan, *Observations concerning the Prevention and Cure of Venereal Disease. Intended to Guard the Ignorant and Unwary against the Baneful Effects of that Insidious Malady* (London, 1796), 29–31.

calomel (mercurous chloride), or corrosive sublimate (bichloride of mercury), or surreptitiously as "life balsams" or "blood purifiers," mercury soon became known both in and out of medical circles as the "Samson of the Materia Medica." During the 1560s, an early mercury prophylaxis known as "A Decoction of the Vulnerary Astringent Woods" required the victims of syphilis to steep their clothes in the liquid and apply specially soaked bandages to their genitals.[56] A popular antisyphilitic of the eighteenth century, Keyser's Mercury Pills, even claimed a poem written in its honor by a Frenchman whose lady friend "had been long in a melancholy situation."

> Illustrious Keyser has at length restor'd
> The beauteous Sylvia to my longing Arms!
> As her Recovery conquers my Despair,
> So thy skill triumphs o'er pale Envy's rage!
> In vain weak Enemies conspire against you,
> Truth's powerful Blaze will dissipate the Cloud
> Fell Malice impotently strives to raise,
> And to eclipse the Glories that adorn you.
> With honest Pride look down on Efforts vain.
> O punish them with still repeated Curses,
> And each be deem'd more wond'rous than the last.
> How many Vot'ries of the Cyprian Queen
> Fin'd in the Prime of Life, a Prey to Ills,
> Pronounced incurable, till you appear'd?
> Like to the vernal Sun, whose strength'ning Rays
> Winter dispel, and give new Springs to Nature;
> You had Contagion cease—her lepr'd Offspring
> Fled at thy great Command—no Vestige foul
> Nor fallow Stain disgrace my Sylvia's Cheek,
> Her dimpled Cheek the Throne of smiling Love.
> All Praise is to heroick Biron due,
> Who for thy Skill procured a proper Sphere
> To counteract that formidable Hydra,
> Fraught with a subtle Virus, Beauty's Bane,
> Blasting the joys that heighten our Existence.
> You've conquer'd—the fell Monster reigns no more.
> Now each glad Hour Love's Raptures we repeat;
> Our warmest Praise attends on Keyser's name!

56. (Anony.), *A Familiar Essay, Explanatory of the Theory and Practice of Prevention of Venereal Contagion*, 106; John S. Haller, Jr., "Samson of the Materia Medica: Medical Theory and the Use and Abuse of Calomel in 19th Century America," *Pharmacy in History*, XIII (1971), 27–34, 67–75.

Keyser, who gave dear Sylvia back to Life,
And makes me happiest of human Race!
Besides the greatful few who loud proclaim
Their Obligations to thy Magic Pills,
How great's the Number! Modesty compels,
In formal Def'rence to their Rank or Station,
With silent Rapture to record thy Cures.
Continue, Sir, to merit of Mankind
Dispensing Health, and Joy to the distres'd.
The greatest Recompence of noble Minds
Is to be conscious of their doing good;
In which exalted Light you stand so high,
Envy'd, unrival'd, and by most rever'd![57]

Physicians readily embraced the mercury treatment, hoping that it would bring a quick end to the venereal scourge; but while it brought relief to some, its many side effects also threw medical circles into the utmost consternation. Some of the confusion surrounding its application grew out of the failure of physicians to determine its exact modus operandi—was it an evacuant as some believed, or a sedative, or perhaps an astringent? The English physician John Hunter theorized that two poisons could not co-exist in the body at the same time; thus, in the case of syphilis, the strong mercurial medicine would expel the lesser syphilitic poison from the system.[58] But others thought that as syphilis acted upon certain elements of the blood and broke them down, mercury seized upon the syphilitic agents, disintegrating them, and expelling them from the system.

All men concede that mercury's the best
Of agents that will cure a tainted breast.
To heat and cold sensitive's mercury,
Absorbing the fires of this vile leprosy
And all the body's flames by its sheer weight,
Dissolving humors that it recreate
The health and with a fine, divided art
Applied to quench the flame right to its heart

57. James Cowper, *A Narrative of the Effects of a Medicine, Newly Discovered by Mr. Keyser, a German Chymist in Paris that Cures the Venereal Disease in Its Most Inveterate and Malignant State, without Salivation or Strict Regime, as Is Now Practiced in France, Both in Private Cases, and in the Military Hospitals* (London, 1760), 57–58.

58. John Hunter, *A Treatise on the Venereal Disease* (Philadelphia, 1818), 7, 312–40.

> And delving deep to every injured part.
> Each acrid mollecule will in its turn
> Seize upon every humor that will burn
> The scourge away by secret energies
> That hide from human eyes their destinies.[59]

According to Hermann Boerhaave, the efficacy of mercury derived from the power of the blood and humors to carry the mercurial particles "through the infected Parts, with such Force as is capable of dividing, attenuating, and at length expelling them by the means of Salivation."[60] More often than not, however, the salivatory cure was worse than the disease, particularly when the mercury treatment brought on a sloughing of the mouth. Medical men in the early decades of the nineteenth century salivated patients with heroic doses of calomel, believing that the patient was effectively doctored only when he salivated, the mouth turned brown in color, or gave off a mercurous odor. Unfortunately for many patients, however, the mercury treatment brought on sponginess and bleeding of the gums, necrosis of the jaw bones, strangulation, irritation of the skin, gangrene, and ulcerated cheeks.[61] "I have seen both cheeks entirely removed by this process," wrote one physician in the 1850s.[62] Another doctor recalled instances when the mercurialized jaw caused "almost the whole bone of the lower jaw cast off, the tongue eroded, the lips, cheek, and chin almost entirely eaten away."[63] Cases were reported of patients whose mouths had become locked by the mercury treatment, forcing the removal of the front teeth so that the patient could suck his food through a quill.[64]

The methods employed to administer mercury varied from pills and ointments, to fumigation and even absorption by the

59. Van Wyck, *The Sinister Shepherd*, 45–46.
60. J. A. Burrows, *A Dissertation on the Nature and Effects of a New Vegetable Remedy, an Acknowledged Specific in All Venereal Scorbutic and Scrophulous Cases* (London, 1780), 14; Arthur Cooper and Berkeley Hill, *The Student's Manual of Venereal Diseases Being a Concise Description of Those Affections and of Their Treatment* (2nd ed.; New York, 1881), 31.
61. Cowper, *A Narrative of the Effects of a Medicine*, xiv; (Anony.), *A Popular Dissertation on the Venereal Diseases*, 4.
62. Samuel Jackson, "The Use of Calomel in the Diseases of Children," *Transactions,* College of Physicians of Philadelphia, II (1853–56), 136.
63. Quoted in *ibid.*, 134.
64. Cowper, *A Narrative of the Effects of a Medicine*, xi–xii.

lungs. The Chinese employed the latter method, mixing mercury with tobacco. Mercurial ointment was sometimes placed in the armpit at night to allow the patient to absorb the mineral during sleep, or was applied between the toes, to be absorbed in walking. Fumigation, which was used in the fifteenth and sixteenth centuries, was re-introduced into English and American medical circles in the nineteenth century by Langston Parker, who employed mercury for its vapor effect.[65] Its therapeutic success was widely acclaimed, and numerous bathing or fumigating parlors were established to provide the service. The syphilitic patient was confined to a room kept at 70 degrees for five or six days, and prepared for fumigation on a diet of water-gruel, aperients, and sarsaparilla. He was then taken to a room of 80 degrees and seated naked on a stool with a robe of oiled or waxed cloth tied around his neck to protect the face and eyes. On the floor under his stool was a spirit lamp over which was placed a china plate containing blue mass, calomel, cinnebar, or gray powder. The fumes of the burning mercury were allowed to cover the body and after the treatment terminated, the patient changed into a pair of flannel underclothes and went to bed. The bath was given several times a week according to the strength of the patient and his ability to tolerate the mercurial effect. When necessary, doctors or parlor specialists localized the fumigation by means of a glass funnel which carried the fumes into the bed of the patient and to particular areas of the body.[66]

From 1910 until 1943 when J. F. Mahoney introduced penicillin in venereal treatment, an arsphenamine called "606" or Salvarsan developed by Paul Ehrlich was the most widely prescribed drug for venereal prophylaxis. The army, however, continued to rely on mercury. Following the announcement by Metchnikoff and Roux that syphilitic infection had been pre-

65. Bumstead, *The Pathology and Treatment of Venereal Diseases,* 493; Acton, *A Complete Practical Treatise on Venereal Diseases,* 334; F. Swinford Edwards, "On Some Points in the Treatment of Syphilis and Gleet," *Clinical Journal,* II (1897), 116–21; Horatio Prater, "The Action of Preventives of Venereal Diseases Considered Physically, Chemically, and Morally," *Lancet,* II (1842–43), 368–74.
66. Bostwick, *A Complete Practical Work on the Nature and Treatment of Venereal Diseases,* 143; James R. Hayden, *A Manual of Venereal Diseases* (New York, 1896), 237.

270 The Physician and Sexuality in Victorian America

vented in clinical experiments with apes with a 30 percent
calomel ointment, Major H. I. Raymond of the Army Medical
Corps succeeded in introducing a German method of prophylaxis at Columbus Barracks, Ohio, in 1906 consisting of
special "K" packets containing an argyrol solution to irrigate
the urethra and a calomel ointment. Navy surgeons introduced
a slight modification consisting of a wash of 1–5000 bichloride
of mercury solution for the penis, an urethral injection of
argyrol or protargol solution, and the application of a calomel
ointment. Sailors were threatened with courtmartial if they
failed to report for disinfection treatment following shore
liberty. These separate prophylaxis methods were later replaced with A and N Protection tubes (3 percent phenol, 3
percent camphor, 30 percent calomel, 32 percent benzoated
lard, and 32 percent lanolin) based on experiments of Colonel
L. M. Maus of the Army Medical Corps in 1910.[67]

Reluctant to rid himself of the ascetic discipline required in
his attempt to become the fittest man, the Victorian male
struggled within society's edict of respectability and the im-
pediments of the Victorian marriage. Anxious to preserve the
decorum of the home circle and the woman's disposition to
denigrate her sexuality, he was frequently led astray by the
impatient desires of his more agreeable habits. The medico-
moral response to his behavior was far less exacting than its
response to masturbation or spermatorrhea. Though considered
a frivolous expenditure of manly vigor, extramarital relationships did not carry the shame of self-abuse, or the threat of
insanity which followed the "unnatural" loss of semen in
sleep. To be sure, there was always the danger of venereal
disease, but society and the medical profession seemed to favor
a silent toleration of promiscuity so long as the act itself was
"natural." Although the Victorian male could seldom overcome
the bodily harm incurred from the gluttony of self-pollution,
he could always resume his ascent to higher evolution after
a momentary pause in the arms of Venus.

67. Bachman, "Venereal Prophylaxis—Past and Present," 602; L. M. Maus,
"The Suppression of Vice Diseases through Personal Prophylaxis and Municipal Control of the Saloon and Courtesan," Chicago Medical Recorder, XXXV
(1913), 21–22; Robert A. Bachmann, "The Problem of Venereal Prophylaxis,"
Medical Record, LXXXII (1913), 195–99.

Chapter VII

THE SILENT FRIENDS

The social queen will lunch at 1 P.M. with an intense headache as her only companion; dress, take a drink of spirituous liquor, or too frequently, a quarter-grain of morphine; go to her drawing-room to entertain pleasantly those for whom she has no other feeling but hatred or envy, dine at 6 P.M. with a man who is supposed to be her protector, but does and says only that which will annoy and distress her. Afterward, at about 10 o'clock, she goes to a party or reception, there spends an evening of excitement mixed with the usual amount of disappointment, returns home in the morning as the sky begins to grow grey in the East, endeavors without much success to secure a few hours' sleep, rises at 10 A.M. with a feeling of exhaustion, and with burning eyes and intense pain in the head endeavors to overcome this feeling with the use of stimulants, takes her usual breakfast of coffee and dry toast and starts out to repeat the yesterday of every day of her life.

H. C. Strong, *Journal*, American Medical Association, 1899

Victorian society typified the aspirations of America at the moment when they were at their highest and when prospects for fulfillment seemed most secure. It was a restless society which overstrained in its efforts to master the continent and empire so recently acquired and rival the industrial energy so recently harnessed. The Victorians were burdened, as no other generation before them, with the weight of their own image. Self-conscious, class-conscious, race-conscious, and nation-conscious, they struggled to gain the highest planes of achievement. Aware of their responsibilities not only to past generations, but to future ones as well, they dutifully bore the obligations with which they were blessed. Children of the industrial age, and descendants of the Enlightenment, they could admit no pessimism, no nihilism, no medieval gloom to impede their steady march onward. White, Anglo-Saxon, and Christian, they saw their destiny ordained by their inheritance; they were the leaders to be followed, the examples of civilization's highest hopes, to be envied, admired, and imitated. This self-image could admit no fault, for their highest duty lay not to themselves, but to future generations. For the Victorian men and women who bore the brunt of this effort, nothing that benefited class, nation, or race was too daring or too difficult.

While the fittest male could always assuage the pressures of the moment by indulging in an assortment of acceptable "vices" outside the home, the Victorian woman had little or no such opportunity. Venerated and ignored, she stood as a silent and mindless tribute to middle-class sophistication, embellishing its legend with both virtue and grace. For those women who had accepted their role without illusion, happiness became a form of wisdom maturing with years, and the will, recognizing the limitation of choice, found peace in resignation. Yet, for as many who struggled to define the excellence of their invented world there were those who wearied of the role and suffered in their despondency. Fragmented by male chauvinism, they admitted almost apologetically the limitations of their sex, preferring quiet brooding to scandalous unconventionality. Insulated by the demands of etiquette from everything but their imaginations, protected from human instincts which had been exaggerated into vices, they sought to redeem the disorder and servitude of their souls in furtive efforts to deaden the mind and will. For those women unable or unwilling to sustain the absurdity of their role, or disappointed with their own reserve of talent, alcohol and narcotics became a compelling escape from their discontent. The impossible demands of a society which had conceived of them ideally as perfect forms, and dealt with them realistically as miscellaneous pleasures, made life a mass of difficulties and a confusion of insoluble problems, hideous with uncertainty. Many plunged into the depths of despair, suffering various forms of mental anguish, sleeplessness, neurasthenia, insane vanity, restlessness, and hysteria. Escape became an obsession—and a curse when money was lacking to procure it. Restricted by the impositions of a culture not her own choosing, the woman became morbid and abnormal, jealous and vain, and tempted by the crudest vices. And in her attempt to escape the closeness of the Victorian parlor, she became enslaved to something far more constricting.

A dark veil of obscurity shrouds the opium and alcohol inebriety of the Victorian woman—a veil whose cloth had been woven by both the victim and the society alike to conceal the failures of those who did not survive the system and its principles. Just as society was most anxious to avoid the reality of drug addiction, since it perhaps implied a serious imperfection in the nature and goals of its institutions, so the Victorian woman strove to remain secretive to avoid society's disfavor and embarrassment. In the foggy recesses of the laudanum bottle and the reluctance of society to recognize its weaker segments, women found obliging conspirators as they tripped the intricate steps of fashionable life. But the physician must also bear part of the burden of responsibility in the Victorian period since it was usually through his prescriptions that the habit was first formed.

Opophagia

Honoring the opium poppy (*papaver somniferum*) with such sobriquets as Manus Dei and Donum Dei, nineteenth-century physicians hailed the dried juice of the poppy as the "sheet anchor" of the materia medica. Although its history goes as far back as the ancient Greeks, whose divinities Hypnos (Sleep), Nyx (Night), and Thanatos (Death) were wreathed with the poppy, the pharmacohistorical importance of opium lies mainly in the Victorian age, which not only witnessed the culmination of the opium trade with China, but also marked the development of morphia and a long list of opium alkaloids. Opium-eating, or "opophagia" as it was sometimes called, reached notoriety in the late nineteenth century, when the annual importation of the poppy increased from 24,000 pounds in 1840 to over 142,000 in 1865, to 416,864 in 1872. Opium was produced principally in India, Turkey (which supplied most of the domestic needs of the United States), and Egypt, but a considerable quantity was also grown in the New England states, California, and Arizona. Most of the domestic market was sent to Philadelphia where, along with the poorer imported grades, it was processed into morphine.[1] Preparations came to the purchaser in a variety of forms. Besides raw gum opium, druggists sold laudanum (tincture of opium), paregoric (camphorated tincture of opium), morphine (sulfate of morphia), McMunn's Elixir (denarcotized laudanum prepared in ether), and Dover's powder (ipecac and opium). In addition to patent and prescription drugs, many homemade cough mixtures, tooth washes, lotions, liniments, enemas, poultices, healing tinctures, and decoctions contained opium. Distilleries (especially those in western Massachusetts and Vermont) added

---

1. Arthur Dickson Wright, "The History of Opium," *Medical Biology Illustrated*, XVIII (1968), 62–70; Henry E. Sigerist, "Laudanum in the Works of Paracelsus," *Bulletin of the History of Medicine*, IX (1941), 530–44; F. M. Sandwith, "Drugs, Old and New," *Medical Magazine*, XXII (1913), 330–36; P. G. Kritikos and S. P. Papadaki, "The History of the Poppy and of Opium and Their Expansion in Antiquity in the Eastern Mediterranean Area," *Bulletin of Narcotics*, XIX (1967), 17–38; O. Marshall, "The Opium Habit in Michigan," *Report of the Board of Health of Lansing*, VI (1878), 70.

opiates to their alcoholic beverages. For the same reason, cocaine and morphine were sometimes even added to soda-fountain beverages and cigarettes in order to stimulate re-purchasing.[2] Victorians applied laudanum to sprains and bruises, poultices of laudanum and hot water for skin inflammations, morphine dissolved in glycerin for irritations of the throat in phthisis, a combination of morphine and cocaine for nasal catarrh and hay fever, opium or its alkaloids for insomnia and neuralgias, and a mixture of opium and tartar emetic for delirium. In cases of colics (renal, hepatic, or uterine), hypodermic injections of morphine were administered by the physician and frequently by the patient himself. Doctors prescribed an opium suppository for diarrhea and dysentery, Dover's powder for night sweats, and uterine wafers containing morphine, introduced into the vagina, for prolapsus uteri and irregular or painful menstruation.[3]

The popularity of opium in all forms of illnesses, and the indiscriminate manner in which it was prescribed and consumed, tempted many Victorians to opium addiction. "It was not for the purpose of creating pleasure, but of mitigating pain in the severest degree," wrote Thomas De Quincey in his *Confessions of an Opium Eater* (1821), "that I first began to use opium as an article of daily diet." Over a period of ten years, De Quincey consumed more than a hogshead of laudanum, taking 8,000 drops daily, or the equivalent of 320 grains of opium.[4] When assigning blame for opium addiction, a number of physicians sanctimoniously directed their criticism against those thousands of men and women who had graduated from "mushroom schools" and practiced the art of healing under the auspices of a "cheap diploma."[5] Surprisingly, how-

2. F. E. Oliver, "The Use and Abuse of Opium," *Report of the State Board of Health of Boston*, III (1872), 167; E. W. Shipman, "The Promiscuous Use of Opium in Vermont," *Transactions*, Vermont State Medical Society (1890), 72–77; Barton W. Stone, "Opiates and Ethics," *Transactions*, Kentucky State Medical Society, n.s., VIII (1900), 180; Alfred H. Allen, "The Analysis of Preparations Containing Opium," *Analyst*, XXXVII (1902), 350–55.

3. Herman D. Marcus, "Opium; Its Use and Abuse," *New International Clinics*, III (1897), 9–10; L. L. Solomon, "Proprietary Medicines; Evils of the Profession," *Transactions*, Kentucky State Medical Society, n.s., VI (1897), 273.

4. Thomas De Quincey, *Confessions of an Opium Eater* (London, 1821), 21.

5. Frank Woodbury, "Physic-Tippling and Medicine-Bibbing—a Warning against Intemperance in the Use of Drugs," *Report of the Board of Health of*

ever, most doctors who discussed the problem in the professional journals placed the blame squarely upon the medical profession. "I am convinced that WE are responsible," wrote J. S. Weatherly, M.D., of Alabama, "in some measure, in a large proportion of cases, for the evil."[6] There were, in fact, few cases of opium addiction which did not originate with a physician's prescription. According to one candid critic, doctors too readily prescribed opium for illnesses which did not require the powerful drug, not only because it gave the patient a false sense of relief but also because the doctor came to be regarded as a "great benefactor" on account of the prescription. "It may be unconscious on his part," wrote another doctor, "and he thinks he is pursuing his duty strictly, but the fact was that the physician had introduced the enchantment of the drug to the innocent victim."[7] After the patient began to enjoy opium's ecstatic effect, he forgot the pain or malady for which it was originally intended and began liberally prescribing for himself in order to seek its comforting properties. "That physician is guilty of a grave crime," C. P. Frost, M.D., of Vermont warned, "who by his thoughtlessness of results, induces the formation of a habit of reliance upon opium, in one who entrusts the care of his health to his charge."[8]

A study by the Massachusetts state board of health in 1872 on the use and abuse of opium concluded that the drug, classified variously as a hypnotic, narcotic, analgesic, antispasmodic, tonic, diaphoretic, and diuretic, was the primary ingredient of doctor's prescriptions and basic to many patent medicines, and that further, women constituted the largest proportion of opium-eaters. The following extracts were from druggists who

---

Pennsylvania, II (1887), 288; Henry L. Swain, "The Attitude of the Profession toward Patent and Proprietary Medicines," *Yale Medical Journal*, VII (1901), 169.

6. J. S. Weatherly, "Increase of the Habit of Opium-Eating," *Transactions, Medical Society of the State of Alabama* (1869), 67; (Anony.), "Confessions of a Young Lady Laudanum Drinker," *Journal of Mental Science*, XXXIV (1889), 550; F. W. Comings, "Opium: Its Uses and Abuses," *Transactions*, Vermont State Medical Society (1895–96), 365.

7. W. W. Johnston, "The Opium Habit," *American Medical Journal*, XXIII (1895), 391.

8. C. P. Frost, "Opium; Its Uses and Abuses," *Transactions*, Vermont State Medical Society, (1869–70), 145.

replied to a questionnaire from the health board on opium abuse.[9]

Ayer—"Those addicted to opium are all females; and most of them contracted the habit from the use of physicians' prescriptions during sickness."

Boston—"Sells less than he did five years ago. Thinks chloral and bromide of potassium are taking the place of opiates."

"Has observed a slight increase in the call for opium, especially in the form of laudanum and paregoric. Cannot explain the cause of such increase."

"For paregoric, there is a greater demand for domestic use; and for morphia, there is an increased call, observed chiefly among the prostitutes of the West End, who take it for the sedative effect."

"Has but one customer and that a noted Temperance lecturer."

Chilmark—"Five cases reported, originating in opiate prescriptions."

Clarksburg—"I think it on the increase, because doctors prescribe it more indiscriminately now than formerly, thus establishing the habit with the patients."

Clinton—"I know of no particular cause for such increase, except the injudicious advice of some physicians."

Dedham—"Several nervous women take opium here."

Eastham—"I think the use of opium has slightly increased, mostly among females."

Everett—"I am of the opinion that the use of opium has increased of late years, it being considered more 'genteel' than alcohol."

Hinsdale—"There are probably half a dozen opium eaters here, all females but one; the habit was originally contracted in these cases by means of the opiate treatment of neuralgia."

Leverett—"One opium eater in town—a woman—who first took the drug for the relief of pain."

Newburyport—"I think the use of opium and its preparations is confined to elderly people. The young and middle-aged are more addicted to tobacco."

Shrewsbury—"Of seven habitual opium eaters within my observation, five began the use by medical prescription, and were unable to leave it off."

Swampscott—"The use of opium in its various forms has materially increased within the last ten years. It is used, in many places, in place of rum."

Westfield—"I have reason to believe this practice exceedingly common

9. Oliver, "The Use and Abuse of Opium," 170–75.

among certain classes of people who crave the effects of the stimulant, but will not risk their reputation for temperance by taking alcoholic beverages."

Worcester—"I have talked with some of our most intelligent apothecaries, who tell me that the use of opium is greatly increased, especially among women. The reasons which one gave are these: The doctors are prescribing it more to their patients, and thus the habit is acquired. There is also the desire for some form of stimulant. Alcoholic stimulants being prohibited, many have resorted to the use of opium."

"Druggists tell me that they sell a great deal more opium and morphia to the people than they used to, and that it is used by women and others who could not take alcoholic liquors without publicity."

The reason for the high incidence of female opium-eaters, according to F. E. Oliver, M.D., author of the Massachusetts report, lay in the life they led. "Doomed, often, to a life of disappointment, and, it may be, of physical and mental inaction, and in the smaller and more remote towns, not unfrequently, to utter seclusion, deprived of all wholesome social diversion," he wrote, "it is not strange that nervous depression, with all its concomitant evils, should sometimes follow—opium being discreetly selected as the safest and most agreeable remedy."[10] Furthermore, Oliver believed that the temperance movement in New England had indirectly influenced the increase of addiction in women. "It is a significant fact," he observed, "that both in England and in this country, the total abstinence movement was almost immediately followed by an increased consumption of opium." The social stigma against women consuming alcoholic beverages had driven many to the more "acceptable" use of opium preparations which were taken under the guise of medicine; indeed, many women who entered the ranks of "teetotalism" and who waged veritable crusades against the tavern habits of their husbands were habitual opium users.[11] As teetotalers, however, they avoided the disdain of husbands and friends by pointing to the delicious syrups, nervines, and tonics made from roots, herbs, and barks, or rich in animal organisms, that supplied all their extra nutrient needs. While receiving the adulation of society for their

10. *Ibid.*, 168; Marcus, "Opium; Its Use and Abuse," 2.

11. Oliver, "The Use and Abuse of Opium," 169; Alonzo Calkins, *Opium and the Opium Appetite* (Philadelphia, 1871), 289–91.

social gospel crusade, they dosed themselves liberally with Brown-Sequard's or Gross's neuralgia pills containing high percentages of morphia, or nipped from a concealed vial of laudanum or paregoric.[12] "It [laudanum] got me into such a state of indifference," confessed one young woman, "that I no longer took the least interest in anything, and did nothing all day but loll on the sofa reading novels, falling asleep every now and then, and drinking tea." "Worse than all," she admitted, "I got so deceitful that no one could tell when I was speaking the truth."[13]

Those desiring an immediate stimulus usually preferred laudanum, consuming it as a substitute for alcohol. Morphine, which could be easily concealed in a variety of sweeteners, was employed by many women because of its smaller bulk and the fact that it acted quickly and with fewer unpleasant effects. It was consumed orally, or taken by hypodermic needle, enema, and even by suppository. One young lady, wrote a Vermont physician, became addicted to the drug in an effort to allay menstrual pains. Soon she was in the habit of using an 85 minim syringe and after filling it and making the puncture, she unscrewed the barrel, leaving the needle in its place and refilling it two or three more times. Addicts would take a teaspoonful of morphia and dissolve it in water by placing the teaspoon over a lighted match. They would then draw up the liquid into a syringe and inject the mixture into an arm or leg. There were cases of fashionable women habituated to morphine who introduced solutions intra rectum by means of a small acuminated glass syringe in order to avoid puncture marks on the arms. In some cases, chloral and even chloroform or ether were added to the morphia. As for paregoric, women were known to consume a quart or more a week, though it was usually a last resort, since it created serious constipation problems when taken in such amounts.[14]

12. Wyman, "Opium-Eating Teetotallers," *Journal of Psychological Medicine and Mental Pathology*, n.s., VII (1881), 74–77; W. D. White, "The Opium Habit; a Narrative of Personal Experience," *St. Louis Clinical Record*, VIII (1881–82), 39–41.

13. (Anony.), "Confessions of a Young Lady Laudanum Drinker," 546–47.

14. Shipman, "The Promiscuous Use of Opium in Vermont," 76; F. M. Hamlin, "The Opium Habit," *Medical Gazette*, IX (1882), 428; Calkins, *Opium and the Opium Appetite*, 57; Marshall, "The Opium Habit in Michigan," 67.

Opium addiction of the Victorian woman was usually carefully concealed within the family circle unless the amount consumed was so large that the effects became clearly visible. Too often, opiates were bought with the frequency that one might buy sleeping pills today and the obviousness of the sale was perhaps just as noticed. In his report to the Michigan board of health, one doctor noted that while physicians were responsible for the majority of opium addictions, they were seldom aware of the numbers of opium-eaters, except perhaps through their business contacts with the local druggist. And the druggist, "from fear of loss of trade, or, as some term it, a violation of confidential business, was often unwilling to furnish any information with regard to it."[15] An auxiliary factor in maintaining the vicious habit, he added, was the comparative ease with which opiates could be obtained from the dispensing apothecary. "The prescription intended for a day, is repeated by the druggist many times, and its use is continued until the habit is formed."[16] In the absence of pharmaceutical regulations, opium-eaters sought their drugs without hindrance, and the apothecary all too often rationalized his sale on the basis of: "If I don't sell it, someone else will." This form of casuistry, commented a New York critic, "is an ugly commentary on the tendencies of the day when conscience can easily be lulled to slumber, and a fresh supply of fuel furnished the flame raging so remorselessly within."[17] The woman who used opium to relieve her "female problems," soon sought its pleasant effects to relieve her neurasthenia, restlessness, and household cares. Before long, her mind would begin "to rise above the paltry things of every-day life, and wander forth in the land of glorious dreams, where everything seems to be possible, and where [she was] always on the eve of accomplishing some great object."[18]

In 1880, Dr. Charles Warrington Earle presented a detailed study of the opium habit in a speech delivered before the West Chicago Medical Society. A physician at the Washington

15. *Ibid.*, 63.
16. *Ibid.*, 70–72.
17. J. B. Mattison, "The Impending Danger," *Medical Record*, XI (1876), 71.
18. Weatherly, "Increase of the Habit of Opium-Eating," 67–68.

Home in Chicago for the care of opium addicts, he interviewed fifty Chicago druggists concerning the number of opium customers, their sex, nativity, age, social relations, marital status, occupation, cause, and type of narcotic. He pointed out that of 235 habitual opium users listed by the druggists, females outnumbered the males three to one. The largest group of females were prostitutes, a fact also noted by both the Michigan and Massachusetts state boards of health and later by the Chicago Vice Commission in 1911. But even after deducting the prostitutes from the number of female addicts, the women still outnumbered the men two to one. By nationality the "native" Americans comprised 160 of the 235. While Germans and Irish preferred beer and whiskey, "native" Americans were fond of easily concealed opium preparations primarily because they did not "incapacitate the victim for business." In addition, opium was a popular pacifier for the self-proclaimed neurasthenic brain-workers who reputedly bore the discomforts of nervousness for the sake of civilization's advance. Of the 235 users, Earle developed a statistical summary.[19]

Although Earle uncovered evidence to suggest that a large number of opium addicts were people who had suffered financial reverses with subsequent loss of standing in their community, he nonetheless found the highest percentage of opium-eaters among the affluent middle class. The majority of male addicts were businessmen while the women, with the exception of prostitutes, were housewives and society ladies.[20] Rather than seek the cause of the housewife's high addiction rate, doctors preferred to focus upon those women who had left the security of the home circle. For them, opophagia seemed an obvious corollary of their inferior mental and physical constitution straining beyond its natural capacity. "Females are more frequently the victims," observed physician F. M. Hamlin in a paper read before the New York Central Medical Association in 1882, "because . . . of their more nervous organization and tendency to hysterical and chronic diseases; and some perhaps use it in preference to alcohol because of its greater

19. C. W. Earle, "The Opium Habit," *Chicago Medical Review*, II (1880), 443.

20. *Ibid.*, 444.

Statistical Summary
of
235 Opium Users

NATIONALITY

Entire number of cases	235
American	160
German	7
Irish	17
Scotch	10
Colored	12
English	6
Scandinavian	5
Unknown	18

AGE (APPROXIMATE)
Males

from 20 to 30 years	5
30 40	19
40 50	7
50 60	11
60 70	1
70 80	1
unknown age	22
Total	66

Females

from 10 to 20 years	2
20 30	18
30 40	39
40 50	22
50 60	14
60 70	4
one-third entire number, prostitutes, probably from 15 to 50	56
unknown age	14
Total	169

OCCUPATION OF 100
Male

Iron merchant	1
Newsdealer	1
Businessmen	5
Physicians	2
Laborer	3
Turner	1
Druggist	1
Bookkeeper	2
Capitalist	2
Clerk	1
Contractor	1
Insurance agent	1
Book agent	1
Railroad men	1
Attorney	1
Unknown	9

Female

Housewives	45
Society ladies	3
Widow	1
Sewing woman	1
Servant	1
Washwoman	2
Prostitutes	5
Unknown	9

KIND OF NARCOTIC

Morphia	120
Tincture opium	30
Paregoric	5
Mc Munn's Elixir	2
Gum opium	50
Dover's powder	1
Unknown	27
Total	235

QUANTITY
Morphia

persons	use from
21	1 to 3 gr. ea. day
17	3 6
12	6 10
10	10 15
12	15 20
7	½ drachms ea. day
6	1 drachms ea. day
20	1 bottle ea. week
5	2 bottles ea. week
1	11 bottles ea. mo.

Tincture of Opium

persons	use
15	1 drachm ea. day
4	3
7	4
12	1 ounce ea. day
4	2
1	3
1	4

Gum Opium

persons	use
3	10 grains ea. day
5	20
9	½ drachm ea. day
12	1
4	2
2	3
1	4

secrecy and less degrading effects." Along with John Harvey Kellogg of the Battle Creek Sanitarium, Hamlin reminded the profession that woman's peculiar nervous complexity, combined with her ambition to get ahead, had much to do with her desire for stimulants, tonics, and restoratives.[21] No one, wrote Margaret Cleaves, M.D., of Iowa, least of all women, expected to remain in the class to which they were born. Schooled in the belief that society was "onward and upward," a mother expected her daughter to "shine socially as a possible mistress of the White House."[22] American social life, even for the young woman, was a ceaseless struggle to better class standing. Although doctors preferred to relate the male's addictive problems to neurasthenia, they tended to associate woman's addiction to "female problems," the demands of fashionable life, or simply her effort to break into the masculine world.

For many women, opium, alcohol, and chloral in prescription drugs and patent medicines were as readily accessible as the beverages their husbands consumed at a local bar, club, or from their own well-stocked cabinets. They had only to turn the pages of their reading material to discover that thousands of their suffering sex were imbibing preparations of Febriline, Hypophophites, Celernia, Sanmetto, and Lactopeptine to relieve their female complaints. The neighborhood druggist's shelves literally bulged with patent and proprietary medicines of unlisted ingredients whose alcoholic or opium content were of hazardous proportions. Rather than pay two dollars for a visit to the local practitioner, they became accustomed to diagnosing their problems from advertisements, then procuring from the local druggist a bottle of Maltine or Wine of Cod-Liver Oil to relieve weakness, Scott's Emulsion for neuralgia, Wyeth's New Enteritis pills (containing arsenite of copper, bichloride of mercury, and morphine) for diarrhea, or Sir James Clark's pills (aloes, hellebore, powdered savin, ergot, iron, solid extracts of tansy and rue) as an abortifacient.[23] The

21. Hamlin, "The Opium Habit," 427.

22. Margaret Cleaves, "Neurasthenia and Its Relations to Diseases of Women," *Transactions,* Iowa State Medical Society, VII (1886), 166.

23. Ely Van de Warker, "The Criminal Use of Proprietary or Advertised Nostrums," *New York Medical Journal,* XVII (1873), 26–27; B. W. Stone,

popularity of patent medicines was basically founded upon human gullibility. A mere perusal of the patent medicine shelf convinced the purchaser that "doctoring" could be simple and inexpensive. Reading the advertisements—the small quantity necessary to effect cure, the certainty of the cure, the large number of diseases which were cured at the same time, the perfect "harmlessness" of the nostrum, and the patronage of distinguished preachers and politicians—the purchaser could not but reflect proudly upon her diagnostic skills. One doctor recalled a young woman who began taking Feeley's Rheumatic Mixture for a neuralgia affliction and not until she had spent nearly six hundred dollars in the consumption of more than a thousand bottles of the nostrum did she finally realize that the medicine (which contained six grains of morphia) had become addictive.[24] Two of the more famous proprietary medicines were Mrs. Winslow's Soothing Syrup and Godfrey's Cordial, both containing large amounts of morphia. Over three-fourths of a million bottles of Winslow's syrup were sold annually in the United States, and literally dozens of citations in medical journals referred to fatal opium poisoning caused by the syrup and others like it.[25]

In a report of the Board of Health of Pennsylvania in 1887, a Philadelphia physician recalled observing a richly dressed woman in a Chestnut Street drugstore request a glass of soda water mixed with bromide of potassium. "She was evidently nervous," he remarked, "but the thought occurred to my mind

---

"Opiates and Ethics," *Transactions,* Kentucky State Medical Association, n.s., VIII (1900), 179; Shipman, "The Promiscuous Use of Opium in Vermont," 76; Hamlin, "The Opium Habit," 428–29; Harry H. Kane, *Drugs that Enslave; the Opium, Morphine, Chloral and Hashish Habits* (Philadelphia, 1881), 42–43.

24. Lewis D. Mason, "Patent and Proprietary Medicines as the Cause of the Alcohol and Opium Habit or Other Forms of Narcomania—with Some Suggestions as to How the Evil May Be Remedied," *Quarterly Journal of Inebriety,* XXV (1903), 3.

25. Oliver, "The Use and Abuse of Opium," 175; Marshall, "The Opium Habit in Michigan," 71; W. F. McNutt, "Mrs. Winslow's Soothing Syrup a Poison," *Pacific Medical and Surgical Journal,* XIV (1872), 62; A. B. Hirsch, "Notes on a Case of Poisoning from Mrs. Winslow's Soothing Syrup," *Lancet and Clinic,* n.s., XIII (1884), 654–56; C. A. Bryce, "A Case of Opium-Poisoning with Dr. Bull's Cough Syrup," *Southern Clinic,* II (1879–80), 399; James E. Reeves, *Bad Health; Its Physical and Moral Causes in American Women* (Wheeling, W.Va., 1875), 18.

that the natural way to overcome nervousness (or nervelessness) would have been to alter the habits of life which produced the morbid condition." In still another drugstore he
noticed a prescription posted behind the counter which called
for a preparation containing chloral. Upon inquiring, he was
informed that the prescription was openly displayed because
of the number of women who requested it.[26] In one town, a
doctor observed "half a dozen ladies come into a drug store
within half an hour and consume a dose of bromides on the
premises." The "hyper-irritability" of the woman's nervous
system had become so prevalent, he wrote, that bromide of
sodium would soon replace common table salt as the dietary
staple in the urban middle-class home.[27]

An interesting sidelight to the chloral habit was related by
Edith Wharton in *The House of Mirth* (1905), depicting the
life of a twenty-nine-year-old woman of social grace, Miss Lily
Bart, who sought marriage and security amid the chaotic mores
of New York middle-class society with its cautious virtues and a
concept of decency defined by the proper material possessions.
Lily Bart was a woman whose interest in the working classes
had been limited to noblesse oblige, of looking "down on them
from above, from the happy altitude of her grace and her
beneficence," and who, finding herself ultimately relegated to
their economic level through a series of social mishaps, died of
an overdose of chloral in a hall bedroom in a New York board-
inghouse. Wharton's depiction of the drugstore scene where
Lily purchased her bottle of chloral reveals more than just the
promiscuous drug abuse of the day.

But what she dreaded most of all was having to pass the chemist's at
the corner of Sixth Avenue. She had meant to take another street: she
had usually done so of late. But today her steps were irresistibly drawn
toward the flaring plate-glass corner; she tried to take the lower crossing,
but a laden dray crowded her back, and she struck across the street
obliquely, reaching the sidewalk just opposite the chemist's door.
Over the counter she caught the eye of the clerk who had waited on

26. Woodbury, "Physic-Tippling and Medicine-Bibbing—a Warning against
Intemperance in the Use of Drugs," 287.
27. A. L. Smith, "What Civilization Is Doing for the Human Female,"
Transactions, Southern Surgical and Gynecological Association, II (1890), 355–
56.

her before, and slipped the prescription into his hand. There could be no question about the prescription: it was a copy of one of Mrs. Hatch's, obligingly furnished by the lady's chemist. Lily was confident that the clerk would fill it without hesitation; yet the nervous dread of a refusal, or even of an expression of doubt, communicated itself to her restless hands as she affected to examine the bottles of perfume stacked on the glass before her.

The clerk had read the prescription without comment; but in the act of handing out the bottle he paused.

"You don't want to increase the dose, you know," he remarked.

Lily's heart contracted. What did he mean by looking at her in that way?

"Of course not," she murmured, holding out her hand.

"That's all right: it's a queer-acting drug. A drop or two more, and off you go—the doctors don't know why."

The dread least he should question her, or keep the bottle back, choked the murmur of acquiescence in her throat; and when at length she emerged safely from the shop she was almost dizzy with the intensity of her relief. The mere touch of the packet thrilled her tired nerves with the delicious promise of a night of sleep, and in the reaction from her momentary fear she felt as if the first fumes of drowsiness were already stealing over her.[28]

Besides opium and chloral, women consumed a variety of sarsaparillas, bitters, and tonics which contained from 17 to 44 percent alcohol; yet in few instances were the purchasers so informed.[29] Patent and proprietary medicines such as Green's Nervura for nerves, Radway's Ready Relief, Oragiene for headache, Hostetter's Bitters, Kilmer's Swamp Root, Warner's Safe Cure, Peruna, and blood purifiers were favorite remedies whose alcoholic content, while not disclosed, did much to lighten the burdens of its unsuspecting users. Doctors who frowned on the temperance crusades of women triumphantly reported cases of agitators who daily dosed themselves with tonics that contained a larger percentage of alcohol than the beverages they denounced so ardently.[30] Beer which contained from 2 to 8 percent alcohol was hardly as intoxicating as Peruna, which contained 28 percent, or Ayer's Sarsaparilla

28. Edith Wharton, *The House of Mirth* (Boston, 1905), 181–82.

29. David Paulson, "Disguised Intemperance; an Exposition of the Patent Medicine Evil," *Bulletin*, Battle Creek Sanitarium Hospital Clinic, XIII (1904), 246.

30. E. B. Lowry, *Herself; Talks with Women concerning Themselves* (Chicago, 1911), 68.

with 26 percent alcohol. The pregnant woman who nipped from her bottle of Hostetter's or Boker's Stomach Bitters to strengthen her nerves consumed four times the alcohol than in the same amount of champagne. "The need felt by a tired wife for Paine's Celery Compound," wrote a doctor seeking to compromise the issue, "is similar to the man's craving for whiskey."[31]

The Massachusetts state board analyst in 1904 listed the following percentages of alcohol content in patent and proprietary medicines, and suggested that intemperance and invalidism among Victorians were all too often the results rather than the causes of the nostrum trade.[32]

MEDICINES	PERCENTAGE OF ALCOHOL BY VOLUME
Lydia Pinkham's Vegetable Compound	20.6
Paine's Celery Compound	21.0
Dr. William's Vegetable Jaundice Bitters	18.5
Whiskol, "a non-intoxicating stimulant"	28.2
Colden's Liquid Beef Tonic "recommended for treatment of alcohol habit"	26.5
Thayer's Compound Extract of Sarsaparilla	21.5
Ayer's Sarsaparilla	26.2
Hood's Sarsaparilla	18.5
Dana's Sarsaparilla	13.5
Allen's Sarsaparilla	13.5
Brown's Sarsaparilla	13.5
Peruna	28.5
Vinol, Wine of Cod-Liver Oil	18.8
Carter's Physical Extract	22.0
Dr. Peter's Kuriko	14.0
Hooker's Wigwam Tonic	20.7
Hoofland's German Tonic	29.3
Howe's Arabian Tonic "not a rum drink"	13.2
Jackson's Golden Seal Tonic	19.6
Mensman's Peptonized Beef Tonic	16.5
Parker's Tonic "purely vegetable"	41.6
Schenck's Seaweed Tonic "entirely harmless"	19.5
Baxter's Mandrake Bitters	16.5
Boker's Stomach Bitters	42.6

31. Myer Solis-Cohen, *Woman: Girlhood, Wifehood, Motherhood; Her Responsibilities and Her Duties at All Periods of Life* (Philadelphia, 1906), 358.
32. (Anony.), "The Alcohol in Secret Nostrums," *Medical World*, XIII (1904), 288.

Burdock Blood Bitters	25.2
Greene's Nervura	17.2
Hartshorn's Bitters	22.2
Kaufman's Sulfur Bitters "contains no alcohol"	20.5
Puritana	20.5
Warner's Safe Tonic Bitters	35.7
Warren's Bilious Bitters	21.5
Faith Whitcomb's Nerve Bitters	20.3

Testimonials, brochures, and "clinical reports" praising the merits of nostrums were handed out with every purchase, explaining their curative claims amid romantic scenes, pastoral landscapes, occasional quiz games, and timely witticisms. In addition, ministers and educational pedagogues supplemented their salaries by giving open and unblushing praise to this form of quackery. Balm of Gilead, a patent medicine which contained 70 percent alcohol, was recommended by a number of "retired clergymen" for those seeking relief from their ills. Religious conferences and revivals in the nineteenth century were often deluged with nostrum vendors seeking recommendations from popular preachers. And having received their endorsements, nostrum sellers began advertising their products with eschatological zeal, promising immediate health and everlasting happiness to the afflicted. "I have often attended the conferences of the Southern Methodist Church of Kentucky," wrote S. J. Harris, M.D., in the *Transactions* of the Kentucky State Medical Society, "and I have actually seen proprietary and patent medicines all around the steps, piled up to such an extent that one could hardly get in or go around without stepping on them."[33] If, as the Reverend Henry Beecher claimed, the cleanliness of Pear's soap was next to godliness, one could only imagine the rejuvenative qualities, both physical and spiritual, of Bromidia or Maltine.

J. B. Mattison of Brooklyn, a leading crusader against opium inebriety in the late nineteenth century, believed that the medical profession had failed to recognize the evils of the promiscuous use of the drug. This was only typified by the remarks of Arthur V. Meigs, M.D., of Philadelphia, who shrugged

---

33. Quoted in Solomon, "Proprietary Medicines; Evils of the Profession," 275.

off the growing concern for opium addiction with the remark that opium-eaters were usually immune to dysentery,
fever, cholera, and rheumatism.[34] In addition, physicians had
failed to guard their patients from dependence on the drug,
leading to its continued use beyond the intended therapeutic
role. By the time the patient became aware of his addiction,
he was usually horrified to find himself unable to abandon it,
falling into grief or seeking the villainous opiumania cures.
"Tossed about by conflicting emotions, preyed upon by dis-
tressing doubts and fears abiding, conscious of his thralldom
and the impotency of his efforts at emancipation, the abject
slave to this galling bondage [went] through life surrounded
by a darkness seemingly impenetrable and at times, down into
the very depths of despondency and gloom." America was in
peril of becoming a "nation of opium inebriates," Mattison
warned. "Tens of thousands of hapless devotees bow at the
shrine of this seductive goddess, and, from the palace and the
poorhouse, the hall and the hovel, are being recruited the increasing host marching downward, with steps, slow but sure,
to death or degradation."[35] In 1878, the *Atlanta Daily Constitution* published a poem entitled "The Opium-Eater" which,
like Mattison's warning, traced the perilous path to self-
destruction.

> Thy curse, O God, has followed me fast,
> In the days and weeks of the shadowy past,
> And the weary years that lie before
> Are ringing loud with the sullen roar
> Of the whistling tide that is carrying me on
> To the starless night, and the cursed dawn
> Of the world beyond. And the opium grave
> Is yawning wide; and there is none to save,
> For mind and will have been swallowed up,
> In the poisoned dregs on the hideous cup
> I have drained so long. And the light of day
> Has shown its last on my lonely way;
> And the hopes of youth that lingered there

34. Arthur V. Meigs, "The Use of Opium in Daily Practice," *New International Clinics*, I (1902), 19–20.

35. J. B. Mattison, "Opium Inebriety," *Medical Record*, XI (1876), 794;
Hamlin, "The Opium Habit," 426; Mattison, "The Impending Danger," 69;
Marcus, "Opium; Its Use and Abuse," 6.

Have given place to a dark despair.
For the poppy wine, with its cursed spell,
Is dragging me down to a lasting hell.
Dragging me down; and the seething wave
Of the waters of lethe my feet will lave,
The shrieks of the damned my ears will greet,
And the soundless thread of hurrying feet,
Fleeing in vain from the burning wrath
Of the merciless friends that bar their path.
Wild as the wail o'er the coffined dead,
Are the burning words of the book unread
That holds my fate. And no hope of day,
Cheers me in my desolate way;
And the voice of the night winds seem to cry,
With a shuddering moan as they pass me by,
"Too late! too late! thou has listened too long
To the lulling strains of the siren's song,
For the witching waves of the poisoned wine
Has bound thy soul in its deadly twine."
Too late! O God! and I dare not pray,
For the light of thy face is turned away.
The curse of thy wrath, and thy angry frown,
To the darkness of night is bearing me down.
Yet the world was bright in the years long dead,
And the Savior smiled as he bowed his head,
And hear the prayer of the innocent rise
To the sinless throne beyond the skies.
The world was bright, but the tempter came
And breathed on me with the breath of flame;
And the tempted fell 'neath the lurid light
Of the mocking eyes, and the ghastly night
Like a pall of darkness settled down
On the broken life; and the weary round
Of the days and weeks, the months, and years
Are filled with the mist of falling tears.

Like other critics of the medical profession, Mattison claimed that over 80 percent of the cases of opium inebriety in the United States were traced to opiate prescriptions made by foolish practitioners unaware of the peculiar susceptibility of Americans to nervous disorders. He also pointed out that far too few physicians made sure that their patients abandoned the drug when the reasons for its administration disappeared. He admitted that prolonged use of opiates after their initial therapeutical purpose was often out of the physician's control, since no law prevented a druggist from filling an opiate prescription as often as it was presented. In order to curb the vice, Mattison suggested that before prescribing opiates, physicians should consider substituting other anodynes, soporifics, and nervines which could accomplish the object more safely than opium. In illnesses where opium was required, he urged doctors to make careful inquiry into the patient's nervous temperament in order to avoid giving it to those who would become easily ensnared by its use. Finally, he warned physicians who prescribed opiates to observe patients more carefully, and under no circumstances allow the patient to administer an opiate to himself with a hypodermic syringe. "Personal employment of this device is fraught with danger," he observed, because "patients almost invariably use it to excess." Doctors should follow closely the course of the patient's use of the drug, and also watch for a period of time after the drug was supposedly abandoned "lest, from some pretext, its use can be resumed clandestinely, and inebriety become established." More important, Mattison hoped for legislation to prohibit a patient from refilling an opium prescription or a druggist from dispensing an opiate without a positive order from a doctor. Such legislation had been enacted by the German government in 1877, and he hoped that the United States would soon follow suit.[36]

Opium Antidotes

To combat opium poisoning, doctors prescribed a variety of antidotes including an emetic of sulfate of zinc or sulfate of copper repeated at short intervals to produce vomiting. Then vegetable acids such as vinegar and lemon juice were administered to the empty stomach, followed by strong coffee, tea, and "cordial stimulants" such as ammonia, musk, and aromatics. Besides this, the patient was kept moving and the surface of the body rubbed or blistered. "We walk patients, pour water upon them, flagellate them with wet towels, and some of us beat them with clubs," wrote H. C. Wood, pro-

36. J. B. Mattison, "The Responsibility of the Profession in the Production of Opium Inebriety," *Medical and Surgical Reporter*, XXXVIII (1878), 102–4.

fessor of therapeutics at the University of Pennsylvania. "I have seen the whole body of a woman almost as black as a man's coat from the beating she had received to keep her awake in narcotic poisoning." Although Wood recognized that extreme measures were sometimes necessary to keep the body functions from complete collapse, he thought that a dry electric brush attached to a powerful battery would in most instances produce sufficient nervous irritation and pain.[37]

While physicians urged opium and alcohol addicts to remedy their problem through enforced abstinence, many sought less drastic solutions—a quest which left them under the dubious influence of advertising quacks and charlatans who preyed upon their weaknesses. Not too surprisingly, the Civil War had precipitated a high incidence of opium addiction growing out of therapeutic practices in army hospitals. (It was there, too, that fashionable southern ladies such as Mary Chestnut gained access to supplies of opium while treating hospital patients.) Opiumania vendors quickly seized advantage of the ready market. In addition to normal advertising in newspapers and magazines, they mailed out pamphlets containing stories of soldiers who had fought bravely in the war and were wounded in battle. Now dependent on opium as a result of treatment, they were on the road to self-destruction until discovering Dr. so-and-so's secret remedy, a concoction developed after years of painstaking effort, which was now being offered to suffering humanity at a fraction of its original cost. Nearly half of the supportive letters in the pamphlet were designed to substantiate the legitimacy of the vendor against the attacks of quackery. In most instances this was achieved by the use of character witnesses who had either known the vendor as an upstanding member of the community or had been supposedly cured by his antidote after the war. The stories were written in gushing Victorian prose that brought tears to the most hardened hearts. On the last page of the pamphlet, there was a list of various opium preparations which most addicts consumed.

37. H. C. Wood, "Opium," *Boston Medical and Surgical Journal*, CXXVIII (1893), 638–39; William G. Smith, *An Inaugural Dissertation on Opium, Embracing Its History, Chemical Analysis, and Use and Abuse as a Medicine* (New York, 1832), 17.

The addict was requested to circle the type used as well as the amount consumed in a given day or week and return the form to the company. Ironically, of course, most nostrums which advertised "relief for the opium-eater" consisted of sulfate of morphia ("the quack's sheet anchor") disguised among herbs and sweeteners. With the information the addict sent, the charlatan prepared an antidote with the appropriate amount of morphia priced in proportion to the strength required to "cure" the victim. The cost of these precious vials ranged from five to forty-five dollars a pint bottle, which was intended to last a month. Tempted with a moderate discount, opium-eaters were encouraged to purchase a "full course," which meant several months' supply.[38]

Opiumania vendors plied their trade with all the mock righteousness of a backsliding Baptist. "I do not advertise or send out circulars," wrote one charlatan, "as there are hundreds of quacks who are doing such low and mean work, I have become disgusted." Another introduced his cure with the remark: "I am sure that there are heartless imposters, destitute alike of position and principle, who are constantly endeavoring to entrap and victimize the anxious, and perhaps too incredulous sufferer. The cunningly devised spurious recommendations of these swindlers are well calculated to deceive the unwary. You will most certainly be swindled by trusting to their representations." Then, hoping to have the confidence of the victim, the vendor proceeded to sell a mixture of opiate equal to the habit. The opium-eater simply continued his addiction under the guise of the antidote, since most of the nostrums were merely solutions of water, glycerin, and morphia colored by aniline. Other antidotes contained quinine, strychnine, cannabis, atropia, hyoscyamia, and chloride of gold. Of some 20 samples of opium antidotes tested by the state analyst of the Massachusetts board of health, 19 contained morphine; the exception was Keeley's Double Chloride of Gold Cure which, incidentally, contained no traces of gold.[39]

38. Oliver, "The Use and Abuse of Opium," 167; Smith, *An Inaugural Dissertation on Opium*, 16; J. B. Mattison, "An Expose of Opium Antidotes," *Atlanta Medical and Surgical Journal*, XV (1877–78), 218.

39. J. B. Mattison, "Opium Antidotes and Their Vendors," *Journal*, American Medical Association, VII (1886), 569–70.

Dr. Beck's Opiumania Cure appeased the opium addict by feeding him ten grains of morphia to an ounce of "cure," at a cost which ranged from three to forty-five dollars. Dr. John Croften Beck supplied his supplicants with a twenty-page brochure praising his product and the philanthropical manner with which he allowed his precious vial to be sold so cheaply. A native of Indiana, he became a professor of medical jurisprudence at the Cincinnati College of Medicine and Surgery in 1858, and in 1862, professor of anatomy and physiology. He was also editor of the *Cincinnati Medical and Surgical News,* and president of the Newport, Kentucky, school board for many years. A dedicated Methodist and Mason, he resolved to cure opiumania and related narcotic addictions. Since "no pecuniary consideration could induce him to encourage a palpable delusion," he spent many years, so he wrote, searching for a definitive cure.[40] Fortified with testimonials, his opiumania cure stood alongside a host of other brazen nostrums in the nineteenth century which assured the addict that his "private problem" could be solved with a minimum of discomfort and shame. Ohio, Indiana, Illinois, Michigan, New York, and New Jersey were states claiming the pioneers in the business of opiumania cures. S. B. Collins of La Porte, Indiana, produced an opium antidote that on analysis was found to contain twenty-five and one-half grains of morphia to the ounce. Mrs. J. A. Drollinger, another producer of an opium antidote from La Porte (and incidentally, the wife of Collins), sold a product containing similar amounts of morphia. Yet Collins claimed that his antidote "is not a substitute for opium"; Drollinger's circular noted that her product "does not contain opium in any of its numerous forms," and Beck also claimed that his cure "has no opium in it."[41]

Ignorance of the addictive qualities of opium, and the lack of standards in preparation and regulation of drugs, surely

40. Quoted in Stanford E. Chaille, "The Opium Habit, and 'Opium-Mania Cures,'" *New Orleans Medical and Surgical Journal,* II (1876), 770, 772; F. Baldwin Morris, *The Panorama of Life, an Experience in Associating and Battling with Opium and Alcoholic Stimulants* (Philadelphia, 1878), i–vi; Mattison, "An Expose of Opium Antidotes," 216–17; B. M. Woolley, *The Opium Habit and Its Cure* (Atlanta, 1879), 13.

41. Mattison, "An Expose of Opium Antidotes," 218–19.

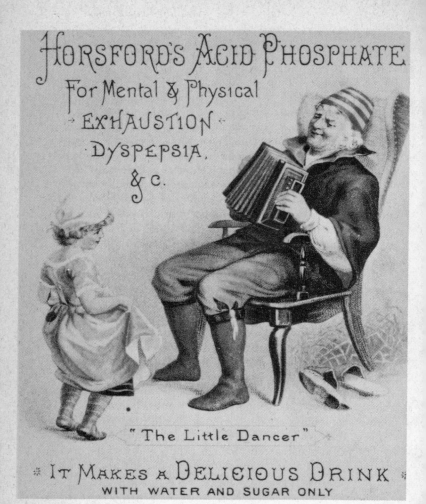

A chromolithographed advertising card given out by druggists (189?) for Horsford's Acid Phosphate. National Library of Medicine, Bethesda.

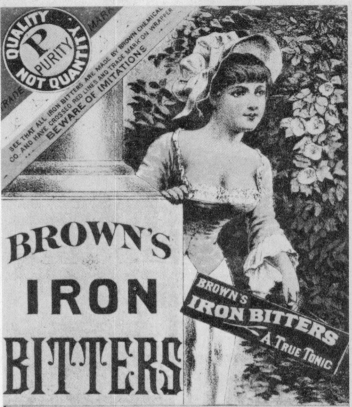

A chromolithographed advertising card given out by druggists (189?) for Brown's Iron Bitters. National Library of Medicine, Bethesda.

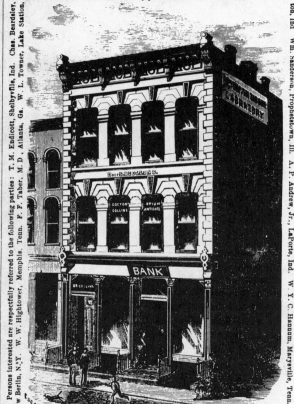

An advertisement from the *American Medical Journal*, 1873.
National Library of Medicine, Bethesda.

dote or Cure has the "air brake" power to arrest this "glass train" in its fearful speed, and with its precious freight, without so much as a shock to endanger the Opium-victim. Then, friend, apply—apply quickly—the powers of this brake before it is too late! too late!

B. M. W.

TO PERSONS WISHING TO ORDER B. M. WOOLLEY'S OPIUM ANTIDOTE OR CURE.

It is necessary to have the following questions plainly and truthfully answered. Be very exact in giving the amount of drug used in 24 hours, or some given time; state in what form and how used—whether taken directly into the stomach or used by hyperdermic injection. If you are not positive of the amount, have some druggist weigh it for you. Never state the amount by guess; by so doing you are liable to cause yourself unnecessary trouble and, perhaps, suffering.

QUESTIONS TO BE ANSWERED.

Age,
Sex,
Married or single,
Occupation,
Present state of health,
Have you palpitation of the heart?
Do you use spirituous liquors?
Do your bowels move regularly?
What caused loss of health?
Length of time you have used Opium?
Cause of habit?
Have you ever taken an Opium Antidote?
If so, whose, and how many bottles or length of time you used it, and the result?
How much opiates were you taking when you began use of antidote, if used?
How long since you quit antidote?
How much Opium, if any, it took to sustain you when you stopped its use, and how much now?
State the exact amount used. If Morphine, the number of grains per day, or the length of time one bottle lasts you. If Gum Opium, the number of grains per day, or the length of time one ounce lasts you. If Laudanum or McMunn's Elixir, the length of time one bottle lasts you, or the number of bottles used per week. (A bottle of Laudanum or Elixir usually contains one ounce, and a bottle of Morphine one drachm or sixty grains.)
Temperament?
(A person who is nervous, quick, sensitive to impressions is of a nervous temperament. One who is stout, full-blooded,

red-faced is of a sanguine temperament. A thin, dark-featured, reticent person is of a bilious temperament, while a pale, fat, sluggish nature, is called phlegmatic, or lymphatic.)
Amount Morphine,
Amount Gum Opium,
Amount Laudanum,
Amount Elixir,
How used,
Name of patient,
P. O. Address,
Nearest Express Office.
It is important that each and every one of the above questions should be fully answered, and as near as possible every symptom, disease or habit each and every patient has been or is now afflicted with should be made known to me, as they are all considered in compounding the medicine for each patient, and are important.
Terms will be given on receipt of a statement of the case, and I will endeavor to make them as reasonable and low, as the nature of the case will admit of.

B. M. WOOLLEY.
P. O. Box 389, Atlanta, Ga.

THE OPIUM HABIT.

IS THERE TOO MUCH SAID UPON THE SUBJECT?

Some persons, and many of apparent conscientious principles and enlarged views, will even scoff at there being any great danger in the habit, and are inclined to speak lightly, if not derisively, of any attempt to check its spreading influence. This is doubtless mainly due to a want on their part of a more perfect knowledge of the figures and facts relating to the subject.

Could the good people of our country for but one day actually see the numerous throng of the Opium-afflicted of this land —could they realize their torments, hear their cries of suffering and earnest entreaties for help, as some have done and are doing—could you but look into their faces, betokening the very gloom of despair and the darkness of their hearts; or witness, it may be, the idiotic smile, offspring of some alluring but sadly delusive dream—such a sound of alarm would go forth as would resound throughout the land, and it would be fraught with such tones of terror, intermingled with sighs of pity as would certainly be heeded where the human heart had not become callous, or the fountains of sympathy and the springs of charity had not forever dried up. Could you but draw aside the curtain of secresy that so universally vails this sad, evil habit and its direful

A facsimile page from B. M. Woolley, *The Opium Habit and Its Cure*, 1879, with instructions to readers on how to order the author's opium antidote or cure. National Library of Medicine, Bethesda.

PRICE LIST.

PRICE FOR A 16-OZ. BOTTLE, OR 2-8-OZ. BOTTLES, A MONTH'S SUPPLY.

Two Drachms Laudanum or Elixir,	or	Eight Grains Gum Opium,	equal	One Grain Morphia.	$3 00
2 to 4¼	. . . .	8 to 16	. . . .	1 to 2	4 00
4¼ “ 7⅓	. . . .	16 “ 24	. . . .	2 “ 3	5 00
7⅓ “ 8⅔	. . . .	24 “ 32	. . . .	3 “ 4	6 00
8⅔ “ 10⅔	. . . .	32 “ 40	. . . .	4 “ 5	6 00
10⅔ “ 12¾	. . . .	40 “ 48	. . . .	5 “ 6	7 00
12½ “ 15	. . . .	48 “ 56	. . . .	6 “ 7	8 00
15 “ 17	. . . .	56 “ 64	. . . .	7 “ 8	9 00
17 “ 19	. . . .	64 “ 72	. . . .	8 “ 9	11 00
19 “ 21⅔	. . . .	72 “ 80	. . . .	9 “ 10	12 00
21⅔ “ 23½	. . . .	80 “ 88	. . . .	10 “ 11	13 00
23½ “ 25½	. . . .	88 “ 96	. . . .	11 “ 12	14 00
25½ “ 27⅔	. . . .	96 “ 104	. . . .	12 “ 13	14 00
27⅔ “ 30	. . . .	104 “ 112	. . . .	13 “ 14	14 00
30 “ 32	. . . .	112 “ 120	. . . .	14 “ 15	15 00
32 “ 34⅓	. . . .	120 “ 128	. . . .	15 “ 16	15 00
34⅓ “ 36¼	. . . .	128 “ 136	. . . .	16 “ 17	15 00
36¼ “ 38½	. . . .	126 “ 144	. . . .	17 “ 18	16 00
38½ “ 40½	. . . .	144 “ 152	. . . .	18 “ 19	16 00
40½ “ 42⅔	. . . .	152 “ 160	. . . .	19 “ 20	17 00
42⅔ “ 53⅓	. . . .	160 “ 200	. . . .	20 “ 25	17 00
53⅓ “ 64	. . . .	200 “ 240	. . . .	25 “ 30	19 00
64 “ 74⅔	. . . .	240 “ 280	. . . .	30 “ 35	20 00
74⅔ “ 85⅓	. . . .	280 “ 320	. . . .	35 “ 40	23 00
85⅓ “ 95	. . . .	320 “ 360	. . . .	40 “ 45	24 00
95 “ 106⅔	. . . .	360 “ 400	. . . .	45 “ 50	25 00
106⅔ “ 117⅓	. . . .	400 “ 440	. . . .	50 “ 55	26 00
117⅓ “ 128	. . . .	440 “ 480- 1 oz.	. .	55 “ 60-1 dr. . .	27 00

By remembering that 60 Grains make 1 Drachm, 8 Drachms make 1 Ounce, and 120 drops of Laudanum or Elixir make 1 Fluid Drachm, the above table will be very easily understood.

Patients using Gum Opium, Laudanum, Elixir of Opium, or other preparations of the drug, must state explicitly the amount of either, and they will be charged according to its equivalent in Morphine.

AN IMPORTANT POINT.

Every patient will please write me, when ordering a second supply, just what day they began use of the first.

A facsimile page from B. M. Woolley, *The Opium Habit and Its Cure,* 1879, showing the price list for his opium antidote. National Library of Medicine, Bethesda.

caused untold misery in the late nineteenth century. Few Victorians were aware of the dangers of continued consumption of their tonics, and unwarned or unnoticed by their physicians, they went on unsuspecting until roused by a sense of their own helplessness. Surely there was a conspicuous lack of wise professional counseling. As physicians increasingly relied on the apparently miraculous powers of this all-purpose drug, they doomed their patients to a life of dependency. Substituting the quick panacea for more arduous diagnosis and treatment, they shared the blame for the addiction and death that so often followed; for, in far too many cases, the easy road of the opium prescription—albeit given innocently, in ignorance of the dangers of the drug—replaced the hard road of involved, painstaking medical treatment. In addition to the large degree of professional responsibility for this opium and alcohol inebriety, nothing prevented the local apothecary from refilling an opiate prescription as often as it was presented and in excess of its legitimate therapeutic use; nor was there legislation to control the contents of the patent and proprietary medicines which went without inspection from manufacturer to consumer. And the manufacturer of the patent medicine was perhaps the most villainous because he exploited the misery of disease by preying upon both the pocketbooks and souls of his victims. His pecuniary interests accounted for the secrecy of the contents of these mixtures and the almost comic innocence with which he advertised their curative powers. Opium, once an effective agent when properly and discreetly applied, became an ogre which devoured the ignorant and unsuspecting.

The industrial revolution, blamed by doctors for the wonderful burden of neurasthenia, was also interpreted as a catalyst in the formation of alcoholism and drug addiction among the weaker elements of the social structure. Industrialism did not determine character but only sorted men into their proper place in the hierarchical scale of society; it did not give qualities to those who had none. The revolution challenged each man to pit himself against the forces of the age, and in so doing, each revealed his own strengths and weaknesses. The increased tempo of the age, the acquisition of greater leisure, the achievements of science and technology, and the subsequent demands upon the individual for greater productivity, greater mastery, and more immediate decisionmaking had resulted in a class of people who found it difficult to keep pace with the new age. For the Victorian male, alcohol, which was easily accessible through an assortment of social avenues, became a welcome stabilizer. The laudanum vial and syringe, on the other hand, became the final resort of those who could not otherwise keep pace with the perilous social struggle. Among Victorian males, only the weakest turned to opiates, for among the psychical outlets available to men, drug addiction was the least acceptable. Although momentary vices like the use of alcohol or prostitution might be tolerated without loss of standing, drug addiction, like homosexuality, was an anathema to the fittest man.

Since the Victorian woman was unable to publicly consume alcohol without social censure, the sly sipping of nervines and tonics for "medicinal" purposes became somehow more respectable. The alarming signs of alcoholism and drug addiction in the woman, however, were not interpreted in the same fashion as they were for men, since medical science had already stigmatized her with an inherently inferior intelligence and weaker constitution. Her susceptibility to alcohol and opium inebriety was, therefore, either a result of her social dissipation—the continuous round of social engagements, card playing, reading of romantic novels, the seduction of her imagination, and her yearning for new luxuries—or of those furtive efforts to assume responsibilities outside her proper sphere. The fact that the largest proportion of women opium addicts, other than prostitutes, were housewives of the fashionable middle class suggested to physicians that drug dependency stemmed from their refusal to maintain their natural position within the proper limits of the home circle.

The problem of drug use in the nineteenth century must not be viewed simply as the tragedy of the individuals involved. The Victorian physician and his patient were both victims of a society whose self-image allowed no false step, and which, unprepared to deal with failure, sought to ignore it. The physician who freely prescribed narcotics to avoid the possibility of a wrong diagnosis or the unpleasant duty of admitting his ignorance operated under the same burdensome self-consciousness that afflicted his patient. The Victorian credo of progress and evolution allowed only ignominy to accompany failure; the limits within which the middle-class society lived admitted no defeat. The surreptitious consumption of narcotics by the Victorians, especially women, served a double purpose: it offered quiet solace, a temporary escape from a reality too difficult to acknowledge, and it provided a hidden recess into which all the disordered or unmanageable elements in the Victorian world could be stowed. Exponent of the thinking of the Gilded Age, the Victorian physician was no more able than his bewildered patient to assess, or to control, the perplexing and paradoxical problems that faced Americans in the late nineteenth century.

Selected Bibliography

THIS BOOK has been researched chiefly from primary sources —books, pamphlets, and journal articles—of the late eighteenth and the nineteenth centuries. Although medical journals were a major source, we have not attempted to include them in our bibliography. The footnotes in each chapter should provide the interested reader with those journal materials which we considered relevant. We have included, however, a complete list of books and pamphlets, as well as certain general works that afford insights into the period and subject as a whole.

Abbott, Jacob. *Gentle Measures in the Management and Training of the Young* (New York, 1872)

Acton, William. *A Complete Practical Treatise on Venereal Diseases, and Their Immediate and Remote Consequences* (London, 1841)

———. *The Functions and Disorders of the Reproductive Organs in Childhood, Youth, Adult Age, and Advanced Life Considered in Their Physiological, Social, and Moral Relations* (3rd Am. ed.; Philadelphia, 1871)

———. *Prostitution, Considered in Its Moral, Social, and Sanitary Aspects, in London and Other Large Cities and Garrison Towns* (London, 1870)

———. *Prostitution in Relation to Public Health* (London, 1851)

Addams, Jane. *The Long Road of Woman's Memory* (New York, 1916)

———. *A New Conscience and an Ancient Evil* (New York, 1912)

———. *Twenty Years at Hull House* (New York, 1910)

Alcott, William A. *Lectures on Life and Health; or, the Laws and Means of Physical Culture* (Boston, 1853)

———. *The Young Husband, or Duties of Man in the Marriage Relation* (Boston, 1839)

Aldous, Joan, and Reuben Hill. *International Bibliography of Research in Marriage and the Family* (Minneapolis, 1967)

Allen, Martha M. *Alcohol, a Dangerous and Unnecessary Medicine* (New York, 1900)

Allen, Nathan. *The Education of Girls, as Connected with Their Growth and Physical Development* (Boston, 1879)

Alsberg, Moritz. *Anthropologie mit Berücksichtigung der Urgeschichte des Menchen* (Stuttgart, 1888)

Amos, Sheldon. *A Comparative Survey of Laws in Force for the Prohibition, Regulation, and Licensing of Vice in England and Other Countries* (London, 1877)

Anderson, Elizabeth G. *Sex in Mind and Education* (London, 1874)

Aristotle (pseud). *Aristotle's Complete Master-Piece in Three Parts, Displaying the Secrets of Nature in the Generation of Man* (Worcester, 1795)

Asbury, Herbert. *The Gangs of New York, an Informal History of the Underworld* (New York, 1927)

Atthill, Lombe. *Clinical Lectures on Diseases Peculiar to Women* (4th ed.; London, 1876)

Bain, Alexander. *Mind and Body. The Theories of Their Relation* (New York, 1873)

Banks, Joseph A., and Olive Banks. *Feminism and Family Planning in Victorian England* (New York, 1964)

Bartholow, Roberts. *On Spermatorrhoea: Its Causes, Symptomatology, Pathology, Prognosis, Diagnosis, and Treatment* (New York, 1866)

Bayley, John C. *Marriage as It Is and as It Should Be* (New York, 1857)

Beard, Charles A., and Mary R. Beard. *The Rise of American Civilization* (New York, 1933)

Beard, George M. *American Nervousness, Its Causes and Consequences* (New York, 1881)

———. *Eating and Drinking; a Popular Manual of Food and Diet in Health and Disease* (New York, 1871)

———. *Electricity in the Treatment of Diseases of the Skin* (New York, 1872)

———. *Other Symptoms of Nervous Exhaustion* (Chicago, 1879)

———. *A Practical Treatise on Nervous Exhaustion* (5th ed.; New York, 1905)

———. *Recent Researches in Electro-Therapeutics* (New York, 1872)

———. *Sexual Neurasthenia, Its Hygiene, Causes, Symptoms, and Treatment with a Chapter on Diet for the Nervous* (New York, 1884)

Beard, Mary R. *On Understanding Women* (New York, 1931)

———. *Woman as Force in History; a Study in Traditions and Realities* (New York, 1946)

Beecher, Catherine Ester. *Letters to the People on Health and Happiness* (New York, 1855)

———. *A Treatise on Domestic Economy, for the Use of Young Ladies at Home, and at School* (New York, 1845)

Bell, Ernest A. *War on the White Slave Trade, a Book Designed to Awaken the Sleeping and to Protect the Innocent* (Chicago, 1909)

Bennett, Cyril. *The Modern Malady; or, Sufferers from "Nerves"* (London, 1890)

Bergeret, Louis F. E. *The Preventive Obstacle; or, Conjugal Onanism. The Danger and Inconveniences to the Individual, to the Family, and to Society, of Frauds in the Accomplishment of the Generative Functions* (New York, 1870)

Besant, Annie. *The Law of Population; Its Consequences, and Its Bearing upon Human Conduct and Morals* (London, n.d.)

————. *Marriage; as It Was, as It Is, and as It Should Be* (New York, 1879)

Bevier, Isabel, and Susannah Usher. *Home Economics Movement* (Boston, 1906)

Bigelow, C. *Sexual Pathology: A Practical and Popular Review of the Principal Diseases of the Reproductive Organs* (Chicago, 1875)

Blackburne, Neville. *Ladies' Chain* (London, 1952)

Blackwell, Elizabeth. *Counsel to Parents on the Moral Education of Their Children* (New York, 1879)

————. *The Human Element in Sex: Being a Medical Enquiry into the Relation of Sexual Physiology and Christian Morality* (London, 1884)

————. *The Sexes throughout Nature* (New York, 1875)

Bliss, W. W. *Woman's Life: A Pen-Picture of Woman's Functions, Frailties, and Follies* (Boston, 1879)

Bloch, Iwan. *The Sexual Life of Our Time in Its Relations to Modern Civilization* (London, 1909)

Bode, Carl. *The Anatomy of American Popular Culture, 1840–1861* (Berkeley, 1959)

Bostwick, Homer. *A Complete Practical Work on the Nature and Treatment of Venereal Diseases, and Other Affections of the Genito-Urinary Organs of the Male and Female* (New York, 1848)

————. *A Treatise on the Nature and Treatment of Seminal Diseases, Impotency, and Other Kindred Affections; with Practical Directions for the Management and Removal of the Cause Producing Them; Together with Hints to Young Men* (New York, 1848)

Bouvier, Sauveur Henri Victor. *Etudes historiques et medicales sur l'usage des corsets* (Paris, 1853)

Brinton, Daniel G. *The Basis of Social Relations* (New York, 1902)

————, and George H. Napheys. *Laws of Health in Relation to the Human Form* (Springfield, Mass., 1870)

Brodum, William. *A Guide to Old Age: Or, a Cure for the Indiscretions of Youth* (London, 1801)

Brown, Herbert R. *The Sentimental Novel in America, 1789–1860* (Durham, N.C., 1940)

Brown, William Symington. *A Clinical Hand-Book on the Diseases of Women* (New York, 1882)

Bryce, James. *The American Commonwealth* (New York, 1888)

Buchan, William. *Observations concerning the Prevention and Cure of Venereal Disease. Intended to Guard the Ignorant and Unwary against the Baneful Effects of that Insidious Malady* (London, 1796)

Bumstead, Freeman Josiah. *The Pathology and Treatment of Venereal Diseases; Including the Results of Recent Investigations upon the Subject* (Philadelphia, 1870)

Buret, Frederic. *Syphilis in the Middle Ages and in Modern Times* (Philadelphia, 1895)

Burrows, J. A. *A Dissertation on the Nature and Effects of a New Vege-*

table Remedy, an Acknowledged Specific in All Venereal Scorbutic and Scrophulous Cases (London, 1780)

Burton, Jean. *Lydia Pinkham Is Her Name* (New York, 1949)

Bushnell, Horace. *Women's Suffrage; the Reform against Nature* (New York, 1869)

Butler, Josephine E. (ed.). *Woman's Work and Woman's Culture* (London, 1869)

Buttenstedt, Karl. *Happiness in Marriage (Revelation in Women): A Nature Study* (Friedrichshagen, 1904)

Calhoun, Arthur W. *A Social History of the American Family from Colonial Times to the Present* (3 vols.; Cleveland, 1917–19)

Calhoun, George R. *Report of the Consulting Surgeon on Spermatorrhoea, or Seminal Weakness, Impotence, the Vice of Onanism, Masturbation, or Self-Abuse, and Other Diseases of the Sexual Organs* (Philadelphia, 1858)

Calkins, Alonzo. *Opium and the Opium Appetite* (Philadelphia, 1871)

Campbell, Harry. *Differences in the Nervous Organization of Man and Woman: Psychological and Pathological* (London, 1891)

Campbell, Hugh. *A Treatise on Nervous Exhaustion and the Diseases Induced by It* (London, 1874)

Camper, Peter. *The Works of the Late Professor Camper* (London, 1794)

Capellmann, Carl. *Facultative Sterility, without Offense to Moral Laws* (Aachen, 1883)

Caplin, Roxey A. *Health and Beauty; or, Corsets and Clothing Constructed in Accordance with the Physiological Laws of the Human Body* (London, 1856)

Capp, William M. *The Daughter: Her Health, Education and Wedlock* (Philadelphia, 1891)

Carden, Maren Lockwood. *Oneida: Utopian Community to Modern Corporation* (Baltimore, 1969)

Cardwell, David P. *The Book of Private Knowledge and Advice, of the Highest Importance to Individuals in the Detection and Cure of "A Certain Disease," (Venereal) Which if Neglected or Improperly Treated, Produces the Most Ruinous Consequences to the Human Constitution* (New York, 1833)

Carpenter, William B. *Principles of Human Physiology* (London, 1842)

Cathell, Daniel W. *Physician Himself and What He Should Add to His Scientific Acquirements* (Boston, 1882)

Chavannes, Albert. *Vital Force and Magnetic Exchange, Their Relation to Each Other and to Life and Happiness* (Knoxville, Tenn., 1888)

Chevalier, Michel. *Society, Manners and Politics in the United States; Being a Series of Letters on North America* (Boston, 1839)

Chideckel, Maurice. *Female Sex Perversion; the Sexually Aberrated Woman as She Is* (New York, 1935)

Chipley, W. S. *A Warning to Fathers, Teachers and Young Men, in Re-*

lation to a Frightful Cause of Insanity and Other Serious Disorders of Youth (Louisville, Ky., 1861)

Christie, Jane J. *The Advance of Woman; from the Earliest Times to the Present* (Philadelphia, 1912)

Christy, Howard C. *The American Girl* (New York, 1906)

Clark, Kate Upson. *Bringing Up Boys; a Study* (New York, 1899)

Clarke, Edward H. *Sex in Education; or, a Fair Chance for Girls* (Boston, 1873)

Cleaves, Margaret. *The Autobiography of a Neurasthene as Told by One of Them and Recorded by Margaret Cleaves* (Boston, 1910)

Cleland, John. *The Relation of Brain to Mind* (Glasgow, 1882)

Coale, William E. *Hints on Health with Familiar Instructions for the Preservation of the Skin, Hair, Teeth, Eyes, etc.* (Boston, 1857)

Coan, Titus M. *Ounces of Prevention* (New York, 1885)

Cobbe, Frances P. *The Duties of Women; a Course of Lectures* (London, 1881)

Cohen, Gustavus. *Helps and Hints to Mothers and Young Wives* (London, 1880)

Comfort, George F., and Anna M. Comfort. *Woman's Education and Woman's Health; Chiefly in Reply to "Sex in Education"* (Syracuse, 1874)

Comstock, Anthony. *Frauds Exposed; or How the People Are Deceived and Robbed, and Youth Corrupted* (New York, 1880)

———. *Traps for the Young* (New York, 1883)

Conwell, Joseph A. *Manhood's Morning; or "Go It While You're Young." A Book to Young Men between 14 and 28 Years of Age* (New Jersey, 1896)

Cook, Clarence. *The House Beautiful; Essays on Beds and Tables, Stools and Candlesticks* (New York, 1878)

Cooper, Arthur, and Berkeley Hill. *The Student's Manual of Venereal Diseases Being a Concise Description of Those Affections and of Their Treatment* (2nd ed.; New York, 1881)

Cornell, William M. *The Beacon: Or, a Warning to Young and Old* (Philadelphia, 1865)

(A Court Physician). *Reproductive Disorders, Spermatorrhoea, Exhausted Brain, etc. Their Nature, Symptoms, Pathology, and Successful Treatment* (London, 1876)

Courtenay, F. B. *On Spermatorrhoea and the Professional Fallacies and Popular Delusions Which Prevail in Relation to Its Nature, Consequences, and Treatment* (London, 1869)

Cowan, John. *The Science of a New Life* (New York, 1871)

Cowper, James. *A Narrative of the Effects of a Medicine, Newly Discovered, by Mr. Keyser, a German Chymist in Paris that Cures the Venereal Disease in Its Most Inveterate and Malignant State, without Salivation or Strict Regime, as Is Now Practiced in France, Both in Private Cases, and in the Military Hospitals* (London, 1760)

Craddock, Ida C. *Right Marital Living* (Chicago, 1899)

————. *The Wedding Night* (Denver, 1900)

Crow, Duncan. *The Victorian Woman* (New York, 1972)

Culverwell, Robert J. *Guide to Health and Long Life: Or What to Eat, Drink, and Avoid; What Exercise to Take, How to Control and Regulate the Passions and Appetites; and on the General Conduct of Life* (2nd ed.; New York, 1849)

————. *Medical Consultations on Morbid Secretions, Stricture, and Irritability of the Urethra; Affections of the Bladder, Prostate Gland, and Other Infirmities of the Reproductive System* (London, 1838)

————. *Porneiopathology. A Popular Treatise on Venereal and Other Diseases of the Male and Female Genital System; with Remarks on Impotence, Onanism, Sterility, Piles, and Gravel, and Prescriptions for Their Treatment* (New York, 1844)

————. *Professional Records. The Institutes of Marriage, Its Intent, Obligations, and Physical and Constitutional Disqualifications* (New York, 1846)

Cunningham, Henry S. *Lectures on the Physiological Laws of Life, Hygiene and a General Outline of Diseases Peculiar to Females, Embracing a Revival of the Rights and Wrongs of Women, and a Treatise on Disease in General, with Explicit Directions How to Nurse, Nourish and Administer Remedies to the Sick* (Indianapolis, 1882)

Cunnington, Cecil W. *Feminine Attitudes in the Nineteenth Century* (New York, 1936)

————, and Phillis Cunnington. *Handbook on English Costume in the Nineteenth Century* (London, 1959)

Dalton, Gerald. *A Practical Manual of Venereal and Generative Diseases* (London, 1913)

Daniels, Henry A. *Book on Stricture, Fistula, Piles, Impotence; Diseases of the Genito-Urinary Organs; Deformities of the Eyes, Nose and Face* (New York, 1873)

Davenport, John. *Aphrodisiacs and Anti-Aphrodisiacs: Three Essays on the Powers of Reproduction; with Some Account of the Judician 'Congress' as Practiced in France during the Seventeenth Century* (London, 1869)

————. *Curiosities Eroticae, Physiologiae; or, Tabooed Subjects Freely Treated* (London, 1875)

Davies, John D. *Phrenology: Fad and Science; a Nineteenth Century American Crusade* (New Haven, 1955)

(Anony.). *Davy's Lac-Elephantis; or, Medicated Milk of Elephants. An Effectual Cure for . . . Venereal Disease, in Both Sexes, with a Plain Prescription* (London, 1815)

Dawson, R. *An Essay on Marriage; Being a Microscopic Investigation into Its Physiological and Physical Relations; with Observations on the Nature, Causes, and Treatment of Spermatorrhoea, and the Various Disorders of the Procreative System in Men* (London, 1845)

Deacon, H. *A Compendious Treatise on the Venereal Disease, Gleets, etc., Divested of the Technical Terms; with the Best Methods of Cure, so Explained as to Render Medical Advice, in the Cure of Most Venereal Cases, Unnecessary. In Which Is Given a Lotion for the Prevention of that Disagreeable Complaint* (London, 1789)

de Beauvoir, Simone. *The Mandarins; a Novel* (New York, 1956)

————. *The Second Sex* (New York, 1952)

Dennett, Mary Ware. *Birth Control Laws, Shall We Keep Them, Change Them, or Abolish Them* (New York, 1926)

De Quincey, Thomas. *Confessions of an Opium Eater* (London, 1821)

Deslandes, Leopold. *Manhood; the Causes of Its Premature Decline, with Directions for Its Perfect Restoration; Addressed to Those Suffering from the Destructive Effects of Excessive Indulgence, Solitary Habits, etc.* (Boston, 1843)

Deutsche, Helene. *The Psychology of Women; a Psychoanalytic Interpretation* (New York, 1944)

(Anony.). *Diana: A Psycho-Fyziological Essay on Sexual Relations for Married Men and Women* (New York, 1882)

Dickinson, Robert L., and Lura Beam. *A Thousand Marriages; a Medical Study of Sex Adjustment* (Baltimore, 1931)

Dingwall, Eric J. *The Girdle of Chastity; a Medico-Historical Study* (London, 1931)

————. *Male Infibulation* (London, 1925)

Ditzion, Sidney. *Marriage, Morals and Sex in America; a History of Ideas* (New York, 1953)

Dix, Tandy L. *The Healthy Infant, a Treatise on the Healthy Procreation of the Human Race, Embracing the Obligations to Offspring; the Management of the Pregnant Female; the Management of the Newly Born; the Management of the Infant; and the Infant in Sickness* (Cincinnati, 1880)

Dixon, Edward H. *The Organic Law of the Sexes. Positive and Negative Electricity, and the Abnormal Conditions that Impair Virility* (New York, 1861)

————. *Some Abnormal Conditions of the Sexual and Pelvic Organs, Which Impair Virility* (New York, n.d.)

————. *A Treatise on Diseases of the Sexual Organs: Adapted to Popular and Professional Reading, and the Exposition of Quackery, Professional and Otherwise* (New York, 1845)

————. *Woman and Her Diseases, from the Cradle to the Grave* (Philadelphia, 1860)

Douglas, G. Archibald. *The Nature and Causes of Impotence in Men, and Barrenness in Women, Explained. With the Methods by Which It May Be Known in Any Case and Whose Part the Imperfection Lies; and Instructions for the Prevention and Remedy* (London, 1758)

Drake, Emma F. (Angell). *What a Woman of Forty-Five Ought to Know* (Philadelphia, 1902)

————. *What a Young Wife Ought to Know* (Philadelphia, 1908)

Dubois, Jean. *The Secret Habits of the Female Sex; Letters Addressed to a Mother on the Evils of Solitude, and Its Seductive Temptations to Young Girls, the Premature Victims of a Pernicious Passion, with All Its Frightful Consequences: Deformity of Mind and Body, Destruction of Beauty, and Entailing Disease and Death; but from Which, by Attention to the Timely Warning Here Given, the Devotee May Be Saved, and Become an Ornament to Society* (New York, 186?)

Duffey, Eliza B. *The Ladies' and Gentlemen's Etiquette: A Complete Manual of the Manners and Dress of American Society* (Philadelphia, 1877)

————. *No Sex in Education; or, an Equal Chance for Both Boys and Girls* (Philadelphia, 1874)

————. *The Relations of the Sexes* (New York, 1876)

Duncan, James Matthews. *On Sterility in Women* (Philadelphia, 1884)

Eastman, Hubbard. *Noyesism Unveiled: A History of the Sect Self-Styled Perfectionists* (Brattleboro, 1849)

Ebbard, Richard J. *How to Restore Life-Giving Energy to Sufferers from Sexual Neurasthenia and Kindred Brain and Nerve Disorders* (London, 1923)

Eldridge, C. S. *Self-Enervation: Its Consequences and Treatment* (Chicago, 1869)

Ellington, George (pseud.). *The Women of New York; or, the Underworld of the Great City* (New York, 1869)

Ellis, Albert. *The Folklore of Sex* (New York, 1961)

————, and Albert Abarbanel (eds.). *The Encyclopedia of Sexual Behavior* (2 vols.; New York, 1961)

Ellis, Havelock. *Man and Woman; a Study of Human Secondary Sexual Characters* (4th ed.; London, 1904)

————. *Study in the Psychology of Sex. The Evolution of Modesty, the Phenomena of Sexual Periodicity, Auto-Eroticism* (Philadelphia, 1900)

Ellis, John. *The Great Evil of the Age, a Medical Warning* (n.p., n.d.)

Engels, Friedrich. *The Origins of the Family, Private Property, and the State* (Chicago, 1902)

Faithfull, Emily. *Three Visits to America* (New York, 1884)

(Anony.). *A Familiar Essay, Explanatory of the Theory and Practice of Prevention of Venereal Contagion, Interspersed with Observations on the Nature and Treatment of Gonorrhoea* (London, 1810)

Farrar, Mrs. John. *The Young Lady's Friend* (New York, 1860)

Figes, Eva. *Patriarchal Attitudes* (London, 1970)

Finck, Henry T. *Romantic Love and Personal Beauty; Their Development, Causal Relations, Historic and National Peculiarities* (New York, 1887)

Finot, Jean. *Problems of the Sexes* (New York, 1913)

Fleming, L. D. *Self-Pollution, the Cause of Youthful Decay: Showing the Dangers and Remedy of Venereal Excess* (New York, 1846)

Flexner, Eleanor. *Century of Struggle; the Woman's Rights Movement in the United States* (Cambridge, 1959)

Foote, Edward B. *Dr. Foote's Reply to the Alphiles, Giving Some Cogent Reasons for Believing that Sexual Continence Is Not Good for the Health* (New York, 1882)

————. *Plain Home Talk about the Human System—the Habits of Men and Women—the Causes and Prevention of Disease—Our Sexual Relations and Social Natures* (New York, 1888)

Forbrush, William B. *The Boy Problem; a Study in Social Pedagogy* (4th ed.; Philadelphia, 1902)

Forel, August. *The Sexual Question; a Scientific, Psychological, Hygienic and Sociological Study for the Cultured Classes* (New York, 1906)

Fowler, Lorenzo N. *Marriage: Its History and Ceremonies; with a Phrenological and Physiological Exposition of Its Character and Design* (17th ed.; New York, 1848)

Fowler, Orson S. *Amativeness: Or Evils and Remedies of Excessive and Perverted Sexuality: Including Warning and Advice to the Married and Single* (New York, 1846)

————. *Creative and Sexual Science: Or Manhood, Womanhood, and Their Mutual Interrelations: Love, Its Laws, Power, etc., Selection, or Mutual Adaption; Courtship, Married Life, and Perfect Children; Their Generation, Endowment, Paternity, Maternity, Bearing, Nursing, and Rearing; Together with Puberty, Boyhood, Girlhood, etc.; Sexual Impairments Restored, Male Vigor and Female Health and Beauty Perpetuated and Augmented, etc., as Taught by Phrenology and Physiology* (Cincinnati, 1870)

————. *Love and Parentage, Applied to the Improvement of Offspring: Including Important Directions and Suggestions to Lovers and the Married concerning the Strongest Ties and the Most Sacred and Momentous Relations of Life* (New York, 1846)

————. *Maternity; or, the Bearing and Nursing of Children including Female Education and Beauty* (New York, 1856)

————. *Matrimony: Or Phrenology and Physiology Applied to the Selection of Congenial Companions for Life: Including Directions to the Married for Living Together Affectionately and Happily* (New York, 1851)

————. *Sexual Science; including Manhood, Womanhood, and Their Mutual Interrelations; Love, Its Laws, Power, etc.* (Philadelphia, 1875)

————. *Tight-Lacing, Founded on Physiology and Phrenology; or, the Evils Inflicted on Mind and Body by Compressing the Organs of Animal Life, Thereby Retarding and Enfeebling the Vital Functions* (New York, 1846)

Fracastoro, Girolamo. *Fracastor Syphilis; or the French Disease* (London, 1935)

Freud, Sigmund. *Modern Sexual Morality and Modern Nervousness* (New York, 1931)

————. *Three Contributions to the Theory of Sex* (New York, 1916)

Friedmann, Marion V. *Olive Schreiner; a Study in Latent Meanings* (Johannesburg, 1954)

Fryer, Peter. *The Birth Controllers* (New York, 1966)

Funcke, Richard E. *A New Revelation of Nature; a Secret of Sexual Life. No More Prostitution* (Hanover, 1906)

Furness, Clifton J. (ed.). *The Genteel Female: An Anthology* (New York, 1931)

Galbraith, Anna M. *The Four Epochs of Woman's Life; a Study in Hygiene* (Philadelphia, 1904)

Galloway, Thomas W. *Love and Marriage; Normal Sex Relations* (New York, 1924)

Gamble, Eliza Burt. *The Evolution of Woman; an Inquiry into the Dogma of Her Inferiority to Man* (New York, 1894)

Gardner, Augustus K. *The Causes and Curative Treatment of Sterility, with a Preliminary Statement of the Physiology of Generation* (New York, 1856)

————. *The Conjugal Relationships as Regards Personal Health and Hereditary Well Being Practically Treated* (Glasgow, 1892)

————. *Conjugal Sins against the Laws of Life and Health and Their Effects upon the Father, Mother and Child* (New York, 1870)

Garnett, Thomas. *A Lecture on the Preservation of Health* (London, 1800)

Garrison, Fielding H. *An Introduction to the History of Medicine* (4th ed.; Philadelphia, 1929)

Gattey, Charles N. *The Bloomer Girls* (New York, 1968)

Geddes, Patrick, and J. Arthur Thomson. *The Evolution of Sex* (London, 1897)

(Anony.). *General Treatise on the Nature and Cause of Disease in the Human Body; Together with Proofs of the Efficacy of Vaughn's Vegetable Lithontriptic Mixture, as a General Restorer of the System, and Purifier of the Blood* (Buffalo, 1845)

Gleason, Mrs. Rachel B. *Talks to My Patients; Hints on Getting Well and Keeping Well* (New York, 1870)

Godfrey, C. B. *An Historical and Practical Treatise on the Venereal Disease* (London, 1797)

Goodell, William. *The Dangers and the Duty of the Hour* (Baltimore, 1881)

Goss and Co. *The Aegis of Life, a Non-Medical Commentary on the Indiscretions Arising from Human Frailty, in Which the Causes, Symptoms, and Baneful Effects of Lues, Venerea, Gonorrhoea, Stricture, Seminal Weakness, etc., Are Explained in a Familiar Way* (London, 1827)

————. *Hygeiana, a Non-Medical Analysis of the Complaints Incidental to Females, in Which Are Offered Some Important Admonitions on the*

Peculiar Debilities Attending Their Circumstances, Sympathies, and Formation (London, 1823)

Gould, George (comp). *Digest of State and Federal Laws Dealing with Prostitution and Other Sex Offences* (New York, 1942)

Graham, James. *New and Curious Treatise of the Nature and Effects of Simple Earth, Water, and Air, when Applied to the Human Body . . . to Which Is Added, an Appendix Containing Pathetic Remonstrances and Advices to Young Persons, and to Old Men against the Abuse of Certain Debilitating and Degrading Pleasures* (London, 1793)

Graham, Sylvester. *A Lecture to Young Men, on Chastity. Intended also for the Serious Consideration of Parents and Guardians* (Boston, 1839)

Gray, George Z. *Husband and Wife; or, the Theory of Marriage and Its Consequences* (Boston, 1885)

Greer, Joseph H. *The Social Evil; Its Cause, Effect and Cure* (Chicago, 1909)

————. *Woman Know Thyself; Female Diseases, Their Prevention and Cure. A Home Book of Tokology, Hygiene and Education for Maidens, Wives and Mothers. A Clean and Clear Exposition of Nature's Laws and Mysteries* (Chicago, 1902)

Gregory, Samuel. *Facts and Important Information for Young Women on the Self-Indulgence of the Sexual Appetite* (Boston, 1857)

Griffith, Dr. *History of the Venereal Disease, with a List of the Disorders Both Venereal and Natural, to Which the Generative Organs Are Subject* (London, 1863)

Grindle, Wesley. *New Medical Revelations, Being a Popular Work on the Reproductive System, Its Debility and Disease* (Philadelphia, 1857)

Gross, Samuel W. *A Practical Treatise on Impotence, Sterility, and Allied Disorders of the Male Sexual Organs* (Philadelphia, 1881)

Guernsey, Henry N. *Plain Talks on Avoided Subjects* (Philadelphia, 1882)

Gunn, Robert A. *The Nature and Treatment of Venereal Diseases; with Numerous Cases, Formulae, and Clinical Observations* (New York, 1874)

Hall, G. Stanley. *Adolescence* (New York, 1904)

Haller, Jr., John S. *Outcasts from Evolution: Scientific Attitudes of Racial Inferiority, 1859–1900* (Urbana, 1971)

Hamilton, Alexander M. *The Anatomy of the Brain* (Edinburgh, 1831)

Hamilton, J. *Nervous-Exhaustion, Hints of Vital Importance to Youth and Manhood* (London, n.d.)

Hammond, William A. *Cerebral Hyperaemia, the Result of Mental Strain or Emotional Disturbance; the So-Called Nervous Prostration or Neurasthenia* (Washington, 1895)

————. *Sexual Impotence in the Male and Female* (Detroit, 1887)

Harland, Marion. *Eve's Daughters; or, Common Sense for Maid, Wife and Mother* (New York, 1882)

Harris, Frank. *My Life and Loves* (New York, 1963)

Harvey, John. *The Restoration of Nervous Exhaustion* (London, 1865)

Hatch, Benjamin F. *The Constitution of Man, Physically, Morally, and Spiritually Considered: Or the Christian Philosopher* (New York, 1866)

Hatfield, Marcus P. *The Physiology and Hygiene of the House in Which We Live* (New York, 1887)

Hayden, James R. *A Manual of Venereal Diseases* (New York, 1896)

Hayes, Albert H. *The Science of Life: Or Self-Preservation. A Medical Treatise on Nervous and Physical Debility, Spermatorrhoea, Impotence, and Sterility* (Boston, 1868)

Heywood, E. H. *Cupid's Yokes; or, the Binding Forces of Conjugal Life. An Essay to Consider Some Moral and Physiological Phases of Love and Marriage, Wherein Is Asserted the Natural Right and Necessity of Sexual Self-Government* (Princeton, Mass., n.d.)

Higginson, Thomas W. *Common Sense about Women* (Boston, 1881)

————. *Women and Men* (New York, 1888)

Himes, Norman E. *A Medical History of Contraception* (Baltimore, 1936)

Himmelfarb, Gertrude. *Victorian Minds* (New York, 1968)

Hiss, A. Emil. *Thesaurus of Proprietary Preparations and Pharmaceutical Specialties* (Chicago, 1898)

Holcombe, William H. *The Sexes Here and Hereafter* (Philadelphia, 1869)

Hollick, Frederick. *A Popular Treatise on Venereal Diseases, in All Their Forms. Embracing Their History, and Probable Origin; Their Consequences, Both to Individuals and to Society; and the Best Modes of Treating Them* (New York, 1852)

Hooker, Worthington. *Physician and Patient; or, a Practical View of the Mutual Duties, Relations and Interests of the Medical Profession and the Community* (New York, 1849)

Houghton, Walter E. *The Victorian Frame of Mind, 1830–1870* (New Haven, Conn., 1957)

Howard, William Lee. *Plain Facts on Sex Hygiene* (New York, 1910)

Howe, Mrs. Julia Ward (ed.). *"Sex in Education"; a Reply to Dr. E. H. Clark's "Sex and Education"* (Boston, 1874)

Hudson, Ellis Herndon. *Treponematosis* (New York, 1946)

Humphreys, Frederick. *Homeopathic Treatment of Diseases of the Sexual System* (New York, 1850)

Hunt, Ezra M. *Hygiene: Its Scope, Its Progress and Its Leading Aims* (Saratoga, N.Y., 1883)

Hunter, Archibald. *Health, Happiness, and Longevity, How Obtained, Embracing Strictures on Diet and Habits* (London, 1885)

Hunter, John. *A Treatise on the Venereal Disease* (Philadelphia, 1818)

Hyde, James N., and Frank H. Montgomery. *A Manual of Syphilis and the Venereal Diseases* (Philadelphia, 1895)

Hyden, James R. *A Manual of Venereal Diseases* (New York, 1896)

Ingersoll, A. J. *In Health* (New York, 1884)

Jackson, Helen Maria (Fiske) Hunt. *Bits of Talk about Home Matters* (Boston, 1873)

Jackson, James Caleb. *American Womanhood: Its Peculiarities and Necessities* (2nd ed.; New York, 1870)

Jacques, Daniel H. *Philosophy of Human Beauty; or Hints towards Physical Perfection* (New York, 1867)

Janney, Oliver E. *The White Slave Traffic in America* (New York, 1911)

Jennings, Samuel K. *The Married Lady's Companion; or, Poor Man's Friend* (New York, 1808)

Johnston, James F. W. *The Chemistry of Common Life* (2 vols.; London, 1855)

Jones, Mrs. C. S., and Henry T. Williams. *Household Elegancies* (New York, 1875)

————, and ————. *Ladies' Fancy Work, Hints and Helps to Home Taste and Recreations* (New York, 1876)

Jones, Ernest. *The Life and Work of Sigmund Freud* (3 vols.; New York, 1953–57)

Jordan, L. H. *Man's Mission on Earth! A Treatise on Nervous Debility and Physical Exhaustion* (New York, 1871)

Jordan, William George. *The Kingship of Self-Control* (New York, 1899)

Jordan and Beck. *The Philosophy of Marriage, Being Four Important Lectures on the Functions and Disorders of the Nervous System and Reproductive Organs* (New York, 1863)

Kahn, Louis J. *Nervous Exhaustion: Its Cause and Cure* (New York, 1876)

Kane, Harry H. *Drugs that Enslave; the Opium, Morphine, Chloral and Hashish Habits* (Philadelphia, 1881)

Kellogg, John H. *Ladies Guide in Health and Disease. Girlhood, Maidenhood, Wifehood, Motherhood* (Des Moines, Iowa, 1883)

————. *Plain Facts about Sexual Life* (Battle Creek, Mich., 1877)

Kenealy, Arabella. *Feminism and Sex Extinction* (London, 1920)

Kett, Joseph F. *The Formation of the American Medical Profession, the Role of Institutions, 1780–1860* (New Haven, Conn., 1968)

Key, Ellen. *Love and Marriage* (London, 1911)

————. *The Woman Movement* (New York, 1912)

Kingsford, Anna. *Health, Beauty, and the Toilet. Letters to Ladies from a Lady Doctor* (New York, 1886)

Kinsey, Alfred C., et al. *Sexual Behavior in the Human Female* (Philadelphia, 1953)

————. *Sexual Behavior in the Human Male* (Philadelphia, 1948)

Kneeland, George T. *Commercialized Prostitution in New York City* (New York, 1913)

Knowlton, Charles. *The Fruits of Philosophy. A Treatise on the Population Question* (Chicago, n.d.)

Kraditor, Aileen S. *The Ideas of the Woman's Suffrage Movement, 1890–1920* (New York, 1965)

Lallemand, Claude-Francois. *A Practical Treatise on the Causes, Symptoms, and Treatment of Spermatorrhoea* (Philadelphia, 1853)

Larmont, Martin. *Medical Advisor and Marriage Guide* (New York, 1859)

Laycock, Thomas. *A Treatise on the Nervous Diseases of Women, Comprising an Inquiry into the Nature, Causes, and Treatment of Spinal and Hysterical Disorders* (London, 1840)

Lerner, Gerda. *The Grimké Sisters from South Carolina: Rebels against Slavery* (Boston, 1967)

Lerner, Max. *America as a Civilization; Life and Thought in the United States Today* (New York, 1957)

(Anony.). *Letters from a Chimney-Corner: A Plea for Pure Homes and Sincere Relations between Men and Women* (Chicago, 1886)

Lewis, Denslow, *The Gynecological Consideration of the Sexual Act* (Chicago, 1900)

Lewis, Dio. *Five Minute Chats with Young Women, and Certain Other Parties* (New York, 1874)

———. *Our Girls* (New York, 1871)

Lewis, H. E. *The Philosophy of Sex* (Burlington, Vt., 1896)

Lifton, Robert J. (ed.). *The Woman in America* (Boston, 1965)

Lindley, E. Marguerite. *Health in the Home* (New York, 1896)

Lindsley, C. A. *The Prescription of Proprietary Medicines for the Sick; Its Demoralizing Effects on the Medical Profession* (New Haven, Conn., 1882)

Little, L. Gilbert. *Nervous Christians* (Nebraska, 1956)

Longstreet, Stephen. *Sportin' House; a History of the New Orleans Sinners and the Birth of Jazz* (Los Angeles, 1965)

Lowry, Edith B. *Herself; Talks with Women concerning Themselves* (Chicago, 1911)

Lundberg, Ferdinand, and Marynia F. Farnham. *Modern Woman: The Lost Sex* (New York, 1947)

Lyman, Henry M., *et al. The Practical Home Physician. A Popular Guide for the Household Management of Disease* (Chicago, 1883)

Lynd, Robert S., and Helen M. Lynd. *Middletown; a Study in American Culture* (New York, 1929)

MacDonald, Arthur. *Girls Who Answer Personals, a Sociologic and Scientific Study of Young Women, Including Letters of American and European Girls in Answer to Personal Advertisements* (Washington, 1897)

———. *Intellectual Women and Matrimony* (Washington, 1896)

McCabe, James D. *New York by Sunlight and Gaslight* (Philadelphia, 1882)

———. *The Secrets of the Great City* (Philadelphia, 1868)

Mann, Arthur. *Yankee Reformers in the Urban Age* (Cambridge, 1954)

Mann, Robert James. *The Philosophy of Reproduction* (London, 1855)

Marcus, Steven. *The Other Victorians: A Study of Sexuality and Pornography in Mid-Nineteenth Century England* (New York, 1964)

Marrs, William Taylor. *Confessions of a Neurasthenic* (Philadelphia, 1908)

Mason, Charlotte M. *Home Education; a Course of Lectures to Ladies* (London, 1896)

Mauriceau, A. M. *The Married Woman's Private Medical Companion* (New York, 1847)

May, Henry F. *The End of American Innocence* (New York, 1959)

May, Rollo. *Love and Will* (New York, 1969)

Mayhew, Henry. *London Labour and London Poor; a Cyclopaedia of the Condition and Earnings of Those that Will Work, Those that Cannot Work, and Those that Will Not Work* (4 vols.; London, 1861–62)

Mead, Margaret. *Male and Female; a Study of the Sexes in a Changing World* (New York, 1955)

Meyer, Donald B. *The Positive Thinkers, a Study of the American Quest for Health and Personal Power from Mary Baker Eddy to Norman Vincent Peale* (New York, 1965)

Meynert, Theodor. *Psychiatry; a Clinical Treatise on the Fore-Brain Based upon a Study of Its Structure, Functions, and Nutrition* (New York, 1885)

Michelet, Jules. *Love* (New York, 1859)

Mill, John Stuart. *The Subjection of Women* (New York, 1874)

Mills, Rebecca. *The Influence of Well-Made Stays on the Health and Beauty of Women, and the Great Injuries Which Ill-Made Ones Inflict* (London, 1841)

Mitchell, Silas Weir. *Doctor and Patient* (Philadelphia, 1888)

Montagu, Ashley. *The Natural Superiority of Women* (New York, 1953)

Moodie, John. *Medical Treatise; with Principles and Observations, to Preserve Chastity and Morality* (Edinburgh, 1848)

Morgan, Anne. *The American Girl; Her Education, Her Responsibility, Her Recreation, Her Future* (New York, 1915)

Morris, F. Baldwin. *The Panorama of Life, an Experience in Associating and Battling with Opium and Alcoholic Stimulants* (Philadelphia, 1878)

Morrow, Prince A. *Social Diseases and Marriage* (New York, 1904)

Muirhead, James F. *The Land of Contrasts; a Briton's View of His American Kin* (New York, 1898)

Myrdal, Gunnar. *An American Dilemma; the Negro Problem and Modern Democracy* (2 vols.; New York, 1944)

Napheys, George Henry. *The Physical Life of a Woman: Advice to the Maiden, Wife, and Mother* (Cincinnati, 1873)

———. *The Transmission of Life. Counsels on the Nature and Hygiene of the Masculine Function* (Philadelphia, 1871)

Newcomer, Mable. *A Century of Higher Education for American Women* (New York, 1959)

Noyes, John Humphrey. *Essay on Scientific Propagation* (New York, n.d.)

———. *Male Continence, or Self Control in Sexual Intercourse* (New York, 1872)

Oleson, Charles W. *Secret Nostrums and Systems of Medicine; a Book of Formulas* (Chicago, 1897)

(Anony.). *Onanism Displayed: Being I. An Enquiry into the True Nature of Onan's Sin II. Of the Modern Onanists III. Of Self-Pollution, Its Causes, and Consequences; with Three Extraordinary Cases of Two Young Gentlemen and a Lady Who Were Very Much Addicted to This Crime IV. Of Nocturnal-Pollutions Natural and Forced V. The Great Sin of Self-Pollution with the Judgment of the Most Eminent Divines upon This Subject VI. A Dissertation concerning Generation with a Curious Description of the Parts and of Their Proper Functions, etc., according to the Latest, and Most Approved Anatomical Discoveries* (2nd ed.; London, 1719)

O'Neill, William L. *Everyone Was Brave: The Rise and Fall of Feminism in America* (Chicago, 1969)

―――. *The Woman Movement; Feminism in the United States and England* (New York, 1969)

Owen, Robert D. *Moral Physiology; or a Brief and Plain Treatise on the Population Question* (London, 1844)

Paget, Sir James. *Clinical Lectures and Essays* (London, 1875)

Palmer, E. R. *Copulation* (Louisville, 1881)

Parker, R. A. *A Yankee Saint. John Humphrey Noyes and the Oneida Community* (New York, 1935)

Parkhurst, Charles H. *My Forty Years in New York* (New York, 1923)

Pattee, F. L. *The Feminine Fifties* (New York, 1940)

Peacock, Thomas B. *Tables of the Weights of the Brain and of Some Other Organs of the Human Body* (London, 1861)

Pearsall, Ronald. *The Worm in the Bud: The World of Victorian Sexuality* (New York, 1969)

Peterson, Houston. *Havelock Ellis: Philosopher of Love* (Boston, 1928)

Phelps, Almira H. L. *The Female Student; or Lectures to Young Ladies on Female Education* (New York, 1836)

(A Physician). *Licentiousness and Its Effects upon Bodily and Mental Health* (New York, 1844)

(A Physician in the Country). *A Short Treatise on Onanism; or, the Detestable Vice of Self-Pollution* (London, 1767)

(A Physician and Sanitarian). *Marriage and Parentage and the Sanitary and Physiological Laws for the Production of Children of Finer Health and Greater Ability* (New York, 1882)

Plater, Felix. *Praxis Medica* (Basileae, 1602)

(Anony.). *A Popular Dissertation on the Venereal Diseases, and Their Sequels; with the Mode of Prevention and Cure* (London, 1818)

Pruner-Bey, Franz. *De la chevelure comme caractéristiques des races humaines d'après des recherches microscopiques* (Paris, 1863)

Puner, Helen Walker. *Freud, His Life and His Mind; a Biography* (New York, 1947)

Pusey, William A. *The History and Epidemiology of Syphilis* (Baltimore, 1933)

Quetelet, Adolph. *A Treatise on Man and the Development of His Faculties* (Edinburgh, 1842)

Reese, Lizette W. *A Victorian Village; Reminiscences of Other Days* (New York, 1929)

Reeves, James E. *Bad Health; Its Physical and Moral Causes in American Women* (Wheeling, W.Va., 1875)

Rentoul, Robert R. *The Dignity of Woman's Health and the Nemesis of Its Neglect* (London, 1890)

Richardson, Joseph G. *Long Life and How to Reach It* (Philadelphia, 1880)

Riegel, Robert E. *American Women; a Story of Social Change* (New Jersey, 1970)

Rockwell, Alphonso D., and George M. Beard. *The Medical Use of Electricity with Special Reference to General Electrization as a Tonic in Neuralgia, Rheumatism, Dyspepsia, Chorea, Paralysis, and Other Affections Associated with General Debility* (New York, 1867)

————, and ————. *A Practical Treatise on the Medical and Surgical Uses of Electricity Including Localized and General Electrization* (New York, 1871)

Root, Harman Knox. *The Lover's Marriage Lighthouse: A Series of Sensible and Scientific Essays on the Subject of Marriage and Free Divorce, and on the Uses, Wants, and Supplies of the Physical, Intellectual, Affectional, and Spiritual Natures of Man and Woman* (New York, 1858)

Rose, Henry. *An Inaugural Dissertation on the Effects of the Passions upon the Body* (Philadelphia, 1794)

Rugoff, Milton. *Prudery and Passion: Sexuality in Victorian America* (New York, 1971)

Russell, William. *An Invalid's Twelve Years' Experience in Search of Health, and a Guide to Health and Strength and the Cure of Weakness and Disease, Theoretically and Practically* (Suffolk, 1891)

Ryan, Michael. *The Philosophy of Marriage, in Its Social, Moral, and Physical Relations* (London, 1839)

————. *Prostitution in London, with a Comparative View of That of Paris and New York* (London, 1839)

Sala, George Augustus. *America Revisited* (London, 1883)

Sanger, William. *The History of Prostitution: Its Extent, Causes, and Effects throughout the World* (New York, 1858)

Santayana, George. *The Genteel Tradition at Bay* (New York, 1931)

————. *The Last Puritan; a Memoir in the Form of a Novel* (London, 1935)

"Saxon." *A Private Letter to Parents, Physicians, and Men Principals of Schools* (Washington, n.d.)

Schlesinger, Arthur M. *Learning How to Behave, a Historical Study of American Etiquette Books* (New York, 1946)

——. *The Rise of the City, 1878–1898* (New York, 1933)

Schreiner, Olive. *Woman and Labor* (New York, 1911)

Schroeder, Aimée Raymond. *Health Notes for Young Wives* (New York, 1895)

Scott, Anne Firor. *The Southern Lady: From Pedestal to Politics, 1830–1930* (Chicago, 1970)

Scott, James F. *The Sexual Instinct, Its Use and Dangers as Affecting Heredity and Morals* (New York, 1899)

Segall, James L. *Sex Life in America, Its Problems and Their Solutions* (New York, 1934)

Seldes, Gilbert V. *The Simmering Century* (New York, 1928)

Sillen, Samuel. *Women against Slavery* (New York, 1955)

Sinclair, Andrew. *The Better Half; the Emancipation of the American Woman* (New York, 1965)

Smith, Henry. *Woman: Her Duties, Relations and Position, a Medical and Social Work* (London, 1875)

Smith, John A. *The Mutations of the Earth* (New York, 1846)

Smith, Page. *Daughters of the Promised Land: Women in American History* (Boston, 1970)

Smith, Paul Jordan. *The Soul of Woman; an Interpretation of the Philosophy of Feminism* (San Francisco, 1916)

Smith, William G. *An Inaugural Dissertation on Opium, Embracing Its History, Chemical Analysis, and Use and Abuse as a Medicine* (New York, 1832)

Solis-Cohen, Myer. *Woman: Girlhood, Wifehood, Motherhood; Her Responsibilities and Her Duties at All Periods of Life* (Philadelphia, 1906)

Sömmerring, Samuel Thomas. *Über die Wirkungen der Schnürbrüste* (Berlin, 1793)

Spencer, Herbert. *Education: Intellectual, Moral, and Physical* (New York, 1900)

——. *Principles of Psychology* (2 vols.; New York, 1910)

——. *Principles of Sociology* (3 vols.; New York, 1910)

——. *The Study of Sociology* (New York, 1896)

Stables, Gordon. *The Girl's Own Book on Health and Beauty* (London, 1891)

Stall, Sylvanus. *What a Man of Forty-Five Ought to Know* (Philadelphia, 1901)

——. *What a Young Boy Ought to Know* (Philadelphia, 1909)

——. *What a Young Husband Ought to Know* (Philadelphia, 1897)

——. *What a Young Man Ought to Know* (Philadelphia, 1897)

Stanton, Elizabeth Cady. *Eighty Years and More; Reminiscences, 1815–1897* (New York, 1898)

Stead, William T. *If Christ Came to Chicago!* (Chicago, 1894)

Steffens, Lincoln. *Autobiography* (New York, 1931)

Stokham, Alice B. *Karezza: Ethics of Marriage* (Chicago, 1896)

————. *The Lover's World: A Wheel of Life* (New York, 1903)

Strakosch, Frances M. *Factors in the Sex Life of 700 Psychopathic Women* (Utica, N.Y., 1934)

Sturgis, F. R. *Sexual Debility in Man* (New York, 1900)

Sudhoff, Karl. *The Earliest Printed Literature on Syphilis* (Florence, 1925)

Talmey, Bernard S. *Woman; a Treatise on the Normal and Pathological Emotions of Feminine Love* (New York, 1906)

Taylor, George H. *The Delusion of Tonics* (New York, 1887)

Thomas, William I. *Sex and Society; Studies in the Social Psychology of Sex* (Chicago, 1907)

Thompson, Eleanor W. *Education for Ladies, 1830–1860; Ideas on Education in Magazines for Women* (New York, 1947)

Thompson, Helen Bradford. *The Mental Traits of Sex; an Experimental Investigation of the Normal Mind in Men and Women* (Chicago, 1903)

Thorburn, John. *Female Education from a Physiological Point of View* (Manchester, Eng., 1884)

Tiedemann, Frederick. *A Systematic Treatise of Comparative Physiology* (London, 1834)

Tilt, Edward J. *On the Preservation of the Health of Women at the Critical Periods of Life* (London, 1851)

Topinard, Paul. *Anthropology* (London, 1878)

Towle, George M. *American Society* (Boston, 1870)

Trollope, Frances. *Domestic Manners of the Americans* (London, 1832)

(Anony.). *The Truth about Love. A Proposed Sexual Morality Based upon the Doctrine of Evolution, and Recent Discoveries in Medical Science* (New York, 1872)

Tyler, Alice F. *Freedom's Ferment: Phases of American Social History to 1860* (Minneapolis, 1944)

Van Wyck, William. *The Sinister Shepherd: A Translation of Girolamo Fracastoro's Syphilidis Sive de Morbo Gallico Libre Tres* (Los Angeles, 1934)

Veblen, Thorstein. *The Theory of the Leisure Class; an Economic Study in the Evolution of Institutions* (New York, 1899)

Venel, M. *Advice to the Nervous and Debilitated of Both Sexes; Containing a Series of Useful and Interesting Information on Subjects of Importance to Married People, or Those on the Eve of Marriage, but Whose Infirmities Are an Insurmountable Bar to Connubial Happiness* (London, 1815)

Vice Commission of Chicago. *The Social Evil of Chicago* (Chicago, 1911)

Vogt, Carl. *Lectures on Man, His Place in Creation, and in the History of the Earth* (London, 1864)

Walker, Alexander. *Beauty; Illustrated Chiefly by an Analysis and Classification of Beauty in Woman* (London, 1836)

————. *Intermarriage: Or the Mode in Which and the Causes Why*

Beauty, Health, and Intellect Result from Certain Unions, and Deformity, Disease, and Insanity from Others (New York, 1839)

———. *Woman Physiologically Considered, as to Mind, Morals, Marriage, Matrimonial Slavery, Infidelity and Divorce* (New York, 1839)

Walker, Donald. *Exercises for Ladies* (London, 1837)

Ware, John. *Hints to Young Men on the True Relation of the Sexes* (Boston, 1850)

Washburn, Robert C. *Life and Times of Lydia E. Pinkham* (New York, 1931)

Wasserstrom, William. *Heiress of All the Ages; Sex and Sentiment in the Genteel Tradition* (Minneapolis, Minn., 1959)

WCTU. *Physiology for Young People* (New York, 1884)

(A Well Wisher to Mankind). *An Essay Addressed to All Parents, Guardians, and Teachers, as Well as to All Orders of Medical Men, upon a Vice, the Bane of the Moral and Physical Constitution of the Youthful of Both Sexes* (London, 1824)

Wenzel, Joseph and Charles. *De Penitiori Structura Cerebri Hominis et Brutorum* (Tubingae, 1812)

West, Geoffrey (pseud.). *The Life of Annie Besant* (London, 1929)

Wharton, Edith. *The House of Mirth* (New York, 1905)

White, William Allen. *Autobiography of William Allen White* (New York, 1946)

Wilcox, Delos F. *Ethical Marriage* (Michigan, 1900)

Willard, Elizabeth O. G. *Sexology as the Philosophy of Life: Implying Social Organization and Government* (Chicago, 1867)

Winick, Charles, and Paul M. Kinsie. *The Lively Commerce: Prostitution in the United States* (Chicago, 1971)

Wood-Allen, Mary. *Marriage; Its Duties and Privileges* (Chicago, 1901)

———. *What a Young Girl Ought to Know* (Philadelphia, 1897)

———. *What a Young Woman Ought to Know* (Philadelphia, 1898)

Woodward, Samuel B. *Hints for the Young in Relation to the Health of Body and Mind* (Boston, 1856)

Woolley, B. M. *The Opium Habit and Its Cure* (Atlanta, 1879)

Woolson, Abba G. *Woman in American Society* (Boston, 1873)

Worcester, Ellwood, Samuel McComb, and Dr. Isidor H. Coriat. *Religion and Medicine; the Moral Control of Nervous Disorders* (New York, 1908)

Youman, Dr. *Dr. Youman's Illustrated Marriage Guide and Confidential Medical Advisor. A Practical Treatise on the Uses and Abuses of the Generative Functions* (n.p., 1876)

Ziff, Larzer. *The American 1890's; Life and Times of a Lost Generation* (New York, 1966)

Index

Aphra Behn   *Oroonoko, or The Royal Slave* (a novel) (Introduction by Lore Metzger)   N702

Margaret Llewellyn Davies, editor   *Life As We Have Known It,* by Co-operative Working Women (Introduction by Virginia Woolf)   N772

Margaret Fuller   *Woman in the Nineteenth Century* (Introduction by Bernard Rosenthal)   N615

George Gissing   *The Odd Women* (a novel)   N610

Margaret Jarman Hagood   *Mothers of the South: Portraiture of the White Tenant Farm Woman* (Introduction by Anne Firor Scott)   N816

John S. Haller and Robin M. Haller   *The Physician and Sexuality in Victorian America*   N845

Karen Horney   *Feminine Psychology*   N686

Raden Adjeng Kartini   *Letters of a Javanese Princess*   N207

Ruth Landes   *The Ojibwa Woman*   N574

Alan Macfarlane   *The Family Life of Ralph Josselin, a Seventeenth Century Clergyman: An Essay in Historical Anthropology*   N849

George Meredith   *Diana of the Crossways* (a novel) (Introduction by Lois Josephs Fowler)   N700

H. F. Peters   *My Sister, My Spouse: A Biography of Lou Andreas-Salomé* (preface by Anaïs Nin)   N478

May Sarton   *Mrs. Stevens Hears the Mermaids Singing* (a novel) (Introduction by Carolyn G. Heilbrun)   N762

May Sarton   *The Small Room* (a novel)   N832

George Bernard Shaw   *An Unsocial Socialist* (a novel) (Introductions by Barbara Bellow Watson and R. F. Dietrich)   N660

Kathryn Kish Sklar   *Catherine Beecher: A Study in American Domesticity*   N812

Julia Cherry Spruill   *Women's Life and Work in the Southern Colonies* (Introduction by Anne Firor Scott)   N662

Barbara Bellow Watson   *A Shavian Guide to the Intelligent Woman*   N640

Mary Wollstonecraft   *Maria, or the Wrongs of Woman* (a novel) (Introduction by Moira Ferguson)   N761

Mary Wollstonecraft   *A Vindication of the Rights of Woman* (Introduction by Charles W. Hagelman, Jr.)   N373